My Cultural Birthrights
& Other Black Gold

My Cultural Birthrights & Other Black Gold
Published by: The Pointe! Image Book Publishing
Boston, MA
dusable2001@yahoo.com

Haroon Rashid, Publisher / Editorial Director
Yvonne Rose/Quality Press.info, Book Packager
Mychea, Text Layout
Cover Fashions by Hakeem Rashid: Hearts Remain/Made to Measure appeal
Cover Photo by Sakeena Tarpley

ALL RIGHTS RESERVED
No part of this book may be reproduced or transmitted in any form or by any means electronic or mechanical, including photocopying, recording or by any information storage and retrieved system without written permission from the authors, except for the inclusion of brief quotations in a review.

The publication is sold with the understanding that the Publisher is not engaged in rendering legal or other professional services. If legal advice or other expert assistance is required, the services of a competent professional person should be sought.

Copyright © 2015 by Haroon Rashid
ISBN #: 9780692611210
Library of Congress Control Number: 2016930045

My Cultural Birthrights & Other Black Gold

Haroon Rashid

The Pointe! Image Book Publishing
Boston, Massachusetts

Dedication

I dedicate this book to my beloved Mother for the unconditional love she has always given me; my brothers & sisters that let me be their big brother while giving me love regardless; my extended family, which is the greatest family in the world; and all my beautiful children.

Let me be the first to say that I also declare my fault and regret for the loss of some of the greatest mothers and women in the world, that were there for me as my partners and or dear friends in life, that stood by me in some of my selfish and foolish manners, while in their lives. I seek refuge in God for my immature behavior and the wrong that I might have done to all or any of them and I accept all the blame for any failure in our lives together. As I accept the wrong for any failures in my individual life, I blame no one and I say to all who were witnesses, it was never you, and it has always been me, not being the man in the moment when it was needed of me the most.

To my children, I also seek their forgiveness for not being the father I could have been while on my world ventures. With God the Father's blessings, I can see how brilliant you all have become in my absence, thanks to your beautiful brilliant mothers.

To my many worldwide friends, I cannot thank you enough for all of your comfort and friendship over the years. This book is dedicated to all of you.

Acknowledgments

Thanks to all of the people who have inspired or encouraged me and that have helped me make this book possible. With the fortune of so many great associates, family and friends I was able to research, catalog and document this novel of my personnel biographical life journey. In my acknowledgements the order of names does not have any special significance over others as it relates to the order that it may be written. If I have missed any of the people that know they have made a contribution in my research and publication of this book please forgive me, and let me know so that I can correct it in the next edition!

Let me start with the one person that I can say was the first who definitely motivated me to write this book. In the beginning there was Mrs. Maria Jossey Owens, a co-founder of the Friends of DuSable NFP. President Barack Obama who recommended that I should use his wife, First lady Michelle Obama, in his place. Her work and services with Friends of DuSable further encouraged me to add in the details of my services of the legacy of Chicago's Founder Jean Baptiste Pointe DuSable in this book. Mr. Douglas Pendarvis, co-founder and Vice President of Friends of DuSable; also Mrs. Jada Goodlett Russell, who was a co-founder of Friends of DuSable; Mr. Pat Patterson, Board member and co-founder of Friends of DuSable; John Low, Board member; Acting President of Friends of DuSable; Mr. Russell Lewis, Friends of DuSable - Board Chair; Mrs. Peggy Montes; Mr. William Walley, Friends of DuSable Treasurer; Andrea Knowles, Friends of DuSable Board member; Mr. Arnold Romeo, Director, Commission of Human Relations Council on African Affairs and Board member, Friends of DuSable; Elsa Tullos, Friends of DuSable Board member; Ms.

Camille Enriques, a Friends of DuSable volunteer Board member; Ms. Hannah Bonecutter, Friends of DuSable Board member; Ms. Aki Antonia, Friends of DuSable Board member; Mr. William Goodlett, writer of a DuSable publication called *Kittihawa & Climbing Bear*.

My family has been my rock and I am indebted to all of them for their ongoing assistance in my goal to complete this book. My first Daughter, Anita Dunn, for her help in editing this book and for being an advisor and family historical consultant; my Son, Mr. Aaron Thompson, a Friends of DuSable volunteer; my Son, Hakeem Rashid, a Friends of DuSable volunteer; Mrs. Ericha Mitchell Merrill, an initial financial sponsor for Friends of DuSable; Mr. Dennis Short, a Friends of DuSable volunteer; my uncle, John S. Jones, advisor and family historical consultant for this book; my cousin, Mrs. Joyce Jones McCormick, advisor and family historical consultant for this book; my cousin, Mr. John Lucky O'Neal, advisor and family historical consultant for this book, my cousin, Denise Baggett, advisor and family historical consultant for this book; my cousin, Mr. James Harris, advisor and family historical consultant for this book; my son, Craig Thompson, advisor and family historical consultant for this book; my cousin, Ms. Latonya Jones; my aunt, Mrs. Essie Mae Butler, advisor and family historical consultant for this book; my sister Ms. Cynthia Pendarvis, advisor and family historical consultant for this book; my brother Mr. Virgil Pendarvis, advisor and family historical consultant for this book my Brother Mr. Joe Pendarvis advisor and family historical consultant for this book; my best friend, Oji Young advisor and consultant for this book.

My gratitude also goes out to: Cardinal Francis George, Chicago Archdioceses; Mark Garski, Director of the Catholic Archdioceses Schools; Mr. Al Washington, CEO, Afam

Products company; Mr. Fred Luster, CEO of Luster's Products Company; Mrs. Linda Rice Johnson of Ebony magazine and Fashion Fair Duke/Ebonie Products; Mr. Paul Dyskstra, CEO, Chicago Cosmetology Association, many of the pictures in this book of the DuSable Bridge ceremony were taken by Mr. Fred Miller, a consultant for Soft Sheen & L'Oreal Products company; Mrs. Gaylin Rose, owner of Gaylinrose Salon; Mr. Reynard Allison, CEO, Enduser Media Productions, advisor and consultant for this book; Mr. Kyle Olejniczak, FOD Marketing Consultant; Dr. Margret Burroughs, Founder of DuSable Museum; Mayor of Chicago, Richard M. Daley; Ms. Erika Summers, Executive Assistant to Mayor Richard M. Daley; Chicago Commission on Human Relations, Commissioner Clarence Woods; Mrs. Bessie L. Neal, President of The DuSable League; Mrs. Virginia Jullian, The DuSable League Historian; Mr. Lonnie Bunch, President Smithsonian African American History Museum; Mr. Leronc Bennett Jr., Laurent historian; Mr. Walter Burnett, Chicago Alderman - 27th.Ward; The Chicago Aldermanic Black Caucus 2010 -19 Members; Mr. Danny K. Davis, U.S. Congressman of Illinois; Imam Wallace D. Muhammad, CEO of The World Community of Islam; Minister Louis Farrakhan, Leader of Nation of Islam; Mr. Barney Muhammad, President, The Actual Facts Research & Survival Center; Mr. Scott Muhammad, DuSable film documentarian; Mr. Kwame Raoul, Illinois State Senator; Mr. Dick Durbin, Illinois U.S. Senator; Mr. Lesley Conde', Consulate General d' Haiti; Mr. Richard Barbeyron, Consul General De France; Mr. Burton Natarus, Chicago Alderman - 42 Ward; Mr. Brendan Reilly, Chicago Alderman - 42 Ward; Mr. Joseph Podlasek, President, American Indian Center, Mrs. Janet Carl Smith, Chicago Dept. of Cultural Affairs; Mrs. Louis Weisberg, Chicago Commissioner of Cultural Affairs; Mr. Homer Bryant, Bryant Ballet Chicago; Mr. Wayne D. Watson, Ph.D., President, Chicago State College; Mr. John Chikow, President & CEO, the Greater North Michigan Avenue Association; Mr. (TY) Tabing, Executive Director, Chicago Loop Alliance; Mr. Michael Towns, President, the Chicago Commission on Human Relations Advisory Council of African Affairs; Dr. Serge Pierre Louis, President, DuSable Haitian Heritage Association; Ms. Antoinette Wright, CEO/ President of the DuSable Museum; Proceeded by Dr. Carol Adams, CEO/ President of the DuSable Museum; Dr. Beniea Davis, Board member of the Chicago Cosmetology Association; Ms. Irma Tranter, President, Chicago Friends of the Parks; Ms. Eleanor Roemer, Legal Consultant for Chicago Friends of the Parks; Mr. Dana Starks, Commissioner, Chicago Commission on Human Relation; Mrs. Yvonne Rose, Editorial Director /Quality Press.info; Mr. Rahni Flowers, CEO, Van Cleef Salon; Professor Dr. Thomas Morsch, Northwestern University Business School Director in Chicago; Ms. Paula Wells, Students Assistant at Northwestern University Business School in Chicago; Mrs. Karen Collins, CEO, Collins Collaboration Consultants.

Contents

i……..Dedication
iii……Acknowledgements
ix……Preface
xiii…..Introduction

Part One: Haroon

1……..Chapter One: Haroon Rashid: In The Spirit Of Harun Al Rashid
9……..Chapter Two: My Parents And Their Lineage
16…...Chapter Three: When I Came Up To Boston
21…...Chapter Four: *The Great Migration (1916-1930)*
39…...Chapter Five: Going Into The United States Marine Corps!
51…...Chapter Six: Back To Boston /Starting My Career
58…...Chapter Seven: Starting My Own Business In Atlanta!
73…...Chapter Eight: The Pendarvis Boxing Enterprise
87…...Chapter Nine: Rashid's Hair Care Center!
94…...Chapter Ten: Three Continent Working Tour: The Caribbean
100….Chapter Eleven: South African / Tour
115….Chapter Twelve: *United Kingdom European / Tour!*
122….Chapter Thirteen: Back To America
133….Chapter Fourteen: When I Moved To New York
146….Chapter Fifteen: The Visionaries Day Spa In Chicago
164….Chapter Sixteen: Back To Van Cleef Salon

Part Two: The Chicago Spirit

176….Chapter Seventeen: My Manifesto Of Change For The Spirit Of Chicago!
183….Chapter Eighteen: Free Blacks In America
186….Chapter Nineteen: The Spirt Of Dusable

PART THREE: AFRICAN AMERICAN HAIR & BEAUTY INDUSTRY THE OTHER BLACK GOLD

250….Chapter Twenty: Knowledge Is Power!
264….Chapter Twenty-One: The History Behind The Hair Industry
278….Chapter Twenty-Two: Ancestors That I Admire
284….Chapter Twenty-Three: Formula For Success
295….Chapter Twenty-Four: African American Mentor Biographies
322….Chapter Twenty-Five: Let's Get Positive

332….In Conclusion
333….About The Author

PREFACE

WHY I WROTE THIS BOOK

I am writing this book to talk about two experiences of my elusive career and my rather interesting, personal life story. Over the years those who know me have told me over and over again that I have had an exciting life and that I should tell my story.

I remember hearing a great African American film writer Spike Lee say that African Americans, in particular, should write or record their history. He said that if they fail to tell their own story then they may leave the chance for others to tell it, and it might not be as truthful or valuable as it should be.

One of my many great mentors Imam Wallace D. Muhammad once told me; "God is the only one that sanctions every life and death that comes into our conscious being." Imagine two extreme experiences: the joy at birth and sadness at death. My mentor said to me, ask yourself the question, "Why is it that 'The Most High', Almighty Creator permits seemingly tragic deaths like murder or terminal accidents for an infant's death? Those are the forms of death that bring so much sadness and pain to people. He answered: "It is to give the true experiences in our life of love and sorrow, to teach us too be grateful and humble, and to make us witness that God alone has the power of our heaven or hell. So we are told in the face of death, to grieve not and to have no fear, for The Most High will walk with thee to replace our sadness."

The truth of the matter is that the act of fear in most cases is a false illusion. That is why we are instructed in scriptures to fear no one but God because anyone that you fear becomes your God, which theoretically translates into your absolute factor. Scriptures further say the Most High is a jealous God and will have us fear no one but Him, even in the act of life or death. God's greatest, existence is in the spirit of love, and providing. These are examples for human and eternal growth, that there is no respect of life or death to the Most High; they are the same elements found in the formulas of creation. It is mankind that measures, but God has no respect of time that is within our human ability of comprehension.

Wisdom is in knowing that to which much has been taken, much will be given; and to whom much that has been given, much is expected.

A true sign of the illusion of life and death can be seen in nature during seasonal changes, a blade of grass sprouts from the earth in a seasonal time then it withers and dies in another season right before our eyes. That most certainly is a sign of life and death in a formula that we can measure and comprehend. But just consider a higher power or formula of life that can measure our experience of a liquid bi-product of earth (sperm) that will develop and then rise from a fetal position in a womb, to an upright being. Then that same form of metamorphism after a time will return to a prostrate position back into the earth, perhaps maybe to return as the blade of grass does to its Mother Earth. Religious scholars say that a day to the Lord is like one thousand years. That being said, our appreciation of time and realty is very primitive.

I hope that there is something in these words that can inspire someone to become better in their life journey, by reading my life examples of the good and bad experiences and knowing some of the facts that are seldom talked about in the hair, health and beauty industry, an industry that has made so many people wealthy and an industry that I have personally spent most of my life working in and enjoying.

This book also tells the story of my blessed life that has taken me to so many places, met many in creditable people and allowed me to experience so many things that most people have not seen or would know very little about in a lifetime. I bare witness that it has been an incredible ride.

I thank God for allowing me to take this journey and share my feelings of love and pride for my family, loved ones and friends.

There are so many people that I owe to whatever I am of importance that it would be a book by itself if I were to go there. But let me start with Almighty God. I am not one of those who do not believe there is an omnipotent power that I will humble my intellectual conscious to. One power, as the Muslim believers would say, Allahu Akbar! Meaning God is greater, bigger wiser. Metaphorically speaking, I will not put God under a microscope like an amoeba to dissect, nor do I want to. I favor the idea that God is bigger, wiser, greater than me, in which is a power I can seek whenever I run out of my range of reality. I will seek my strength from that which is greater than mankind or creation; yes, I can live with that.

INTRODUCTION

*L*et me tell you a little about my long and interesting career, in hopes that you will see some of the good and bad things that might give you a broader understanding of my most exciting and very rewarding life. Also my adventures and prospective of the hair and beauty industry as I know it, and an important understanding of why I am writing this story. **Started June 19, 1998 Finished June19, 2015:**

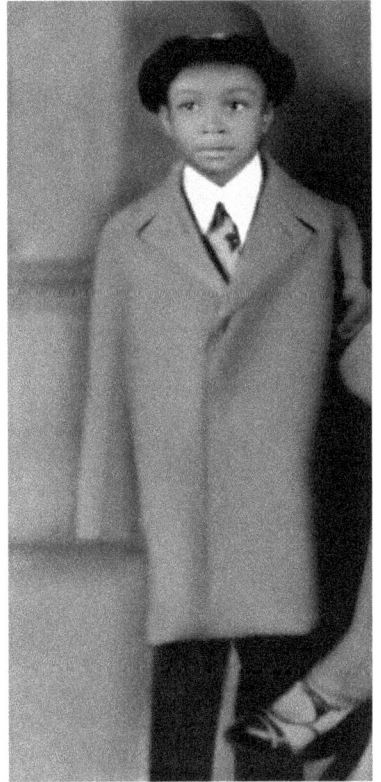

Aaron Bernard Thompson Jr. AKA Haroon Rashid

I was born Aaron Bernard Thompson Jr. on June 19, 1945 in Jacksonville Florida.

Ironically, I later in life found a common relationship to the date of my birth and the Juneteenth African American slave's celebration being on the same day.

From: *Wikipedia, the free encyclopedia*

Juneteenth Freedom Day or Emancipation Day:

Though Abraham Lincoln issued the Emancipation Proclamation on September 22, 1862, with an effective date of January 1, 1863; it had minimal immediate effect on most slaves' day-to-day lives, particularly in Texas, which was almost entirely under Confederate control. Texas was resistant to the Emancipation Proclamation, and though slavery was very prevalent in East Texas, it was not as common in the Western areas of Texas, particularly the Hill Country, where most German-Americans were opposed to the practice. Juneteenth commemorates June 18 and 19, 1865. June 18 is the day Union General Gordon Granger and 2,000 federal troops arrived in Galveston, Texas, to take possession of the state and enforce the emancipation of its slaves. On June 19, 1865, legend has it while standing on the balcony of Galveston's Ashton Villa, Granger read the contents of "General Order No. 3": The people of Texas are informed that, in accordance with a proclamation from the Executive of the United States, all slaves are free. This involves an absolute equality of personal rights and rights of property between former masters and slaves, and the connection heretofore existing between them becomes that between employer and hired labor. The freedmen are advised to remain quietly at their present homes and work for wages. They are informed that they will not be allowed to collect at military posts and that they will not be supported in idleness either there or elsewhere. That day has since become known as Juneteenth, a name derived from a portmanteau of the words June and nineteenth.

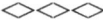

As a result of knowing that information I would often say to myself and others as a way to explain my perception of my character that I was born to be free and consequently I would never consciously capitulate or accept living out of a so-called slavery mentality. In that regard I do declare that I am a **SOVEREIGN HUMAN BEING** that will only recognize those that respect my absolute Equal Human Rights by any other human being. **I have been asked so many times what does my name Haroon Rashid,**

mean and does it have a history? The answer to that obviously is yes, on a personal level Haroon means Aaron as translated in English, the 1st Priest among the Hebrew People: Rashid is interpreted in the Persian cultural history as meaning the 98 of the 100 listed attributes of (Allah) it means Intelligent or the one that Gives Right Guidance. The surnames for the ancient Persians or Muslim people would likely always be one of the attributes of Allah, to be given or chosen as a template or description for the character of anyone who will use the names. So I always take a position that at any given time that I may be the only leader in a room and will adjust myself accordantly.

Once I received that name under the directions that, because of my well-known character and services that had been documented and observed by two of my great leaders and mentors at that time, The honorable Elijah Muhammad and his successor and son Imam Wallace Deen Muhammad, as the one that officially gave me the right to ascribe to my SOVERIGN name as Haroon Rashid: in the spirit of Harun AL Rashid.

Within powers of my limitations I will always honor my name and my sovereign identity that I have been honored to now pass on to my present and future descendants.

This information will explain that question of: "Who was my name derived from?" I will tell who and why in Chapter One.

~ Harun al-Rashid

Part One

HAROON RASHID

Chapter One

Haroon Rashid:
In the spirit of harun al rashid

I have included this information from Wikimedia Commons that has media related to Harun al-Rashid. However, I personally believe that the starting statement that he was the fifth Arab Abbasid Caliph that encompassed modern Iraq and if that is true it is very fascinating because Abbasside caliphate during Haroon's reign encompassed at least modern day Iran, Iraq, Saudi Arabia, Syria and parts of northern Africa.

Wikisource has original works written by or about: Harun al Rashid, Brentjes Sonja (2007). "Hārūn al-Rashīd". In Thomas Hockey et al. the Biographical Encyclopedia of Harun al-Rashid from Wikipedia, the free encyclopedia for the 12th-century caliph with the same epithet, see Al-Rashid (12th century).

Harun al-Rashid Harun-Charlemagne.jpg Harun al-Rashid receiving a delegation sent by Charlemagne at his court Caliph of the Abbasid Caliphate Reign 14 September 786 – 24 March 809 Predecessor al-Hadi Successor al-Amin Spouse Zubaidah Issue Muhammad, Caliph al-Amin Abdullah, Caliph al-Ma'mun Abbas, Caliph al-Mu'tasim Qasim

Sukaynahf full name Kunya? Given name: Harun Laqab: al-Rashid, Dynasty Abbasid: father al-Mahdi, mother al-Khayzuran, born 17 March 763 Rey, Abbasid Caliphate died 24 March 809 (aged 46) Tus, Abbasid Caliphate burial Tus

[1]
Harun al-Rashid (Arabic: هارون الرشيد}; Hārūn ar-Rashīd; English: Aaron the Upright, Aaron the Just, or Aaron the Rightly Guided)

(17 March 763 or February 766 — 24 March 809) was the fifth Abbasid Caliph. His rule encompassed modern Iraq. His actual birth date is debatable, and various sources give dates from 763 to 766.

Al-Rashid ruled from 786 to 809, and his time was marked by scientific, cultural, and religious prosperity. Islamic art and Islamic music also flourished significantly during his reign. He established the legendary library Bayt al-Hikma ("House of Wisdom").

Since Harun: was intellectually, politically, and militarily resourceful, his life and his court have been the subject of many tales. Some are claimed to be factual, but most are believed to be fictitious. An example of what is factual is the story of the clock that was among various presents that Harun had sent to Charlemagne. The presents were carried by the returning Frankish mission that came to offer Harun friendship in 799. Charlemagne and his retinue deemed the clock to be a conjuration for the sounds it emanated and the tricks it displayed every time an hour ticked.

[2]

Among what is known to be fictional is The Book of One Thousand and One Nights, which contains many stories that are fantasized by Harun's magnificent court and even Harun al-Rashid himself.

[3]

Hārūn was born in Rey. He was the son of al-Mahdi, the third Abbasid caliph (ruled 775 – 785), and al-Khayzuran, a former slave girl from Yemen, and a woman of strong personality who greatly influenced affairs of state in the reigns of her husband and sons. Hārūn was strongly influenced by the will of his mother in the governance of the empire until her death in 789. His vizier (chief minister) Yahya the Barmakid, Yahya's sons (especially

Ja'far ibn Yahya), and other Barmakids generally controlled the administration.

The Barmakids were a Persian family (from Balkh) which dated back to the Barmak of Magi, who had become very powerful under al-Mahdi. Yahya had helped Hārūn in obtaining the caliphate, and he and his sons were in high favor until 798, when the caliph threw them in prison and confiscated their land. Muhammad ibn Jarir al-Tabari dates this in 803 and lists various accounts for the cause: Yahya's entering the Caliph's presence without permission, Yahya's opposition to Muhammad ibn al Layth who later gained Harun's favour, Ja'far release of Yahya ibn Abdallah ibn Hasan whom Harun had imprisoned.

During the reign of the Harun al-Rashid, the city of Baghdad began to flourish as a center of knowledge, culture and trade.

The fall of the Barmakids is far more likely due to their behaving in a manner that Harun found disrespectful (such as entering his court unannounced) and making decisions in matters of state without first consulting him. Al-Fadl ibn al-Rabi succeeded Yahya the Barmakid as Harun's chief minister.

Hārūn became caliph when he was in his early twenties. Before that, in 780 and again in 782, he had already nominally led campaigns against the Caliphate's traditional enemy, the Byzantine Empire. The latter expedition was a huge undertaking, and even reached the Asian suburbs of Constantinople. On the day of accession, his son al-Ma'mun was born, and al-Amin some little time later: the latter was the son of Zubaida, a granddaughter of al-Mansur (founder of the city of Baghdad); so he took precedence over the former, whose mother was a Persian. He began his reign by appointing very able ministers, who carried on the work of the government so well that they greatly improved the condition of the people.

[4]

A silver dirham minted in Madinat al-Salam (Bagdad) in 170 AH (786 CE). At the reverse, the inner marginal inscription says: "By order of the slave of God, Harun, and Commander of the Faithful."

It was under Hārūn ar-Rashīd that Baghdad flourished into the most splendid city of its period. Tribute was paid by many rulers to the caliph, and these funds were used on architecture, the arts and a luxurious life at court.

In 796, Hārūn decided to move his court and the government to Ar Raqqah at the middle Euphrates. Here he spent 12 years, most of his reign. Only once did he return to Baghdad for a short visit. Several reasons might have influenced the decision to move to ar-Raqqa. It was close to the Byzantine border. The communication lines via the Euphrates to Baghdad and via the Balikh River to the north and via Palmyra to Damascus were excellent. The agriculture was flourishing to support the new Imperial center. And from Raqqa any rebellion in Syria and the middle Euphrates area could be controlled. Abu al-Faraj al-Isfahani pictures in his anthology of poems the splendid life in his court. In ar-Raqqah the Barmekids managed the fate of the empire, and heirs, al-Amin and al-Ma'mun grew up.

Due to the Thousand-and-One Nights tales, Harun al-Rashid turned into a legendary figure obscuring his true historic personality. In fact, his reign initiated the political disintegration of the Abbasid caliphate. Syria was inhabited by tribes with Umayyad sympathies and remained the bitter enemy of the Abbasids, while Egypt witnessed uprisings against Abbasids due to maladministration and arbitrary taxation. The Umayyads had been established in Spain in 755, the Idrisids in Morocco in 788, and the Aghlabids in Ifriqiya (modern Tunisia) in 800. Besides, unrest flared up in

Yemen, and the Kharijites rose in rebellion in Daylam, Kerman, Fars and Sistan. Revolts also broke out in Khorasan, and al-Rashid waged many campaigns against the Byzantines.

For the administration of the whole empire, he fell back on his mentor and longtime associate Yahya bin Khalid bin Barmak. Rashid appointed him as his vizier with full executive powers, and, for seventeen years, this man Yahya and his sons served Rashid faithfully in whatever assignment he entrusted to them.

[5]
Al-Rashid appointed Ali bin Isa bin Mahan as the governor of Khorasan. He tried to bring to heel the princes and chieftains of the region, and to re-impose the full authority of the central government on them. This new policy met with fierce resistance and provoked numerous uprisings in the region. A major revolt led by Rafi ibn al-Layth was started in Samarqand which forced Harun al-Rashid to move to Khorasan. He first removed and arrested Ali bin Isa bin Mahan but the revolt continued unchecked. Harun al-Rashid died very soon when he reached Sanabad village in Tus and was buried in the nearby summer palace of Humayd ibn Qahtaba, the former Abbasid governor in Khorasan.

Al-Rashid virtually dismembered the empire by apportioning it between his two son's al-Amin and al-Ma'mun (with his third son, al-Qasim, being belatedly added after them). Very soon it became clear that by dividing the empire, Rashid had actually helped to set the opposing parties against one another, and had provided them with sufficient resources to become independent of each other. After the death of Harun al-Rashid, civil war broke out in the empire between his two sons, al-Amin and al-Ma'mun, which spiraled into a prolonged period of turmoil and warfare throughout the Caliphate, ending only with Ma'mun's final triumph in 827.

Both Einhard and Notker the Stammerer refer to envoys travelling between Harun's and Charlemagne's courts, amicable discussions concerning Christian access to the Holy Land and the exchange of gifts. Notker mentions Charlemagne sent Harun Spanish horses, colourful Frisian cloaks and impressive hunting dogs. In 802 Harun sent Charlemagne a present consisting of silks, brass candelabra, perfume, balsam, ivory chessmen, a colossal tent with many-colored curtains, an elephant named Abul-Abbas, and a water clock that marked the hours by dropping bronze balls into a bowl, as mechanical knights—one for each hour—emerged from little doors, which shut behind them. The presents were unprecedented in Western Europe and may have influenced Carolingian art.

When the Byzantine empress Irene was deposed, Nikephoros I became emperor and refused to pay tribute to Harun, saying that Irene should have been receiving the tribute the whole time. News of this angered Harun, who wrote a message on the back of the Roman Emperor's letter and said "In the name of God the most merciful, From Amir al-Mu'minin Harun al-Rashid, commander of the faithful, to Nikephoros, dog of the Romans. Thou shalt not hear, thou shalt behold my reply". After campaigns in Asia Minor, Nikephoros was forced to conclude a treaty, with humiliating terms.

[6][7]
Harun made the pilgrimage to Mecca several times, e.g., 793, 795, 797, 802 and last in 803. Tabari concludes his account of Harun's reign with these words: "It has been said that when Harun al-Rashid died, there were nine hundred million odd (dirhams) in the state treasury."

Al-Rashid sent embassies to the Chinese Tang dynasty and established good relations with them.

[8][9] He was called "A-lun" in the Chinese T'ang Annals.

[10]
In 807 Caliph Harun al-Rashid issued a decree that Jews wear a yellow belt and that Christians wear a blue belt.

[11]
In 808, Harun went to settle the insurrection of Rafi ibn al-Layth in Transoxania, became ill, and died in 809. He was buried under the palace of Hamid ibn Qahtabi, the governor of Khurasan. The location later became known as Mashhad ("The Place of Martyrdom") because of the martyrdom of Imam ar-Ridha in 818. Another tradition maintains that the tomb of Harun was razed in the Mongol raids of 1220, by forces under the command of Genghis Khan.

Anecdotes

Many anecdotes attached themselves to the person of Harun al-Rashid in the centuries following his rule. Saadi of Shiraz inserted a number of them into his Gulistan, in one telling how Harun enjoined his son to forgiveness.

Al-Masudi relates a number of interesting anecdotes in The Meadows of Gold illuminating the character of this caliph. For example, he recounts Harun's delight when his horse came in first, closely followed by al-Ma'mun's, at a race Harun held at Raqqa. Al-Masudi tells the story of Harun setting his poets a challenging task. When others failed to please him, Miskin of Medina succeeded superbly well: The poet then launched into a moving account of how much it had cost him to learn that song. Harun laughed saying he knew not which more was entertaining, the song or the story. He rewarded the poet

[12]
There is also the tale of Harun asking Ishaq ibn Ibrahim to keep singing. The musician did until the caliph fell asleep. Then,

strangely, a handsome young man appeared, snatched the musician's lute, sang a very moving piece (al-Masudi quotes it), and left. On awakening and being informed of this, Harun said Ishaq ibn Ibrahim had received a supernatural visitation.

Harun, like a number of caliphs, is given an anecdote connecting a poem with his death. Shortly before he died, he is said to have been reading some lines by Abu al-Atahiya about the transitory nature of the power and pleasures of this world.

Chapter Two

My Parents
And their lineage

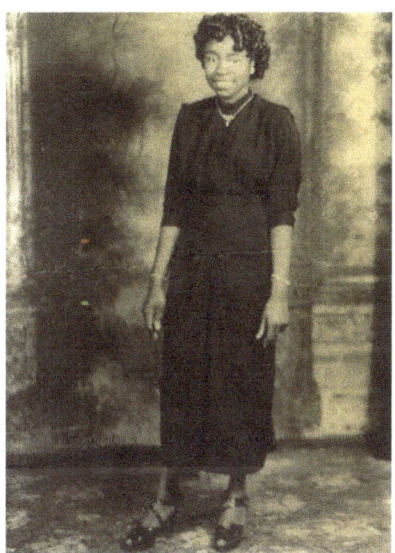
Mom: Marie Thompson Pendarvis

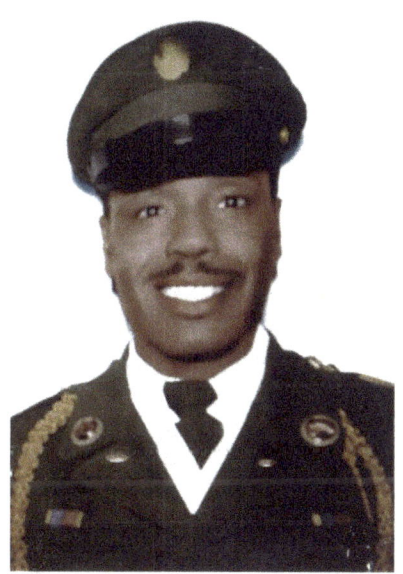
Dad: Aaron Smith

My mother Marie Thompson and my dad **Aaron Smith** had me when they both were very young; my mom was a domestic worker, at that time. My dad was active in the United States Army during the war against Japan when I was born. They both were born and raised in Jacksonville, Florida. My mother's mother, Pearl Amakar Corley, was a well-known seamstress in South Carolina where she was born. At a very young age, Mama Pearl was taught her skills that were passed down to her by her mother, Mama Essie Amakar who was the matriarch and entrepreneur of the family. It was considered a miracle by most that Mama Pearl's mother, Mama Essie was so well respected for her talents as a seamstress, and that even after she later became blind, she still was able to sew and do excellent work with the help of her daughter Pearl. It has been said that, as the second oldest, Mama Pearl was so close to her mother and that by her helping her mother perfected her work as a seamstress during that time; and it enabled her to become a master in the craft herself. My grandmother, Mama Pearl Corley, on my mother's side was one of 23 siblings and she died when I was a just a child. I have very vague memories of her in Florida when I lived there, because I was so young before I left to live in Boston.

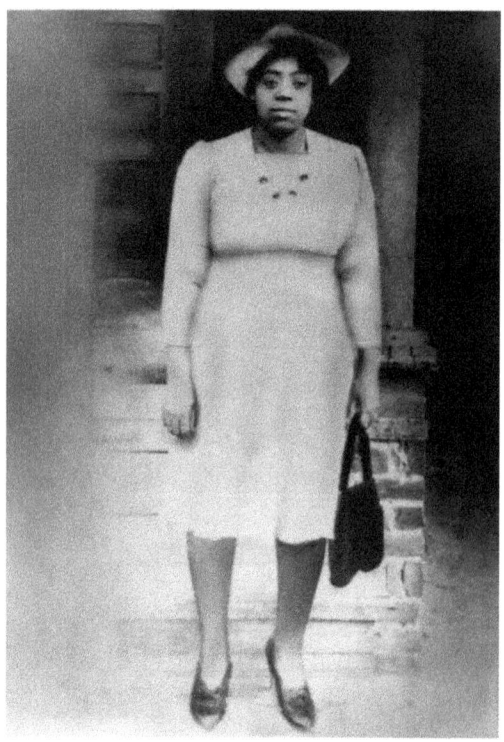

Grandmother Pearl Amakar Corley

I do remember the great love I had from my family and especially my mother's mother before she died, when I was just three years old. So it was my dad's parents, who I referred to as Daddy Amos and Mother Carrie Smith, who were the only immediate grandparents that I had alive in my life when I was a young child, other than my great grandmother on my mother's side of the family, who we all affectionately called Mama. I loved all of my grandparents because they all gave me so much special love and attention. Each summer during school breaks I would travel from Boston to Jacksonville to visit my grandparents. Daddy Amos was a middle class entrepreneur who owned several row houses in Jacksonville that he rented out to tenants; he also had a business of selling wood chips and coal for heating and cooking to a large amount of clients. He would sometimes let me help him bag the materials as he would stack them in one of his pickup trucks. Daddy Amos retired as a factory worker from a box container and manufacturing company in Jacksonville, Florida before he died.

Mother Carrie was a very religious housewife as well as a successful AVON products salesperson. She had clients all over Jacksonville. Mother Carrie was the AVON lady that loved to dress formal, even in the heat of the day, and if I or my brother and sisters would go out in the public with her, she made sure that we were well dressed to the maximum. As children, it was a known fact that every weekend we would get to go downtown Jacksonville to shop and sometimes we would travel with her as she would go door to door and sell to her many AVON clients as she negotiated her sales.

The Smiths were well-respected Christians in the neighborhood where they lived and many of the neighbors would come to both of them for advice or help from Mama Carrie or Daddy Amos. Whenever we would walk the block with them in the neighborhood everyone that would be on the porches - men, women and children - would greet them, "Hey Miss Carrie or Mr. Amos" and sometimes it would take an hour to just go one block because of the intercommunication and bonding among the neighbors in the neighborhood. I soon got to know every one of them and they knew me as well. If they witnessed any bad behavior from me or my brother and sisters they would warn me, and in some cases send me immediately to my grandparents; but that did not happen too often because I loved my grandparents and did not want to disappoint or embarrass them.

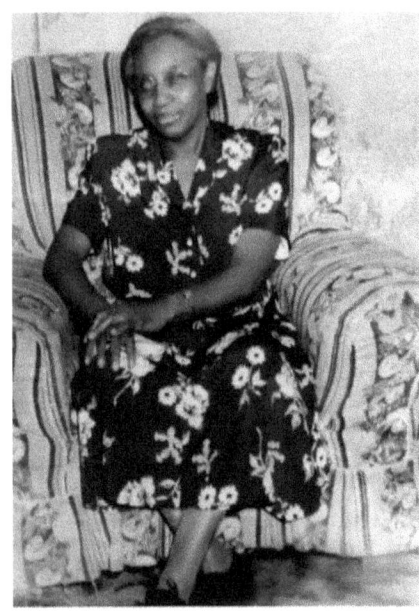

Great-grandmother Essie Boyde Amakar, Jones

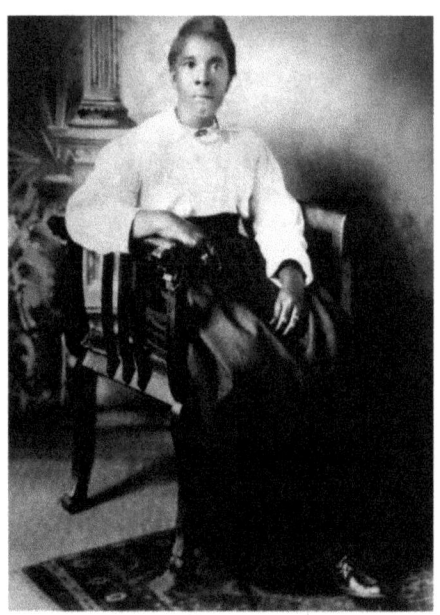

Great great -Grandmother Emma Amakar

My great- grandmother on my mother's side Mrs. Essie Boyde Amakar Jones was born and lived in Orangeburg South Carolina. She had been married two times in her life, her first husband Mr. David Amakar died, after having two children with Mama Essie, Pearl Amakar Corley & Sarah Amakar Harris. She remarried and her second husband, Mr. Isaac Israel Jones who was a Baptist preacher at that time, left and moved to Jacksonville Florida. Soon after Mama came to Florida, she lost her vision and was blind the rest of her life.

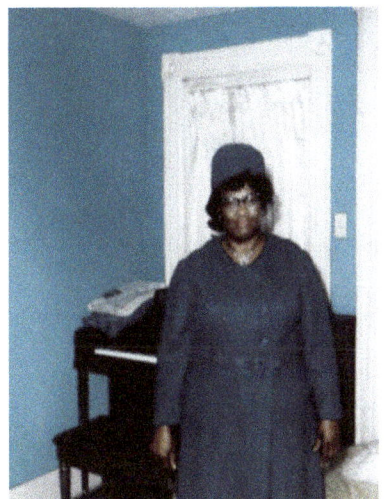
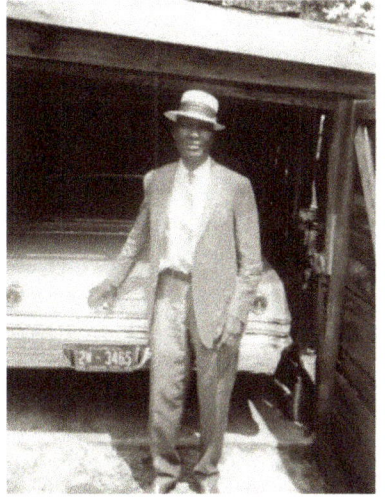

Grandmother: Carrie Smith   *Grandfather: Amos Smith*

Ethnically speaking Mama's dad was of mixed race and her mother was a Cherokee Indian. As a child I can remember being fascinated by her long waist-length gray hair; I loved her and always wanted to be around her. I was her first great-grandchild; and to me she was so beautiful, soft-spoken and extremely smart.

After moving to Boston, I can remember when I was around seven years old; I was allowed to take Mama around the neighborhood that was then called the South End, which is a section of Boston where most of the African Americans lived that had migrated from the south at that time. I was so attached to Mama that when she would go to church every Sunday, I would escort her. I can remember that when she would get (the holy spirit) in church and she would get up praising and, not knowing what was wrong with her, I would get so scared that she was hurting and would cry until someone would come to convince me she was alright.

Even though my dad and my mother never got married, my grandmother, Mother Carrie Smith and my grandfather, Daddy Amos Smith, on my dad's side treated me and my mother with a lot of love. In the late thirties and early forties, when I was just five-years-old I moved to Boston to join with others in my mom's large family that started migrating from Florida in the late thirties and forties.

My dad and my mother never married, but my mother did meet a man that, at the time, was a porter on the railroad and he was responsible for many of the family members riding the railways as means of transportation out of the south and migrating to Canada, Boston and New York in the early 1940's.

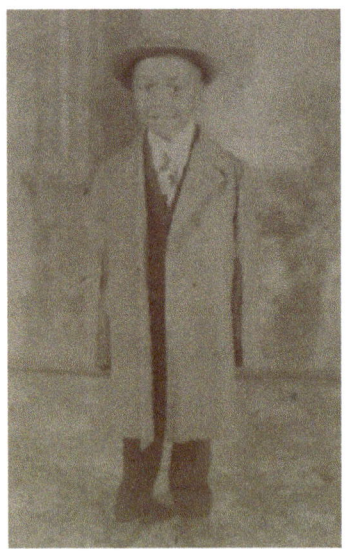
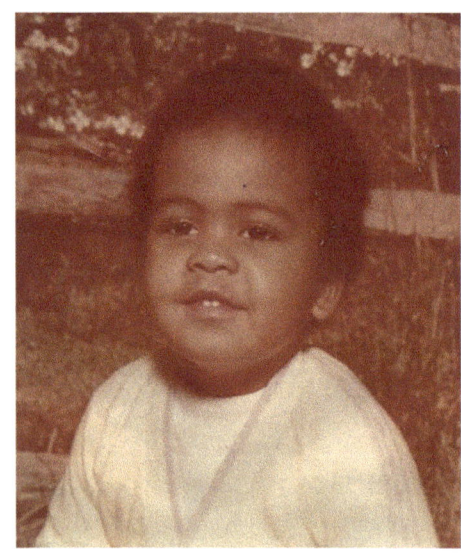

Aaron Bernard Thompson Jr.   *Brother: Joe Pendarvis*

My Mother got married after I was about two or three years old, to Mr. Leonard Pendarvis, she soon had my brother Douglas Pendarvis in Jacksonville; but unfortunately things were not working out for their marriage and she decided that she wanted to move with the rest of her family that was slowly migrating to Boston. Soon after moving to Boston, my mother and step father had one more child together, my sister Cynthia Pendarvis, before they finally separated due to irreconcilable differences. Later we were blessed with my youngest brother Joe Pendarvis, who was adopted by my mom as a baby and became a beloved member of our family, as well as the academically stable business-minded one of the siblings. After Joe joined the Massachusetts National Guard he went on to become a Non Commission Officer in the financial division in the Metro New England District. He and I are the only ones of the siblings that entered into the military and we proudly and humorously would often compare the differences of the Marine Corps and the National Guard.

Chapter Three

When I Came Up To Boston

While talking about my journey coming to Boston, I learned that the plan was my Aunt Viola Jones Drummer would take me with her by train and I would stay with her until my mom could get things together and then later come herself.

My Aunt Viola Drummer was a remarkable woman, who soon after graduating in 1941 from the Public Stanton High School in Jacksonville Florida, graduated from a cosmetology school. She soon became the family cosmetologist and barber, as well as the trail blazer for many other family members, including myself, in the field of cultural services. Aunt Vie, as all my younger cousins referred to her as, would often tell the story about how I was one of the first children in the family to come up directly from the south when she brought my favorite cousin Joyce Jones and me with her to Boston.

She would often remind me of an incident that happened while we were traveling. When we got to New York City from Florida while waiting in Grand Central Station for a train to Boston, I wandered away from my Aunt Viola and Uncle Charlie Drummer, who was minding me at the time. A strange white man managed to get my attention and started walking off with me. While I was happily singing gospel songs and skipping along with this stranger my Aunt Vie said she was afraid that he was trying to kidnap me.

My Uncle Charlie stopped the man and we made it on to Boston without further incident. After that dangerous and scary experience Aunt Vie would always remind me that I was a child who loved to travel and would wander off in a minute if not watched.

That singular interest in the phenomenon of traveling has always spiked a curiosity in me of the nature and history of migration or metaphorically speaking, what is on the other side of the mountain or river?

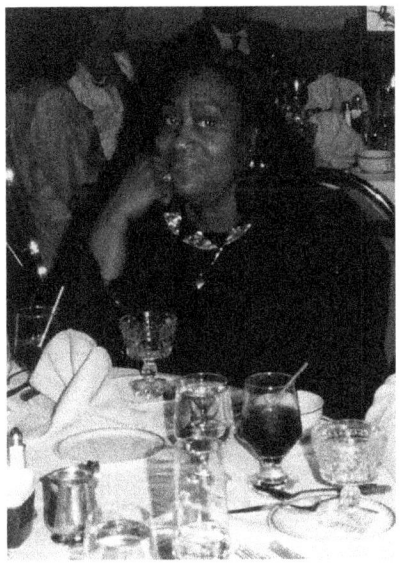
Aunt Viola Drummer

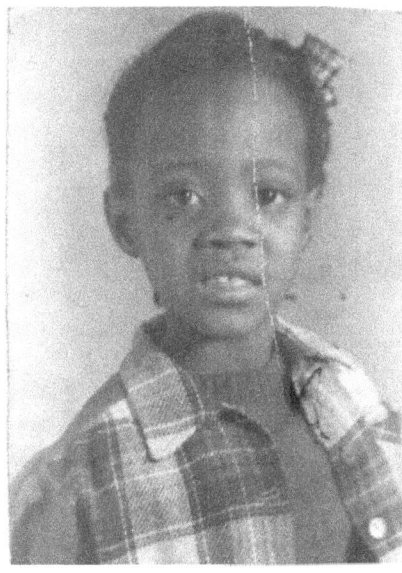
Cousin Joyce Jones

My step-father Mr. Leonard Pendarvis, like most working class African American men and women in the forties and fifties, would make every attempt to dress as formal and professionally as their experience would allow them to achieve. Dress suit, ties, polished shoes and top hats, even in their homes if they knew that they would be captured in a picture.

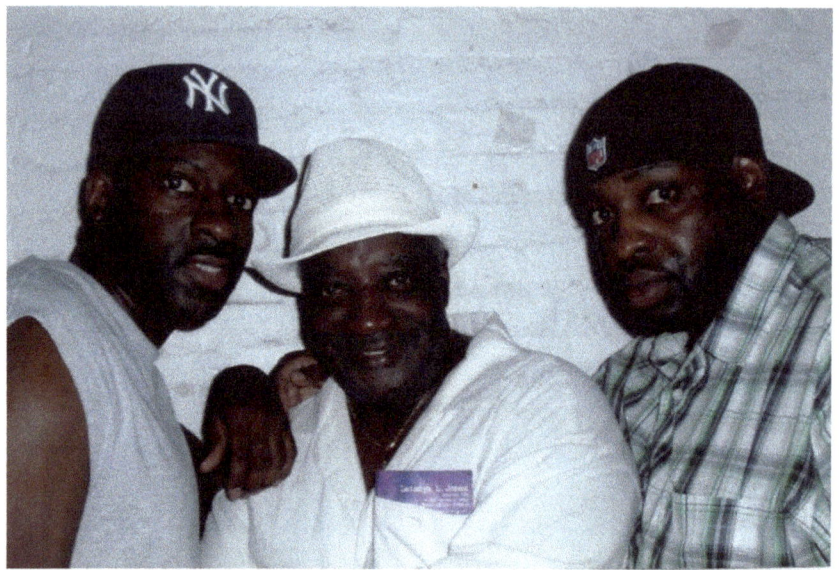

My brothers Kennard, Douglas and Virgil Pendarvis

Of his biological children, besides my brother Douglas Pendarvis and my sister Cynthia Pendarvis, I have three other brothers: Leonard Pendarvis Jr., Kennard Pendarvis, and Virgil Pendarvis. My step-father was an honorable man that did everything he could to help my Mom and the family the best way that he knew how.

He prided himself in maintaining a fatherly interest in his children and set examples of strong working ethics; however when he would demonstrate his casual or leisure moments he did it with a lot of style. Pops, as he was called by his children, was a railroad porter which in those days was considered as a very important working class, African American job for men. Historically, these men were basically responsible for most of the means of traveling for so many African Americans during the great migration from the South to the North. My family was very indebted to the service and support from Pops.

MY CULTURAL BIRTH RIGHTS

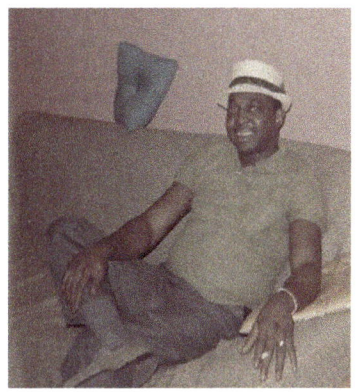
Mr. Leonard Pendarvis

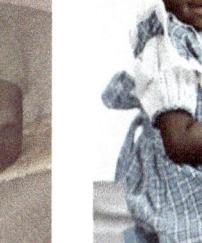
Sister; Cynthia Pendarvis

After my Mother finally came to Boston by train she brought with her my great-grandmother, Mama Essie Amakar Jones; my brother Douglas; and one of my favorite cousins, Juanita Walker.

Douglas was the second and my Sister Cynthia the third of my stepfather's children; and after my mom had finally moved to Boston they and I would travel back and forth to visit my Grandparents, Mother Carrie and Daddy Amos. Visiting my family in Florida was always great for me.

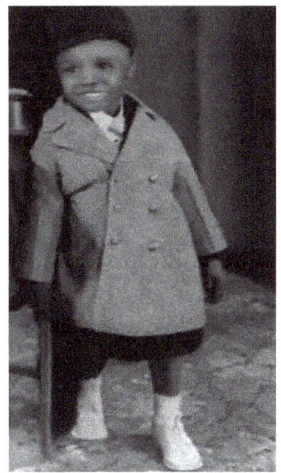
My Brother: Douglas Pendarvis

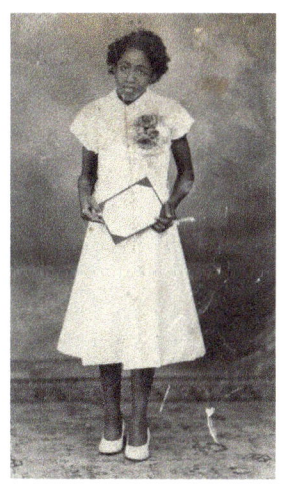
Cousin: Juanita Walker

Later, my family would use the porter service that would escort us as youths, without the company of our parents, from Grand Central Station in New York City all the way to Jacksonville, Florida.

Chapter Four

The Great Migration (1916-1930)

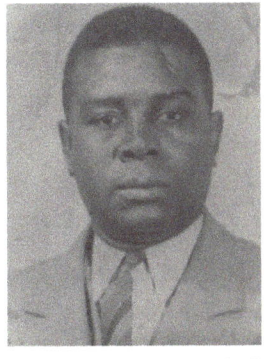

Uncle Marion Jones

This is my micro version of some of my research and thoughts on the subject of migration of African Americans from the South to the North. In my family's case we can trace one family member, my Uncle Marion Jones and his immediate family members, moved from Jacksonville, Florida to St. John's New Brunswick Canada in the early nineteen thirties. Then in 1937 Uncle Marion Jones moved his family members to Boston, paving the way for others like Aunt Vie and the rest of my family that followed.

During that time, even before my Aunt Vie brought my cousin Joyce and me to Boston, two of my uncles, Buster and Son as the family called them, were both in the Merchant Marines. While traveling around the Northeastern area and knowing that their brother Marion had moved to Boston they would go there to visit him and his family before any of the rest of their siblings would eventually go to Boston.

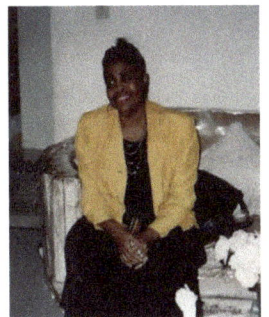

Aunt Essie Mae Jones Butler

It was also known that my grandmother Pearl and my Aunt Essie Mae Jones Butler had also come to Boston to visit her brother Marion. It is said that she might have stayed in Boston, but she was the oldest female of her siblings and her mother had gone blind since moving from Orangeburg, South Carolina to Jacksonville Florida. Even though blind, Mama was still sewing clothes, with the help of her oldest daughter, my grandmother Pearl, whom she had taught the skills of the trade. That being said, visiting Boston before going back to Jacksonville helped encourage other family members to eventually move to Boston, including Mama. Unfortunately, my grandmother died early from serious health issues.

The family migration had begun to expand beyond the South and move more into the North: Baltimore, Washington D.C., Philadelphia. Newark New Jersey, New York and Boston. The great migration had already begun in my family and like most African Americans, we never looked back.

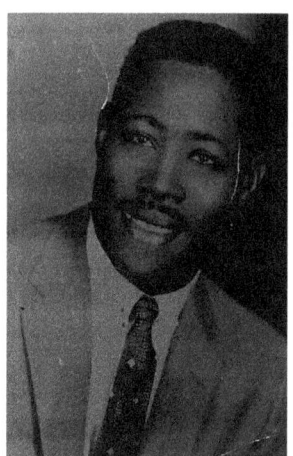

Uncle Son: Willie Jones

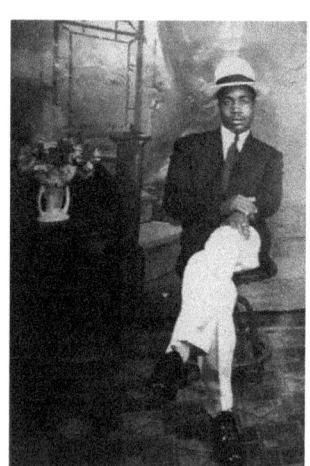

Uncle Buster: John S. Jones

Some 1.5 million people moved north between 1916 and 1930 during the Great Migration when the war industry offered industrial jobs to African Americans. Thus began the transformation of the African-American population from a predominantly rural to a predominantly urban people. It is of special interest to know that in most major cites the first home and residency for African Americans was in the downtown district of those cites. As the middle class American Caucasians or the affluent moved up, the poor and African Americans were forced out of the center of most large cities as the Caucasians kept the best location of the cites, the heart of the cities for themselves. My family followed in the tradition of many African American southerners during that time in American history. Around 1930- 1955 the migration increased in vast numbers as our family members began to settle in Boston.

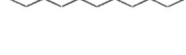

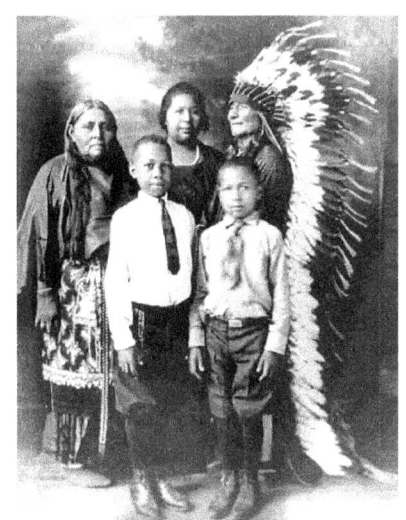

Picture from Google search Images of "The Trail of Tears; the American Black Indians

As I mentioned, ethnically speaking Mama's dad was of mixed race and her mother was a Cherokee Indian which technically made her a black Indian.

This was the story that I was taught about my family's early migrations and its relationship to the American Indians Trail of Tears. It was always for me a question that was left to explain: *what is a Seminole Indian and how does that relate to my family and their reason to leave one of the most racist States in America, South Carolina and to go further south into another racist environment?*

Beginning with an important question of what is the make-up of a Seminole Indian Tribe?

In 2008 I had been invited as a guest speaker and gave a lector at an American Indian Tribal Consul meeting. It was there that I had the pleasure to experience the lesions of wisdom by an honorary Tribal Chief and Wiseman named Billy Wildfire.

He was a guest speaker that spoke on behalf the North American, Mexican and Canadian Tribal Chief's about the different Indian bands and tribal concerns.

It was located at the Forest Band Reservation and Casino on the Forest Band National Park in Wisconsin. I was there representing the Friends of DuSable Not for Profit as a guest speaker and I was asked to speak on the legacy of Chicago's Founder Mr. Jean Baptiste Pointe DuSable.

History has shown that hypothetically speaking Mr. DuSable was actively performing as the First Mayor in the City of Chicago: when it was then called Eschicago.

Mr. DuSable was a man of African and European decent and married to a full Native American Pottawatomi woman named Kittihawa, later after being converted into the Catholic Church she then became Catherine.

Together they had two children a boy Jean and a girl Susanne making their children to become the first multi-cultural diverse experience in the region and one of their grandchildren being born in Chicago further known as the first Black Indian's.

My mission was to update the narrative of the First People in relationship to multi-cultural global diversity of the African Indigoes people.

The fact of the matter is that the Seminole people were a mixture of trans-tribal bands of Indians, of many different Indian Tribes and Bands that found reason to unite as one; and they were then called Seminoles.

It was also known at that time that many of the bands of Indians had biracial children, who were born from interracial marriages with Native American Indians, also known as The First People. My family connection to the Cherokee nation was heavily populated in the North and South Carolina region near the slave plantations.

It was also well known and commonplace that when a runaway slave would escape off the slave plantations many of them would escape to the safe haven of some Indian Reservations for freedom, while there they would intermingle and marry, thusly producing the first multicultural experiences on the reservations, the American Black Indians.

It has been said by many Native American Wiseman that there had been many brutal wars fought to protect the children of the Black Indians and their parents from their former slave masters that would consider their children as their sovereign property and would demand for their return back into slavery on their plantations.

That is one of the reasons why many of the Black Indians became Seminoles, they were protected and fought many brutal wars to that end and was a nexus in the historical journey of the Native Americans-Trail of Tears.

Hypothetically speaking my family had journeyed on the Trail of Tears from the State of South Carolina to Florida seeking to escape the slavery conditions of South Carolina and was able to fine some opportunities along the way to then settle in the city of

Jacksonville Florida and then ultimately latter finally migrate and to eventually permanently settle in Boston Massachusetts.

It has been well documented that slavery was prevalent between 1630 until 1783 which was the year that slavery was abolished in Massachusetts. However little is known or talked about the cynical beastly actions of the European settlers in New England and the United Kingdom British leadership on human slave traffic exchanges. History has revealed that many of the Native Americans were the first to be enslaved in Massachusetts and how that caused a big problem for the barbaric settlers in that the Native Americans were so much more familiar with their natural terrain.

Because of that fact, the new settlers, upon their captivity of the Native Americans to be their slaves for labor, found it difficult to contain them as domestic or field slaves.

So they made agreements with England that they would trade Native Americans as slaves into the United Kingdom in exchange for the African slaves in England, which they captured during the notorious Trilateral Slave Trade era involving (Africa, Europe and the Americas); that would disable ether the two nationalities of their natural habitat from the ability to feel comfortable to escape into a potential unfamiliar environment.

It is also well known that some Native Americans negotiated for their own freedom with the European settlers and slave owners by being bounty hunters and that some of them were even slave owners themselves with their own plantations.

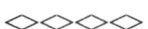

The migration of African Americans, or the so-called "Negro", to the north was very popular in those days, as southerners desired to leave the segregation in the south for a better life of opportunities in the north. Along the east coast, New York, Boston, Baltimore, Newark, Hartford, Providence, Washington D.C., and Philadelphia were the most popular cities that many African Americans migrated to.

Other known great northern cities for this great Migration were: Chicago, Detroit, Milwaukee, Gary, Indianapolis, St. Louis, Seattle, or Cleveland; they too had similar opportunities for African Americans.

New York was famous for entertainment, fashion, and great department stores, merchandise industries and factories in great numbers; also in those days New York City offered better paying jobs. The New York population grew, and the five boroughs of New York City were developed in Manhattan, Queens, Brooklyn, the Bronx, and Staten Island. The big boom of populations started after the Civil War that spurned the great migration from the South.

History shows that around the early 1600-1700's most of the African American slaves that first lived in New York on the Island of Manhattan, in the down town section near the World Trade Center district. In fact, in the late 1990's while a contracting construction company was digging up a section of land in lower Manhattan, they dug up an ancient African American burial ground that gave evidence of the presence of an African American community that lived in that area. Many within the African American community in New York demanded the construction stopped until there was a clear presence of forensic scientists and African spiritual leaders that would preserve the remains and give a proper African burial libation ceremony to honor the dead and their remains. The body remains were eventually sent to Howard University to be further researched and preserved by African American forensic scientists.

The other city of choice on the East Coast was Boston because it was the city for educational opportunism and the pilot city for the freemason culture in America. Boston had the first Masonic lodge and headquarters in America. It started for the purpose of instituting a so-called high class culture to make a people that wanted class and were willing to learn in a method of extreme secrecy the knowledge to aristocracy. In the city of Cambridge, which is separated by the Charles River from Boston, is housed the first College or University in America known as Harvard University, which started as a Theologian College.

History tells us that King James of England was the father of the British slave trade and that he commissioned Sir John Hawkins for that purpose. It is interesting that King James around the early 1600's also commissioned an action to diligently revise the Christian Bible to the King James Version of the Bible and soon after those colonies, then cities like Boston, in America were being developed.

Many of these citizens were the unwanted mischievous misfits that came from Southern Europe, and were being gathered up and exiled to the New England colony area. The city of Boston developed quickly and soon had the first Public Park, the first Public Museum, first Public Transportation System and the first Public Schools. All were models designed by Great Brittan immigrants to be called to this day the Hub of the American culture in New England.

In the tradition of the early American cities demography: what is known as Beacon Hill in downtown Boston, was the first location and area that African Americans lived in. Boston, like

New York, Philadelphia or Chicago, as the city grew was developed into sections such as Back Bay, Roxbury, East Boston, South Boston, Dorchester and Mattapan. Each section was populated with the different nationalities that immigrated or migrated to Boston and most of the African Americans were brought there as slaves or servants in the inner-city areas.

Growing Up In Boston

My family is very close knit; we always stayed close to each other and looked out for each other. My best friends growing up in Boston were my cousins; and I felt good, knowing that I belonged to a large family. I would go every summer to visit my father's parents and my grandparents in Florida. While there, I can remember feeling that I was special, and I believed my grandparents were some highly moral, Jesus loving people, and to me they were living a good life. My grandmother's father was a holiness evangelist minister from North Carolina. He brought his family to Jacksonville, Florida to help spread the Christian gospel.

There was a similar circumstance on my mother's side of the family as well. That is why when I was born I was given the name of my father which was Aaron, meaning the first priest of the Hebrews and the brother of the Hebrew prophet Moses.

I always felt pressured that my grandparents' desire for me was to become a Christian preacher and that I never could find the motivation to do that. I know that I surprised them and maybe disappointed them when I later became a Muslim minister.

My Grandparents were a hard-working, middle class couple, my granddad owned several row houses that he rented out, and he worked for a cardboard Container Company until his retirement.

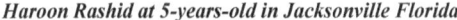

Haroon Rashid at 5-years-old in Jacksonville Florida

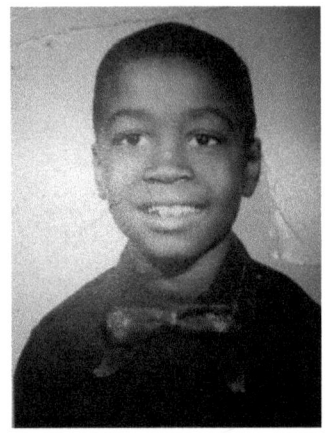

When I was 5-years-old my grandmother put that ensemble together on me while I visited her down there in Jacksonville Florida on a summer vacation and she took this picture. I love the bow tie but the collars, well that is another thing all by itself; however, it was the thought that counted. Maybe that's why whenever I would come back home after my yearly summer vacations to Boston and prepare for the new school year, along with my new wardrobe of suits, shoes and pants; I would always have lots of new white shirts with my initials A.T. monogrammed on the shirt collars. I loved my grandmother, Mother Carrie.

I would have chores to do in the houses, helping my granddad as he would paint or fix up one of those houses every summer when I would visit them. I had a sister, my dad's daughter, whose name is Sandra Smith and lots of cousins and friends that lived there. I would have a great time all summer and I would look forward to returning each year. I especially looked forward to visiting my baby sister Sandra whom I loved to see each year.

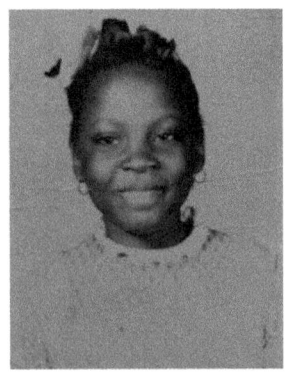

My Sister Sandra Smith

It was while going back and forth to Florida that I learned my first motto. When I was a young boy, I had a crush on my grandparents' neighbor's daughter, Patti.

She would always quote to me when she sensed I was trying to flirt with her, but I would not say anything. Patti would tell me, **"Say what you mean and mean what you say"**. To this day I still can be heard saying those profound words to people.

One of the other things that were most exciting about going and coming from Florida was the bragging rights that I would have among my friends at school. I truly think that began my taste for grooming and style, which I grew up with.

I grew up in Boston in an era when having your clothes custom-made, especially if you had the means to get them, was a special trend among African American youths that knew where to get their clothes reasonably made. There were plenty of stores that catered to fashionable stylish youths in those days just for that purpose. It created a kind of friendly competition among African American youths, based on who could create the best items. Strangely many Caucasian boys in those days would wear jeans that would sag and expose their underwear, which was the clear difference between the two cultural styles in those days.

I always felt that my peers and I had more class and taste, as we were considered as being over the top by our Caucasian classmates or friends and we laughed at them as being clueless about what we simply called as cool style and fashion. It is sometimes laughable how the young African Americans in the 21st century wound up trending after that genre of the 20th century Caucasian youths. I can remember getting my pants and shirts custom made as a teenager. My hats were custom made and had my name monogrammed on the inside brim. I remember shopping in those days at the then famous Filene's Basement department store in Boston for designer shoes, topcoats and accessories with one of my cousins James Harris, as teens to finish off the looks of our custom pieces.

James and I both later became hair stylists; James' specialty was hair fashion designs. I know now that we were preparing ourselves as youth for the business of cultural grooming, and we did not even know it then. The good thing about growing up in Boston was that the city is so culturally orientated that it is a breeding ground for cultural development. There are museums, libraries, colleges and universities all over the six-mile by six-mile square city boarder of Boston, and as a youth I was encouraged, by word of mouth, to go to one or all of those facilities. I have always loved visiting the museums and the options to sit in on classes in one of the many colleges and universities to gain extra knowledge.

Most of my friends in some way had an enthusiastic appreciation for art, whether it was painting, drawing, singing, dancing, writing, lecturing or fashion; and everyone competed in some friendly way. To the best of my knowledge, I began having an interest in art at the eighth grade level while in junior high school, at the Patrick T. Campbell School in Boston, Massac-Massachusetts. The Campbell was a very diverse school at that time because the community was still made up with a broad multicultural neighborhood. There was a large presence of Jewish students, Synagogues and businesses in the area at that time. We lived on Quincy Street, which was two blocks from the school and I prided myself in knowing all the students that had talents in the arts. I personally was taking drum lessons, arts and science, and my favorite was vocal music and dance.

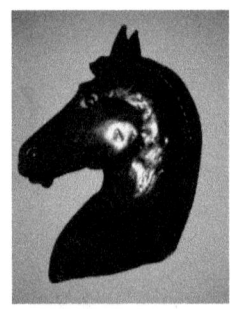

Wood carved sculptor of a Trojan horse 9th. Grade

In the ninth grade I represented the arts and crafts department for my school as part of our graduation ceremony from Junior High on to

High school. My arts craft that I created was a wood carved sculptured redemption of the symbolic American Bald Eagle with its wings spread and its claws holding twelve arrows.

I thought that the sculpture was alright, but I knew I could do better. My mother naturally said she liked my art piece and it was good to her, I found myself constantly defending what was friendly, teasing jokes among my friends about my art.

One of my close friends Lenny Thomson would playfully tease me and say that it looked like a buzzard holding bones; but that did not make me mad because I knew he was just teasing me. So when his older sister said to me that my artwork was so nice and she asked me if she could have it, I gave it to her. I liked her and it was a way to say to Lenny it cannot be that bad, your big sister likes it. Anyway I knew it was pretty good, after all I represented my school's arts and craft department, and was given a free tuition summer course in sculpturing at the Massachusetts College of Arts at the 9th grade level. I also carved a solid oak wood Trojan horse from scratch that I gave to my Mother and it is still in her house today.

It was at the Massachusetts College of Arts that I learned the basics of sculpturing & the science of artistic form and shaping. My instructor showed me how to find and develop head forms, dimensions, and shapes by molding, using clay and wire. That knowledge would help me later as some people would say to become an excellent hair cutter.

I went on to Boston Trade High School, because I knew that I wanted to work with arts and crafts in some way. There I tried to study the tool and die making trade; even though I was good at it, the idea of dirty and cut up hands was not appealing to me. The School was directly across the street from the Wentworth Institute of Technology an Aeronautical Engineer College. I had ideas at times that I would apply there after graduating from high school. But it never happened that way. In High School as well as Junior High, I ran track and loved it. I also was very good at it; in fact, later when I became a Marine I ran for the United States Marines Corpse track team as a sprinter. Again I did not get beat too often when I was in a track meet match.

The other thing that was popular for me in the sixties was singing. If you could a hold a note, most young kids were on a corner singing or trying to get discovered in Boston. I had a pretty good voice, so I found myself in and out of a lot of local singing groups singing at teen concerts. Boston was a city rich with talent. Of the many singing groups that I was in, we would travel to Providence, Rhode Island; Stanford Connecticut; and all throughout the Cape in Massachusetts to compete with other groups; and we had built a good reputation. I think that experience also prepared me later for an ability to understand stage presence, which made me later become a good platform artist in the hair industry, and a Minister in the Nation of Islam later on in my life.

I was sixteen when I started with other friends in an attempt at having a singing career; we were pretty good, we called ourselves the "Four Flares". We did not have our own style we just would copy certain groups that held the attention of an audience.

I remember one day we were singing in a church hall that was used for weekend teen recreations and concerts. On this occasion the group was singing a song and we reached a part in the song that I sang a high long note; we watched a group of girls grab their crouches and fall down on the bottom of the stage. That is when we knew we were hot and we had what it took to make it happen. Unfortunately, girls distracted us, or the neighborhood street gangs did. That was rampaged in Boston and that changed the courses in our lives. Gangs were very popular, but they were for the most part a bragging right competition in the neighborhood.

I can remember that the way the city of Boston broke up the local street gangs was by infiltrating them and getting the names of most of the members. They then listed them in the center page of the Boston Globe daily newspaper. That did it, when our parents saw our names in the paper we got yanked out and disciplined. The hard-core members stayed together but the majority of us - Black, White and Latino - calmed down and quit the gangs.

Besides those distractions for me, it was when I met my first spouse Marlene Scott. She was smart, petite, and beautiful also a singer like me. We soon fell in love with each other, and what might have been just two youth experimenting with feelings turned into a very serious situation.

Because she was a Jehovah's Witness, and I was not, our seeing each other was considered by her family as taboo. It got her put out of her home by her parents, and excommunicated from her church. Since I knew nothing about the Jehovah's Witnesses I was very frightened for Marlene. We were just very young teenagers. So I made probably one of the biggest decisions that I could at that time to find a place for my girlfriend to stay and to help support her.

Since I did not know where to go, I took her to my mother and made up a story to provide a shelter for her. Marlene was born in New York, and grew up in Boston. I told my mother that Marlene was part of a singing group from New York, and was stranded in Boston until she could make arraignments to go back to New York. Up until then we never had sex, just a lot of heated passion between each other, Marlene was still a virgin, so this situation made it convenient for me to sneak in the room where she was sleeping and that was the beginning of our sexual romance. After that, we were more determined to be together. Unfortunately, my mother realized that something was wrong with my story after the first day had passed, so I began to look for a place for both of us. I felt responsible for her and I wanted her to be all right.

Butch Ruffin, who was one of my best friends and also a fellow singer in the vocal group somehow helped me to find a furnished room, but unfortunately it came without electricity or heat. Fortunately, it was in the summer months so we managed to get by without those conveniences. In the beginning we used our over coats that served as blankets or sheets for the first few nights that we lived together. Even though I left my mother's house, my mom was so compassionate and confident that I would get it together, that she allowed me to come back and forth to her house until we both, in a short time, found jobs to make things work out. I would take a loaf of bread, peanut butter and jelly, and a sheet or blanket for our bed; and that is was how we lived for about a month.

I had plenty of meaningless jobs during that month, but the one thing that I was exposed to that fascinated me the most was my Aunt Viola's beauty business and my Uncle Buster's barbershop. I found myself always around one of them and I watched them enough to pick up knowledge on how to do some things. I convinced my mother and my Aunt Viola, when I was about sixteen years old, to press and curl my hair. I kept insisting that my singing career was going to take off because we were good and I needed to look the part. I convinced her and she did it pretty much because I pleaded. I wanted to wear my hair straight, just like the famous singer among youth of that era, David Ruffin. He was a singer in a famous group for Motown Music Corporation called the Temptations, and since I was copying his style of singing in the group I wanted to look like him as well. My aunts and mother did not think I could take the pain of a strong hair relaxer, so they compromised with me; she pressed and curled my hair. I wore my hair short on the sides and a curly hairstyle for a while. One day my Uncle Buster decided that he wanted to use me as one of his male hair relaxer models to advertise his talents and he was very good at it; soon all of my friends and peers wanted the look that he gave me.

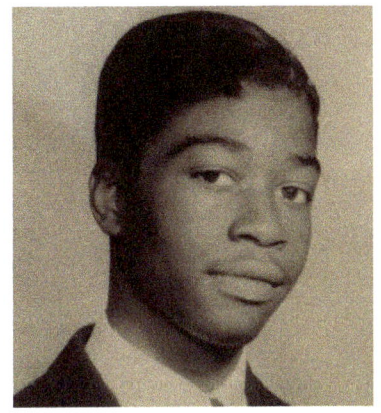

Haroon at sixteen years' old

Uncle Buster opened up a whole new vision in me and it was then that I not only liked how it was working for me, I decided that I could do it myself so I bought myself a home barber kit and began cutting relaxing and finger waving some of my friends' hair. That helped me make a little money, but I basically would have done it for free because of the fun and enjoyment that I had in doing them, also I was testing my new cultural art skills without even knowing it.

Soon Marlene and I found another apartment that was better than the one we were living in, now with utilities and living essentials. Marlene got a job working for an entertainment manager and radio celebrity on W.I.L.D. radio station in Boston, he was called Mambo Willie. She was a receptionist at his office in Roxbury, not far from where we lived. She would always say to me that he was constantly asking her to go out with him on a date or flirting with her. The fact that I was jealous over what I thought might have been threatening to me, and the fact Marlene told me that she might have been pregnant, made me feel very insecure and anxious to find a better way to provide for her.

It was around that same time, three of my best friends decided to join the United States Marine Corps: William Mabels, whom we called Peas, Leonard Thomson or Lenny, and Melvin Sharpe also known as Sharpe. By the time I found out about it Peas and Lenny had already been sworn in. But Sharpe somehow failed the test to enter the Marines and had decided to take it again. This time he talked me into going with him on what was called the buddy plan, meaning we would both be together throughout the whole four years active and two years inactive stint. I thought at least I could earn steady money for Marlene and my child, and travel all over the world as they promised, with one of my best friends. In the back of my mind, even though I never had a relationship with my father other than through his loving parents, the one vision of him that I had at that time was his picture in a military uniform and somehow I was proud of that.

Chapter Five

Going Into The United States Marine Corps

The only problem was since I was quitting High School as a junior I had just turned seventeen and was obviously too young to join the military unlike my friends that were a year or two older than me. So I forged my birth certificate Even though my mother objected to my joining the service, she still supported my decision to do what was right for my new problem of being a father. So she signed a parental release form for me to go in. There was one other problem, Sharpe failed the entrance examination again, and was turned down from entering the Marine Corps again. Since I had passed the physical exam and test, that meant I was going in the Marines by myself without the buddy plan.

Even though, if I had known officially that if I had not taken the oath I would not have been required to go in. But because it was a way of resolving the problem that I had put myself and Marlene in, I kissed my then girlfriend, said goodbye to my family, and was off to Paris Island, South Carolina.

Boot Camp in Parris Island South Carolina

On the East coast, Marine Corps recruits are sent to Parris Island, South Carolina and that place had a reputation of being the toughest place in all of the United States military recruit boot camps of any branch of service to be trained in at that time.

It is an Island surrounded by swamps and infested by mosquitoes, gnats, and snakes; however, you would learn to live with them, because as a discipline many of the fresh or new recruits were put on so-called mosquito *burying details* if they were caught killing one that bit them while they were standing at attention. This detail would require you to find the insect that they killed dig a hole with your back pack shovel, six feet by six feet, bury the insect, and then say a military prayer for the bug. I personally witnessed many recruits that, after realizing what they had gotten themselves into, tried to run away (AWOL) at night; and some died in the surrounding swamps trying. However, to the best of my knowledge for the sixteen weeks that I was there no one ever got away.

The four and a half years I spent in the military was rough as hell, it was like a punishment for lying about my age to get in there in the first place. Right from the beginning at boot camp as I was getting my first distribution of military clothes, a Drill Sergeant had us all standing in front of this long table with our arms, and hands by our sides looking straight forward. We were bald headed with a fresh military haircut, from which I was harassed by the barber because I was wearing one of my uncle Busters famous hairdos as they were called, which was faded sides and relaxed top with finger waves. That was the style in Boston at that time, and I was one of my uncle's best models to advertise his work, so I was as they say wearing it. So after a strip of clothes and forced shower while standing their naked, this drill sergeant was standing on top of the table going from one end to the other, cursing out loud and screaming at everybody. For some reason I looked up at him with a look like *what is your problem*? He caught my glance and came over to me and said, "Who in the hell are you looking at screw, are you eye-fucking me, sun shine?" I do not know why, but I grabbed at his tie to yank it, and was about to kick his ass for calling me a racist name until I felt this fist hit me on the side of my head. When I came to my senses, I was in a psycho-observation ward. After they're examining me they sent me to what was called a motivation barracks. When I got there the Drill Sergeant told me, "It is not often we get a Nigger from Boston in the motivational barracks, but when we get through with you in here boy, you will be motivated! Do you hear me, screw?"

I knew right then that I had made a big mistake and I had to get out of the problem that I had made for myself in joining the Marines. Unfortunately, I ended up spending four and half years in the military. Although I tried to get out, it became the best experience as a young boy to grow up around older experienced men. But at that time, I was scared. I wrote my mother and asked her to tell somebody, any officials, that I had lied about my age, and to get me out of there. She said no, you felt you were man enough to lie about your age, to join, so she said to me, "Be a man and stick it out," because she was not going to contribute any further to my lies that put me there in the first place.

After getting in the Marines, I just hoped that I would find a way to see my friends Lenny or Peas while I was in there. I did run into Peas very briefly after boot camp in Charleston, South Carolina. I had just arrived when he was leaving; Charleston was a place where many Marines that were trained in Parris Island boot camp in South Carolina were sent. It was a rest and recuperation period location that was called liberty. All Marine cadets' boot camp graduates received this time off before going to the specified training at Camp Geiger, South Carolina, which was the advance special training camp. This camp was designed to assign and train new recruits for their Military Official Status (MOS).

That was the last I saw of Peas or Lenny until I was about to get out of the service four and a half years later. After sixteen weeks of boot camp training, I finally went home to Boston on leave.

While at home for those thirty days Marlene and I got married, it was a small wedding by a neighborhood preacher in his house, me in my uniform and Marlene in a maternity dress, because by then she was showing with our daughter Anita Marie. My Mother and her lifelong companion, Mr. Leroy, were our witnesses for our marriage and, by this time, Marlene had already moved in with my mother until our first child Anita was born.

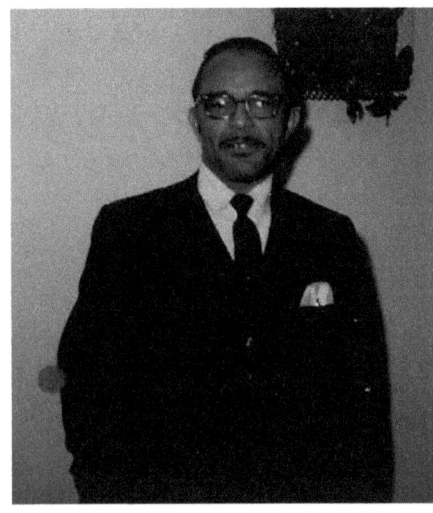

Mr. Leroy Jessie Milton, our Father figure

My First Base Assignment at Camp Lejune North Carolina

When I got off leave or liberty I was sent to my first base at Camp Lejune North Carolina to my permanent military home base. Marlene and I missed each other so much that I was taking every leave I could to get back to Boston to be with her.

Sometimes I was even hitchhiking from North Carolina through some of the most racist southern roads in America, just to be with Marlene; so we knew that I had to find a way for us to get together.

After two years in the Corps Marlene and I had two children that were born in Boston - Anita, and Aaron. We finally moved together and were living at Camp Lejune North Carolina in a trailer camp for enlisted personnel couples.

My job description was artillery gunner I was trained to operate a 155-millimeter howitzer cannon. This weapon was attached to a truck that carried its own fire team of men. It was also the kind of job description that was most likely to be in a battle zone. There was a lot of prejudice and racism on the military bases, especially troops that were in, or coming from Viet Nam. It was so bad that an African American named Sergeant Major Huff was assigned to the African American enlisted men to encourage us not to engage in any racial activities.

It is important to know that this was the sixties and social unrest was on the rise in America; the civil rights movements were affecting military personnel, as well as civilians. It was too late for me to avoid the civil rights or black pride movements because I had already been influenced by my family in Boston that were very active in the nation of Islam. I would listen with great respect to Huey P. Newton, Malcolm X., and Muhammad Ali; they were my mentors and heroes then. Sergeant Major Huff and other African American officers gave me advice that I should get a Military Operational Status (MOS) that would give me rank, a clearance or special training.

While cutting the hair of an African American Officer, he told me I should start applying for a transfer to a security duty opportunity on one of the Navy Bases. He said I would likely get a clearance, and that generally would keep me out of the war zone. It was also well known that the Viet Cong was using the African American revolutionary experience to put doubt in some of the African American soldiers in combat by using propaganda about why were African Americans fighting them in a unjust war while in America African Americans were being discriminated against and treated unequal to whites. So there was that extra pressure on my behalf because I was so young in the military at that time.

Soon after Marlene came with my children, Anita and Aaron, to be with me in North Carolina, we were living in a trailer on the military enlisted housing camp. That was when I saw the need for more income. It was then and there that I started cutting hair for the guys at the trailer camp and in my barracks, while I was applying for a transfer to a security base. At first, it was just the African American soldiers' hair that I would cut, but soon I was doing anyone that asked me.

When I went into the Marines, America was at peace; there were no wars, so for me, I thought it was good timing to travel all over the world as I was promised when I joined. But as soon as I was officially enlisted, a conflict broke out in Cuba, Santa Domingo, Panama and Viet Nam. Of course, because the Marines are attached to the Navy, whenever we would travel it was always on a ship. Of course, while aboard I would make it my business to let the word get out that I was available to cut hair. Because of that I always had a little extra money to send home, or buy something to bring home.

By the time I got out of boot camp the Cuban Crisis had blown up, and we were sent to Guantanamo Bay Cuba to be on standby for a military strike. President Kennedy was under pressure to invade Cuba to put back into power the exiled so-called Cuban businessman that immigrated to Miami. President Kennedy also had the military ready to defend America against threats from President Fidel Castro of Cuba, and President Mikhail Gorbachev of Russia. Kennedy was told that Russia had given Cuba nuclear missiles that were ready to be launched at Miami, Washington D.C. and New York City. That action caused a series of defense and counter-defense activities in the world; fortunately, every one stood down and we were taken out of combat-ready status and sent home.

My next combat tour of duty was the Santa Domingo uprising, as it was called; we were made ready to strike. We were then put on ships and sent to Santa Domingo. When we landed, our presence was so forceful that the Santa Domingo government backed down. Again we came back to the second Marine Battalion Camp Lejune in Jacksonville, North Carolina.

We were home two months before being deployed to Panama for Jungle training. We landed on the Island in a city called Coco Solo. Then we performed an exercise to force march from one end of the Island to the other, while being attacked by Marine recon patrol along the way, as part of the exercise. We finally ended in the Panama jungle, where we were taught how to live in a jungle. Our food and water was taken, and our sleeping equipment. We were shown how to eat in the jungle; we were blindfolded and placed in front of samples of foods to eat. When we took the blindfold off, we discovered we had eaten monkey, squirrels, worms and bug meats, grass, coconut leaves and palm tree leaves. You can imagine when I saw what we ate I wanted to throw up.

I also went to Vargas, Puerto Rico as part of an artillery-training mission at a Marine base in Puerto Rico. We were there three weeks - two weeks' combat in training, one week of liberty in San Juan. In San Juan it was a city full of military personnel; old San Juan was off limits to us because solders were known to get robbed there. I made friends in San Juan because I was African American. I was told that they preferred showing me, their brother, the Island rather than the EL Diablo Blancos, as white people were secretly called at that time.

It was during the New Year's Eve celebration that I was at a night club in San Juan while on liberty and since I was still under age and pretty much the only military person in uniform that was not buying drinks, in fact, I was left to watch the other soldiers and civilians having a ball. When midnight came around a group of Puerto Rican young women came to me and said to me that they were "New Ricans" meaning that they were Puerto Ricans from New York and that they wanted to show me a good time away from the EL Diablo Blancos, and so that is what I did. That was the best party that I had, the entire time in the military. I was convinced after that experience, that New Yorkers were my kind of people and that in America the culture of New York was one that, no matter where I went internationally, was the premiere city of interest that people from around the world were fascinated with and would proudly associate themselves with if they could make the case.

McAlester Oklahoma, Naval Ammunition Depot

Subconsciously that experience also started a hidden bond and love for Puerto Rican people within me and I vowed that I would always go back to Puerto Rico.

At the end of two years in North Carolina I was about to get deployed to go on a Mediterranean cruise to Morocco, Spain, France and Italy; but instead I got transferred to McAlester Oklahoma, Naval Ammunition Depot. Marlene was not able to come with me because there was not enough housing space available for non-commissioned soldiers' families on the base at the time, and I could not afford to live off the base with my income.

So we agreed for Marlene and the children to stay at my mother's house once again, while she took on another job to help raise more money; and then we would try later for her to come to Oklahoma so that we could be together.

Soon after I was stationed in Oklahoma, Marlene got pregnant again and we were now a family of three, with the new birth of Carmen.

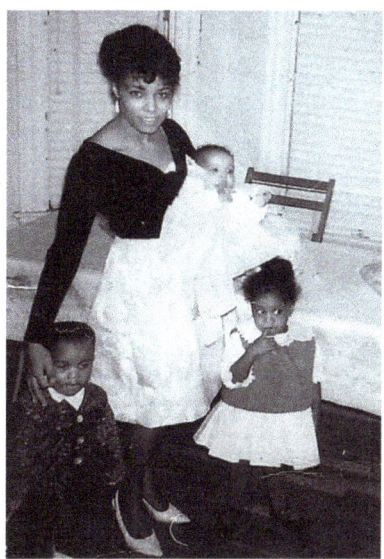
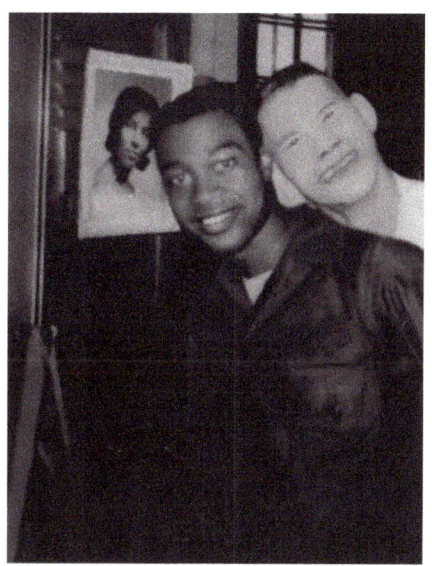

Marlene, Anita, Aaron and Carmen *Me and my military comrade and best friend*

In Oklahoma I was part of a small company of Marines that was trained to secure and protect a Navy special ammunition base. I was given a background check and my clearance authorized me for stationary guard and patrol. The base was isolated from the nearest city, which was McAlester, near the border of Texas.

There were a lot of Native Americans and African Americans in McAlester, and the town was rural and full of military soldiers and bars. Everyone in the town was depending on the base for income, or a military man or women that could improve their lives in some way, or to just take them away. Oklahoma was a racist State so were the cities; in McAlester there was one club for the African American service people. Socializing was hard there because of the limited places you had to meet or make friends, but we made the best of those conditions.

After a year there, I met two women that became more than friends while I was there; it turned out they were cousins. It was wrong in every way dealing with them, but not being able to get back and forth like I did living in North Carolina to see Marlene, I started seeking companionship and things happened. I really liked them both for different reasons. I wonder what would have happened if I did not lose track of them, because I found out that they both had given birth from me around the same time.

While on that base, I went back to cutting hair to earn some extra money. One day while cutting hair in the barracks the Company Officer came in and told me, since the base barber had left there was a need for a barber. He asked if I would be interested in becoming the base barber. I immediately accepted the opportunity to earn more money. Now I found myself as the only person cutting all types of hair, and never had gone to a barber or beauty school. I was working with the knowledge I had retained from watching my uncle Buster in Boston.

In Oklahoma being a Marine had begun to seem easier for me; I received a promotion in my rank, which helped increase my income. As I got less time to serve in the military or was, as it was called "getting short", meaning my military time was running out. Many alleged opportunities began to arrive to me, I was offered more rank and a bonus of cash money if I would re-sign up for two to four more years, but I wanted to get out so that I could do something with my family. The single thing that sealed my mind to get out was the war in Viet Nam, every one that I knew that went there never made it back. It definitely appeared to most Marines at that time we were not wining that war. I felt lucky that I was not sent on a tour of duty in Viet Nam. I believed it was because I was attached to a Special weapons security base, which was run by the Navy and secured by Marines. With a security status, even though I was working at the barbershop, I still was assigned as a security guard, which cleared me for base duty.

I saw some of friends on the base that wanted to go so bad that they made appeals to be deployed to combat duty and they were sent only to die soon after they went, like my Marine comrade in the picture with me, who did not survive a Month in combat.

After I had served three and a half years of the four years I was enlisted for; I was told that I would be mandatory extended six more months so that I would have enough time to meet the minimum requirements for combat tour of duty in Viet Nam, which was one year. Needless to say, I did not like that at all; I felt that I had already given three and a half years of volunteer enlistment on my part to serve and protect. I felt the need to go home and protect my family and I was not willing to volunteer more time away from them and better the chances of being killed in the process. I verbally objected. I wrote the Secretary of Military Justice Services, my Congressperson for the state of Massachusetts and a list of others whom I thought would help me with my appeal. Unfortunately, none of them could do anything, including Senator Kennedy. So I was enlisted for six more months.

I remember the company officer calling me in and asking why was I writing letters complaining to politicians. I explained how unfair I thought the whole process was to me. Of course, he told me to act like a Marine and stop complaining; but I knew too many of my friends that went to Viet Nam that never came back to their families. I did not regret what I was doing, but I stopped writing because I was told there was nothing I could do about it because all the marines that came in at the time I came in were given the same extension.

My complaints began to create a bad attitude toward me from other non-commissioned officers, especially those that had re-signed more years for a higher rank or money. Before I started complaining, I thought one of those men was a friend of mine. He was a Native American from Oklahoma, a Sergeant, and I was at that time a corporal in rank. The good thing was that all the complaining I did seemed to have had an effect on decisions by upper authorities not to send me on a tour of duty in Viet Nam. But that seemed to anger a lot of my peers and others, pretty much because I seemed happy that I was short, meaning that my time to get out was near.

I had less than a year left, so I found myself being so happy, that the closer I got to my departure date I began selling off my extra season uniforms knowing that I would never be using them again. One incident, while I was selling one of my dress uniforms was when that so-called friend of mine started complaining that I was out of order for selling my uniform. One thing lead to another! I felt he was getting personal and I told him if he wanted to take it to the back of the barracks that would be fine with me; otherwise he would need to get off my back. When I least expected it, he sucker punched me and we started fighting until others broke us apart. I was still angry when we separated, looking at each other; but when he started grinning and I felt blood running down my face, I got mad. While he stood there looking at me and smiling, I went to my wall locker, got my rifle, took the barrel of the rifle, walked over to him and cracked him on the side of the head. He took off. When I went to the dispensary to tend to my wound I was visited by two Military Police; they arrested me and I was put in the brig for two days until I could see the Company Officer. I ended up losing my rank and put on restriction for a week.

I did not care at that time because I knew I was getting out and it seemed I got a lot of respect from the rest of the non-commissioned officers after that incident.

Chapter Six

Back To Boston - Starting My Career

When I finally finished my tour Marlene and I had three children - Anita, Aaron, and Carmen - but we had a very fragile marriage. Our being separated for such a long time, opened a window for seeing other people while married, on both of our parts. It put a strain on our marriage as we tried to work through our problems, but a year later we were unfortunately getting a divorced.

Marlene then moved to Los Angeles, California but a few months before she left we got together once again and had our final child together- Craig; but neither of us knew at the time before she left with the children and started a new life that he was my child. She was always a beautiful, smart and a good woman; I only wish that we both could have been stronger at the time because she was a good friend before things went wrong.

I will always love her for the beautiful exciting times we had growing up together and the beautiful children that came out of the relationship.

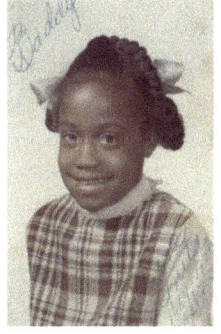

Anita Thompson

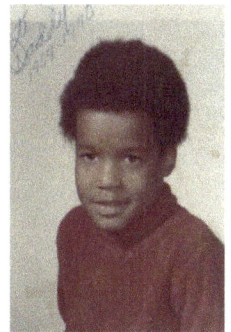

Aaron Thompson

One of the things that I found myself being attracted to get involved with when I got back was the 1960's new black revolutionary spirit that existed in America at that time and also in me, when I got out of the Marines. The most vocal African American activists among the youths at that time were the black Panthers, I too soon after, started going to the Black Panther Party meetings, and eventually joined the movement.

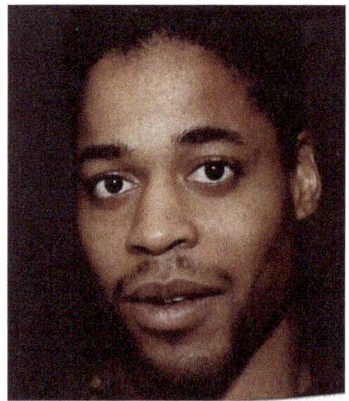
Craig Thompson

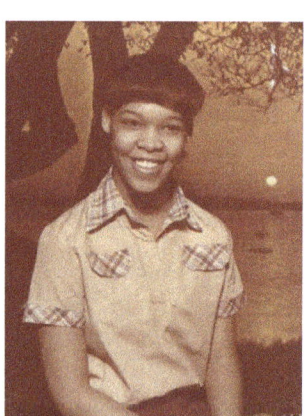
Carmen Thompson

However, I would frequently visit the Black Topographical Research Center; it was a center that distributed geographical information about conditions of African Americans geographical cultural environment in the major cities nationwide. It was at the Topographical Research centers that I was able to understand many of the African American infrastructural demographics in their neighborhoods, which ultimately was designed to control and contain human beings like rats in cages or prisoners in prison.

I admired the courage of the youth at that time to defy the system, mostly because young Americans during and after Viet Nam wanted a change in global politics after the war that in part I played a role in.

I felt disappointed that I had spent four and a half years in the military only to come home to anger from everyone around me for me being stupid enough to join the military, as was reminded to me often. There was no welcome back home solder for me. Even though I was proud to have been in the military, I felt foolish because by then I knew that the war was a farce.

Unfortunately, I learned quickly that there was something wrong with the Black Panthers also. After traveling throughout New England, going to rally after rallies with them, I began to see certain leaders were asking members to do or go on, what I felt, were suicide-type missions and I told them about it. I objected to the notion of untrained civilian citizens testing the disciplined military services with radical civil disobedient tactics. I knew that the Military had just enforced a strategic offence for that, because I was trained not long before I left on what was called Riot Control defense techniques and that was an available National Guards service technique that was ready and very effective to be deployed at any time. I warned them of deadly consequences and began to wonder why there was such insistence on that gullible logic when there was clear evidence that people would get hurt unnecessarily. I pulled back from the Black Panthers after that and began to focus on my career. I maintained support as much as I could, but I lost respect for what I began to see in the local leadership's missions and ambitions. My theory at that time, if I could not see and respect a disciplined body of leadership I did not want to risk doing more harm than good by enabling risky and or radical strategies.

I wanted to be relevant and I had already championed men like Malcolm X and Muhammad Ali as heroes and mentors to admire. To emulate their courage and dedication to the African Diaspora, much of what was drilled in me by Marine Corps Sergeant Major Huff, that intervened with me in regards to preventing me from being radicalized by the American black revolutionary movements, and was beginning to have a very permanent reverse effect on me. Then after that, it became a search for the right cultural fit for me, which I felt would enable my spirit to search and research my African Diaspora, wherever I found myself: with the ultimate purpose to either look for, or project my understanding of strong leadership for the communities that I resided in. Whether it was in America or anywhere in the world that I might happen to be, I will always honor America.

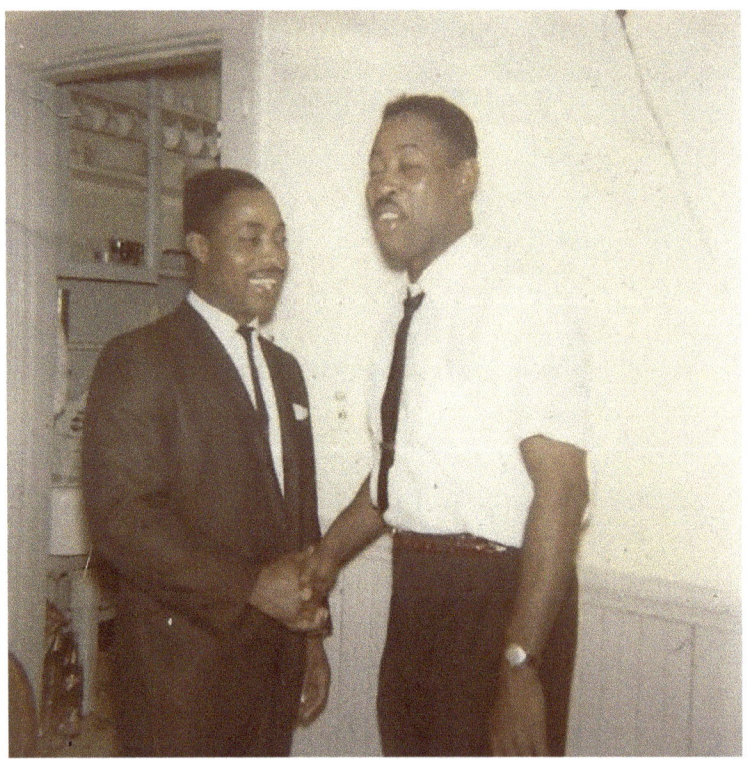

Uncle Buster/John S. Jones & Uncle Son / Willie Jones

I up started my career as a Barber in my uncle's barbershop. I used what was called my GI bill loan to go to Vaughn Barber

College in Boston; it was an Italian school that took pride in mastering scissors over comb cutting, rather than clipper cutting. They used to say what if the electricity would go out; if you were good with your scissors skills, you would always make money. After graduating, I went to Buster and asked to go to work but there were no chairs empty at that time so he suggested that I go to beauty school because he was expanding his shop to add more chairs and make room for me.

Uncle Buster told me that he was in the process of expanding the space in the barbershop and he suggested that I should use the GI educational loan guaranty once again to enroll in Wilfred Beauty Academy; it was the best beauty school in Boston at that time. He felt that it would increase my skill set and give me an advantage in the trade.

I excelled very easily at the school because of my cutting skills. It was at Wilfred that I met would be leaders in the hair industry like Richard Bonner who would become the founder of the West Coast beauty show that was called Black Gold Beauty Show in Los Angeles, California. It was also there that I talked my cousin to come to Wilfred to get his beauty license, since he was already working in beauty salons and building a reputation as a teenager doing women's hair. He agreed and he has become one of the most important people in the hair industry; since then James Harris became an internationally recognized Hair Fashion Consultant and Stylist.

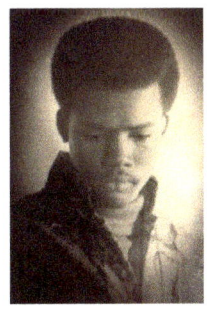

My Cousin Mr. James Harris

This is a picture of one of my favorite cousins Mr. James Harris, when we both were young in the hair and beauty business. He was my first

Afro haircut model in a photo shoot that I was the hairstylist for back in the late sixties.

Immediately after getting out of school, and working in my Uncle Buster's shop. James Harris my cousin, my uncle, and the staff of Sportsman did very well. We had most of the in crowd or celebrities in Boston coming to us; it was an upper and lower level barber shop and beauty salon. I was doing so well I bought my first car in less than a year; it was a fairly new Jaguar XKE. Our family business was the talk of the town. When I came out of beauty school it was at a time when African Americans were wearing Afro hairstyles. Everyone wanted to identify with the Afro look including Caucasians; and to add to the demand and problem was that African Americans were wearing their hair in a straight hairstyle by using hair relaxers, which made it seem impossible to achieve an Afro. That texture of hair would not stand out like an Afro; in fact it would have to be cut off and start over to let new hair grow out. We called them T.W.A's meaning Teeny Weenie Afros. It was from that demand that we created a technique to give this look, it was using gels and oils on clean hair and wrapping sections of the hair on what was called Spooly's into a pin curl method putting a person under the hair dryer until dry, then picking out and styling the hair.

We had people lined up - black and white women and men - and it became our number one moneymaker. Soon other barbers and beauticians heard about what we were doing and began asking us how we did it and would we show them. We started a product line known as Natural U. Afro Revert Kit. The Company was Sportsman Pyramid cosmetic; we did trade shows and workshops for barbers and beauticians. We manufactured shampoos, gels, Spooly's and Afro picks. We traveled all over New England, New York, Philadelphia, North Carolina, Chicago, and Florida. We were doing a great business, building reputations as individual hair celebrities across the country.

It was through that traveling that I became aware of the beautiful city of Atlanta, Georgia working the Bronner Brothers Hair Show. The Afro kit was a unique product at the time because it served a market that was in demand by the clients of chemically treated hair who wanted to wear a natural or Afro. In a very short time that market changed, because everyone who was wearing a relaxer was letting their hair grow natural and wearing an Afro. Sportsman Pyramid Cosmetics did not move with the change, so unfortunately my uncle sold the company to Gillette Company in Boston.

Chapter Seven

Starting My Own Business In Atlanta

I went back to Atlanta from Boston after being there once before with my uncle Buster, my cousin James Harris and business associate Tony Briggs to work at the Bronner Brothers Beauty Trade show as we were introducing our Natural U Products line hair products.

I had already established a great respect and friendship with Mr. Nathaniel H. Bronner Senior, so I went to him and asked about working with him in some way. At that time, he had a large building on the corner of Ashby Street and Auburn Avenue. In this mall-like building there was a beauty supply, beauty salon, barbershop and other retail businesses. Mr. Bronner asked me to work in the barbershop cutting hair. I accepted it and would even give his two sons haircuts, Nathaniel Jr. and Bernard. Things were not working out for me there because of my leaning so strong in my Afro centric cultural beliefs. Mr. Bronner was a moderate conservative and my personality did not fit at that time, so with respect for him I decided to move on.

Mr. Bronner knew of a man that had a barbershop not far from his business and he recommended that I might want to talk to him, since his shop was on the Atlanta University campus location and that I might be able to take advantage of the walking traffic in that area.

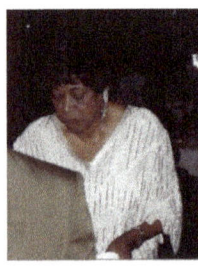

My Cousin: Dr. Anna Grant,
Dean of Social Science at
Morehouse University

One of the main reasons that I felt somewhat comfortable in the Atlanta area was because I knew that I had a family member there who was a great contact if I needed to go to her, Dr. Anna Grant, Dean of Social Science at the prestigious Morehouse University eventually became very helpful to me in balancing my social political thoughts from time to time, as I journeyed back and forth from Boston to Atlanta.

As a young man, I was impressed by Atlanta because there were many young and successful African American entrepreneurs. So I moved there to get my own business in the city that was called "The Little Apple"; but my destiny would not allow that to happen there until several years later. However, I still did hair, but mostly men's haircuts in different barbershops throughout Atlanta. Since I was living in an apartment next to the Morehouse campus, it made it easy for me to solicit customers; but I was experimenting with other business venture ideas as well.

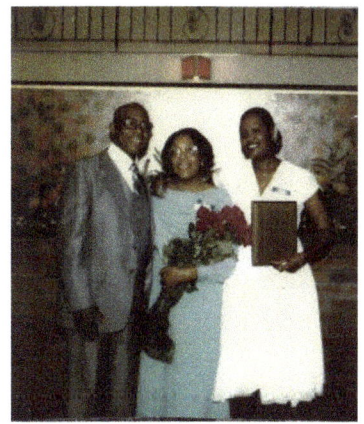

Uncle Willie & Aunt Sarah Harris & Cousin Yvonne Stewart

Growing up in Boston as a young kid I experienced working in my Aunt Sarah, and Uncle Willie's restaurant, as did most of my siblings and family members. It was called T&W restaurant, named after two family members - Thomas, the baker and Willie the chef. After they both became Muslims, it later became Shabazz restaurant under the leadership of the Honorable Elijah Muhammad, and guidance of Minister Malcolm X and later Minister Louis Farrakhan.

When Minister Malcolm X. was silenced by Elijah Muhammad from speaking for the Nation of Islam because of disagreements of comments that Malcolm had made, it is said that Uncle Willie, Aunt Sarah and my Cousin Yvonne were all put out of the nation because of the close relationships that they had with El Hadj Malik Shabazz (Malcolm X) and Sister Betty Shabazz and because they continued to communicate with Brother Minister Malcolm X after he was silenced. They were forced to give up their restaurant, as it was then considered "Nation of Islam" property, and because of that they never went back to the Nation of Islam.

Uncle Willie and Aunt Sarah went on to have a very successful restaurant business outside of the Nation of Islam. After leaving the Nation of Islam, they started over with a new restaurant idea, using the kosher or Halal type foods in their menus and they called it the Unity Lunch in Boston. Many of the family members had worked at the Unity Lunch, including my Mom, who worked there until it finally closed several years later. Unity Lunch was one of the main providers for weekend breakfasts at the prestigious Northeastern University/Black Student Union dormitory in Boston.

With me being exposed to that type of entrepreneurship as a youth, it motivated me to try my own restaurant business in Atlanta.

At the time I had a friend who was a young entrepreneur from Houston Texas, and we convinced each other that we could and wanted to go into business together, so we put our money together found a place to rent in Atlanta, on Bankhead Highway, which by coincidence was the same street that Muhammad Temple #15 was on. We bought produce and meats from the Nation of Islam Muslim Farm in Georgia and tried to run a small restaurant venture.

My partner began to feel uncomfortable with my interest in purchasing our food supply from the Muslims, so we both gave up on the idea of a partnership. My mother and Aunt Sarah also convinced me to give up on the idea of a restaurant venture because they both thought that it would be too risky and difficult making the business work. I went back to cutting Hair in a barbershop on Ashby Street near the Morehouse University and Spellman campus site.

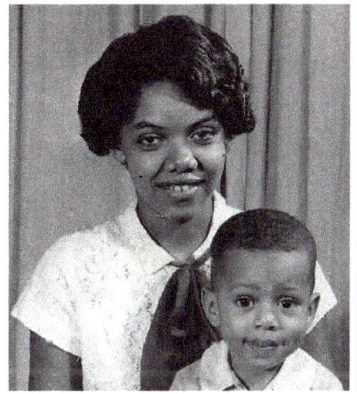 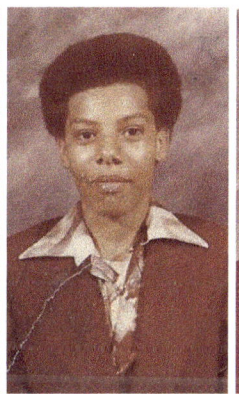 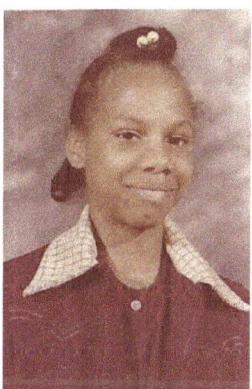

Sheila La Costa Rashid & Karl Rashid   *Karl Rashid*   *Dawn Rashid*

Sheila La Costa and I were both young artists in Atlanta: she was from Chicago and I was from Boston. I was working as a freelance barber one day in an Afrocentric Bookstore in the Atlanta University campus site, and she was an Afrocentric jewelry maker and entrepreneur at the same location. I met Sheila while walking from the store one day, I saw this beautiful woman coming toward me with a big red Afro. She looked like Angela Davis, at a distance, and as much as men like me in those days loved Angela Davis, I knew I had to talk to her. We became friends and I found out that she had two children living with her. They were beautiful kids - a boy, Carl and a girl, Dawn - and she had just moved to Atlanta from Chicago.

It was also in Atlanta that I became fully aware for the first time of my personal interest in a religious experience.

There was a young Muslim named Brother James, who was nicknamed Sticky, because once he made up his mind he was going to bring you to the Temple he would put on his beautiful smile and charm and stick with you until you were there. Brother James became attracted to me because I put in the window of the barber shop that was facing the Morehouse College tennis court, so that many of the students could visibly see the large posters of Malcolm X, Dr. Martin Luther King, and Huey P. Newton, Angela Davis and Muhammad Ali. Students would always visit because I stood out as a revolutionist in the area. The shop became a conversation piece among my peers and that action really made Sticky very anxious to recruit me into the Nation of Islam. It also caused my cousin, Dr. Anna Grant, who was the only female on the staff at Morehouse and who was a new face of diversity of the great Dr. Benjamin Mays, who made the decision to hire her as the first female staffer and Dean at Morehouse, to advise me on the sociopolitical limits of my activism.

At that time because of the Black Nationalist spirit, especially on Atlanta College campus, which consisted of: Morris Brown, Atlanta University, Morehouse College, Spellman College, Clark College and the Atlanta Theological Institute, the Afrocentric genre was what many of the young African Americans wanted to identify with, African names. So when I arrived in Atlanta, I referred to myself as Brother Abu Ali. I found out later that I was of special interest to Sticky because I was calling myself by a Muslim name, and I was not a Muslim. I chose the name from people that I admired. Abu was a friend from Boston; he and his family had a reputation in Boston as leading African American businessmen in the Boston neighborhood. They owned a black bookstore called A Nubian Notion and a Barbershop Called Breu Bremau. That is one of the reasons I felt a kinship to Abu, we were in the same business. I took my last name Ali from my hero, Muhammad Ali.

One of the other things that I was doing was building a reputation of being a Robin Hood like character with the drug dealers, "taking away the weed from the white hippy drug dealers and giving it to the poor black consumers that wanted it." That action got out to Sticky, which made him more determined to rescue me into the Nation to channel my activism in a more constructive manner. That, along with a few more things I was doing, worried Sheila; so she convinced me to go to a meeting with Sticky and her one time.

When we went to the Temple, the minister seemed to be talking directly to me. He spoke about slave names and how the slave masters' children had mentally branded the slaves like they would physically brand the animals that they owned with their surname as a property claim. He said that Negroes are proud to be called by their slave masters' names. He preached that the greatest tool of volunteered slavery was for the slave to try to identify with his master's culture and hate his own by giving over themselves to false pride of the slave master's birthright. I was already aware of this theory, my name of use was Abu Ali; but then he went into the theory of how some people out of ignorance or no knowledge of self would take on names just to claim one without even knowing what it means. He then looked at me and said, like Abu Ali.

After his speech, he asked if anyone was ready to join the Nation of Islam. I did not budge, but I watched Sheila walk right past me and go up to join, I must admit I was shocked because I still was not ready to join myself. After that night, we both went back home. Sheila called me to meet her in the restroom, I then witnessed her pour a kilo of weed into the toilet as she pleaded with me that we should join together and no longer should practice the crazy Robin Hood game that I was doing.

I rejected her for a while, but eventually I gave into the notion of becoming a member of the NOI and wound up joining the movement; and soon after, we got married

I was told that I would receive an acceptance letter from the messenger himself in Chicago; but what I received instead was a letter from The Messenger Honorable Elijah Muhammad saying that I should not shame myself by using a name that has no meaning to who I really am. He said that I should wait on Allah to give me a name that gives honor to who I am. So I was given the name Aaron X instead of Aaron Thompson the X meant unknown factor until I became creditable or worthy, then Allah would give me a Holy name. That letter, at that time, more than anything else set me on a course to build a character of creditability for myself and my people in a more dignified way.

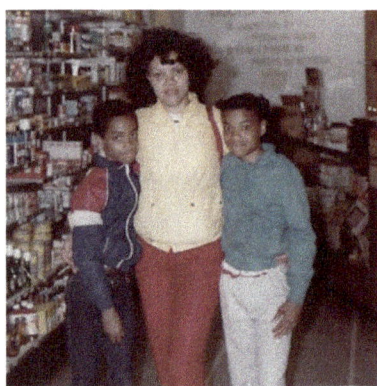
Hakeem, Sheila & Darya Rashid

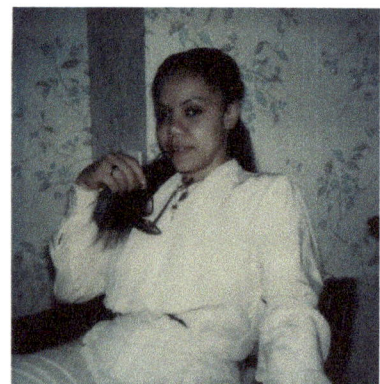
Sheila Rashid

I felt that if I would continue the practice as a professional hairstylist, somehow touching women other than my wife was wrong. So I would only cut the men's hair as a favor, more or less, and eventually got out of the hair business altogether. After getting more involved in the Nation of Islam, and because of my former military experience, I started to move up the ranks among the men and soon became a squad leader. Sheila and I both decided that it was time to leave Atlanta, go to Boston and try living in a city among my family ties.

We left Atlanta and moved to Boston. We had two children: Darya Venia and Hakeem Ibn Harun Rashid, along with Karl and Dawn; our family was beginning to grow. Learning religious discipline as young converts in the Nation of Islam under the teaching of the Honorable Elijah Muhammad was exciting and intellectually rewarding. I joined the student Minister class in Boston. I took on new job challenges to make ends meet. I had most of my old hair clients asking me to do their hair, but I refused to get back into it. My first job was working as a bank teller during the day and also as a security guard at night.

While I was working in the bank, a Jewish man, who was a customer of the Bank, took to me and asked if I would be interested in working as a salesman. He owned a company that sold office equipment and supplies. Since I was doing so well selling the Muhammad Speaks newspaper in my spare time, I felt that I could do well in sales. I was not making the money working the two jobs that we thought I should have to make ends meet for my family, so I quit the bank job.

As a salesman for the office supply company, I was doing well. But my curiosity about how things were run in Chicago at the headquarters was developing in both of us, so we decided that it was time to go to Chicago and pursue my desire to be a Minister in the Nation of Islam. Going to Chicago, Illinois, which also happens to be Sheila's hometown, I felt would give me the chance to meet her family and learn more about the Nation of Islam.

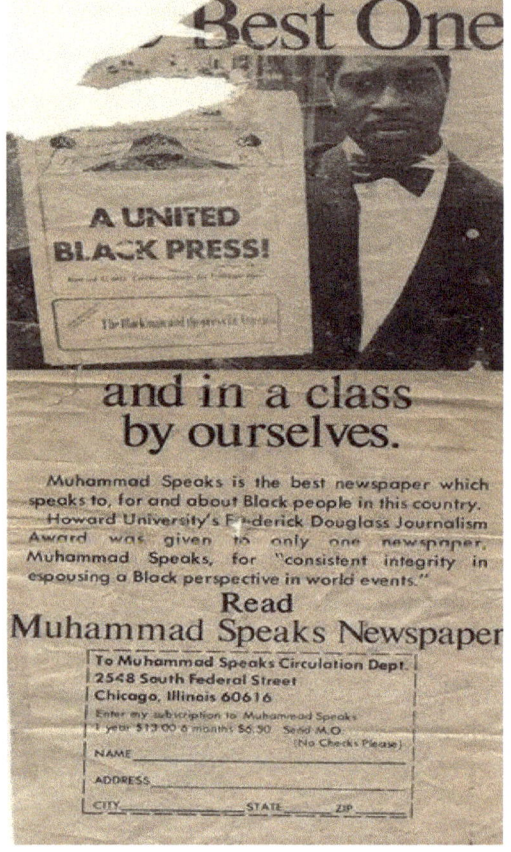

Muhammad Speaks Newspaper Top Salesman Advertisement

Eventually we moved to Chicago, where my first job was at the Muhammad Speaks Newspaper plant. I was a pressman. I was very proud to have a role in printing words of my leader and teacher, the Honorable Elijah Muhammad; however, I knew that I came to Chicago primarily to be a leader in the Nation. I grew in the ranks in Chicago to become one of the top newspaper salesmen and I was chosen to be the face of the advertisement for the Muhammad Speaks newspaper.

While working as a pressman I got a call to join the elite security team of the Nation of Islam to protect the Messenger, and the Nation's property. This was a job that I had plenty of experience from during my stint in the U.S.M.C. I followed up on the student minister's classes that I had started in Boston, now in Chicago.

Again I moved up the ranks in the NOI until the death of my first real mentor, the Honorable Elijah Muhammad. I also used my military GI bill to buy my first house on the south side of Chicago in the south shore community three blocks from the National Headquarters of the Nation of Islam.

As a minister in the nation, I was a member of an elite group of ministers that felt the Chicago headquarters for the NOI was the most important area for teaching and learning the messenger's words. The satellite ministers, as we were called, opened up seven satellite Temples around the city. We took a no nonsense attitude in those neighborhoods where we were assigned to teach, to convert people to come into the NOI. I opened a Temple in Roseland on 115th and Wentworth Street; I had created a staff and built a congregation of over one hundred people. My area was as far south as 138th street in the (Artgeld Gardens housing projects), East to the Eden expressway, North to 103 Street, and west to Halsted (Morgan Park) I was living in one of the best times in my life and full of excitement.

I had Olive Harvey College as part of my territory. One day a student came to me and asked me if I could get Muhammad Ali to come to the school as a guest speaker during Black History Month, so I asked his people if he would and got him to come. When he came to the event, he was sick from a cold but after his patent speech when we were about to leave, a very big sister got in front of Ali and begged him, Ali please! Please! She pleaded for a hug. Even though he was not feeling well he said okay and hugged her, like on clue a line of girls and women lined up about fifty strong for their chances and he hugged every last one of them. I said to myself what a compassionate man this brother is.

During that time, I also would go to Cook County correction facility every Saturday morning to talk to inmates, and to every church, organization, school, and social group in my territory to talk about black love, and unity. I also developed a great relationship with the orthodox Muslim in my territory; we had great respect for each other's missions and differences.

When the Honorable Elijah Muhammad died I, as did many others did not take the death of Mr. Muhammad well. He was like the father figure that I did not have, my mentor, the only person that I believed unquestionably. About a year before the death of messenger Muhammad, one of his sons that had not been actively involved in the Nation of Islam since I joined came back to take over leadership. We were told that his father had asked him to come back and lead us to the next level of the Nation's mission to make us more mainstream Muslims. His name was Wallace Deen Muhammad. When Imam Wallace Deen Muhammad spoke, much like Malcolm X when I heard him for the first time, I was totally enchanted by his wisdom.

Then one-day Imam Muhammad called all the satellite ministers together for the first time, we thought to enlighten us and encourage us to learn more. He greeted us and then he turned to me and asked me what my name was. I told him my name was Brother Minister Aaron 2X. He said to me he had heard of the work that I was doing in the Roseland community and was proud of my service; so from now on, I should call myself Haroon Rashid, it is a name that would suit me better. I was so excited because I had been waiting since the day I received my acceptance letter from the Honorable Elijah Muhammad for this day to receive a Holy Name; I was overjoyed. All of the other satellite ministers started chanting, almost screaming *All Praises Are Due to the Honorable Elijah Muhammad.*

It was a sign they knew that they too would likely be honored to receive their Holy names, and he did go down the list and gave them their new names. Of course, I was extremely honored that he started with me first.

However, with the new changes in the structure of the leadership, I began to change my views on a lot of things. Some of those things affected my marriage, and Sheila and I were starting to go in different directions. I wanted to get reacquainted with my personal family and decided to step back from leadership, and go back into the world as it was called to relearn my people and family.

I stayed in Chicago two more years before I moved to Jacksonville, Florida. I went there to live with my grandmother, she called me knowing from my mother what was going on with me and asked me to come stay with her for a while because she was alone and sick and needed me to help her.

It was there that I went back to barber school at the Florida Hair Styling Academy, got my license and practiced working in the barbershops, and beauty salons in Jacksonville. After I got my career started again, while there I used that time to reacclimate myself to my family in Jacksonville. While I was there, my grandmother made sure she did all that she could to convert me back into the faith of Christianity! I would go with her every Sunday to the church that she worshiped and served in, pretty much to appease her; but after all that I had previously gone through for well over a decade I was taking a sabbatical.

While there, I did travel throughout Florida to get a feel for my family's roots in the state and I found that it was very different now as an adult. With my new vision on the southern racist culture, I felt lot of pity and anger for my people living an apathetic culture in the South and I knew that it was time for me to go back to Boston to finish what I had started as a young hair artist.

I knew that, since I had spent most of my early career as a Barber, I would have to get back under some masters in the trade of cosmetology, even though I was educated in the cosmetology skills. I tried a couple of the local barbershops before I found one of my friends that I went to beauty school with; she had a beauty salon not far from the barber shop that I first worked in. She took me under her wings to help me prefect my skills again doing women's hair to the perfection that I needed to do what I wanted in Boston and in the industry.

Stacy Beauty Salon

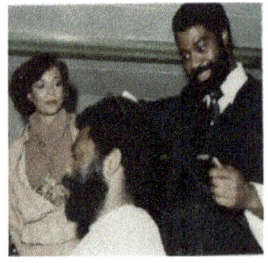

Ms. Stacy Jones and Haroon cutting a client's hair

I went to work at ***Stacy Beauty Salon,*** Stacy J. as we called her. Stacy Jones and I went to beauty school together, when I first came out of the service. We attended the Wilfred Academy Cosmetology School on Temple Court, located in downtown Boston directly across from the historical Boston Commons Park. We became great friends, and we had a great time as peers and students while there. Stacy would soon after school invest into a salon in a progressive area of Boston known as the South End. Stacy was also well-known in Boston as a beautiful socialite with lots of friends and a great social network.

It was also well known that she had a close friendship with the popular basketball Hall of Famer Mr. Bill Russell of the Boston Celtics when he was the owner of a restaurant and night club called Slade's, which was one block north of her eventual beauty salon. I eventually left Stacy's, at a request of some manufacturers, to become an advance educator in a beauty school in Dorchester.

After leaving Stacy, I worked in a beauty school and salon that was called the **La Parisienne Beauty Academy** for a short period of time. But because it was a beauty school and salon in the neighborhood, it somehow did not fit for me; especially after spending my educational experience in the downtown Boston area, I learned to enjoy that diverse feel for clientele downtown.

Olive's Beauty Salon

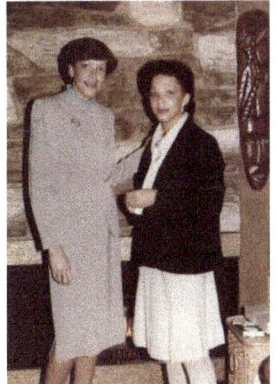

My friend Norma Hughes & her daughter

One day I was talking with my neighbor, a hair stylist named Norma Hughes about my career and concerns at the time. Norma was working at a salon that she thought would be a great fit for me and suggested that I visit her there. I did, and it was an immediate love and respect when I met and found my new friend Olive Benson.

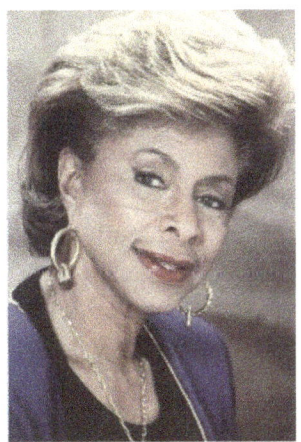 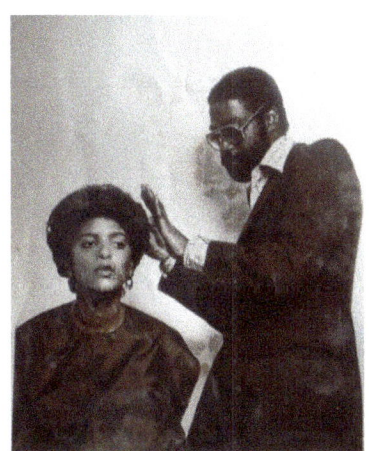

Ms. Olive Lee Benson, of Olive's Beauty Salon: Photoshoot preparation at Olive's

The last beauty Salon that I worked at while in Boston was Olive's Beauty Salon. It was uniquely located in the heart of the upscale business and tourist area of downtown Boston on Boylston Street, facing the Lord & Taylor Department store. Olive became a great inspiration and friend to me. She encouraged me to join multi-cultural hair and beauty organizations as well as to know and stay up on the hair and fashion trends.

I was privileged to travel around the country with Olive as a platform artist and educator. We traveled throughout the country as a hair styling educational team and I eventually purchased one of her salons in Atlanta. Olive was a legend in her time across multicultural lines. She was the educational advisor for every major ethnic product company in America during her life services to the beauty industry. She was the second women only to one of the pioneers of the African American beauty business, the great Madam C. J. Walker, to have a signature product line in her name. L'Oréal of Paris invested in her name brand by creating a chemical relaxer system called the Olive Benson line of products. She, also along with my cousin Mr. James Harris, created an advance educational training concept and program called the Hair Metric System. I loved her like a big sister and would try to protect her like a bodyguard when needed.

During that same time, while my beauty career was taking off, my brother and I ventured into a totally new enterprise that took off very successfully.

Chapter Eight

The Pendarvis Boxing Enterprise

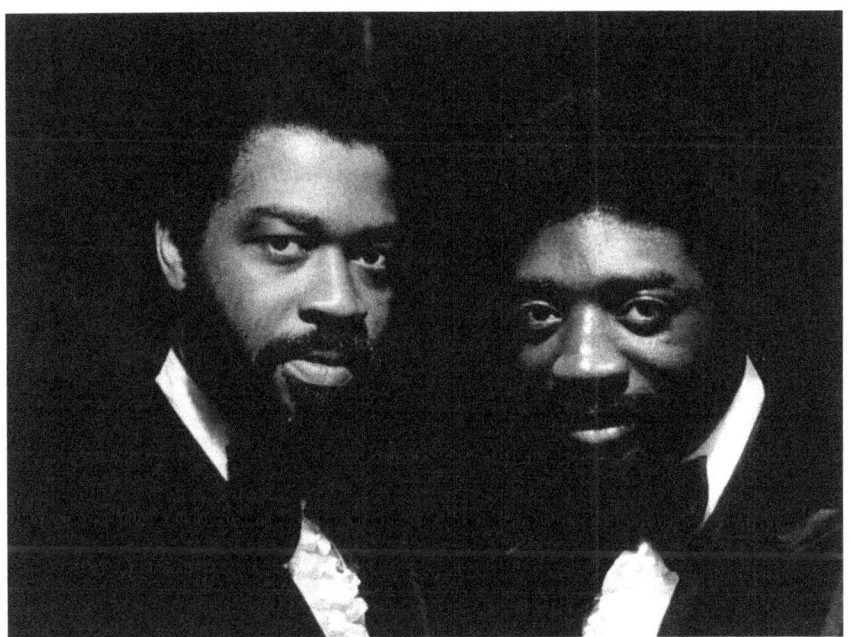

Haroon Rashid Vice President & Douglas Pendarvis President:

My brother, Douglas Pendarvis and I got into the professional boxing business when he was working for WBZ-TV as a news editor. He began to also get involved in the professional boxing industry.

For a short period, Doug was a sparring partner with The Marvelous Marvin Hagler and soon after decided to get into the business of boxing as opposed to getting the ring. It was at that point, in 1985, that Doug and I started the Pendarvis Boxing Enterprise. Doug said the thing that got him interested in the game of boxing is that while living in the city of Brockton he kept noticing this bald headed black guy running through the streets and he thought that the guy was crazy. It turns out that he had just fought a boxing great called Sugar Ray Seals. The fight was aired on television and they were having a victory party at a club called Pete and Mary. Doug attended and he met Marvin's Mother, Malayn Hagler, who introduced him to Marvin and they instantly became friends.

While at WBZ-TV, Doug started introducing Marvin to the management and staff at the television station. At that time, WBZ was doing a lot of cultural network events and Doug would bring Marvin along with him. After becoming friends Doug would go with Marvin to his gym, talking and working him, while watching him spar and train. Doug immediately became a part of his entourage alongside Marvin's managers and trainers, Goody and Pat Petronelli. Doug has said that, after seeing what was going on with Marvin, he developed a desire to be a boxing promoter to support the Petronelli Brothers. In doing that, he discovered he would need insurance for the fighter, a security bond and a financial statement. He had gone to the boxing commission and they refused to give him a license because he did not have any of the things that were required. So Doug was forced to complete the requirements by getting the insurance and then bringing his problem to Lovell Dyett, a producer of WBZ-TV to explain why Lords of London would give him the insurance, but at a cost of $15,000 wherein the other boxing promoters were being charged only $48.00 for the whole show. After that show was aired Doug got a call from the security of the boxing commissioner telling him that they now had good news for him that they would give him the same price as the other promoters and that how he was able secure the insurance? Next he had to find someone that would loan him the money, which he did through a personal friend's bonding company for the amount of $50,000. Finally, he needed a financial statement that would show he had a fifty thousand dollar passport loan in the Unity Bank of Boston and after that they granted him his promoter's license. He then felt ready to help promote secure fights for Marvin. Doug felt that he could now help because he did not like the fact that because Marvin was a left-hand boxer he was getting overlooked by the boxing promoters to match him for fights. He figured that if he could somehow become a boxing promoter that he could change things around and that would make the difference for Marvin to get booked and win some fights.

At the time Marvin was being promoted by a boxing promoter called Rip Vallinti, who was the main promoter in Boston at the Boston Gardens. When Doug asked Rip if he would partner with him to promote some fights in the Gardens and said that he had the blessings of the Petronelli brothers, Rip refused and Doug had to go around him.

Rip also had an objection to me because of my name and the fact that I knew Muhammad Ali. Rip disliked Ali because Ali refused to come to do a fight for him in the Boston Gardens and Rip bragged about his dislike for Ali to us. Ali was the premier boxer at that time and an iconic hero for me, so I did not want anything to do with Rip after he revealed himself to me in that way.

I personally liked the Petronelli brothers though and I got along with them with a great deal of respect and they liked Doug and would do whatever they could to help get the Pendarvis Boxing Enterprise up and running.

Doug took helping Marvin very seriously after knowing that he would only be able to help him as a friend and supporter, so he studied him and gave him and the Petronelli Brothers whatever assistance that he could in making sure that Marvin had a legitimate chance of success. By the time that Pendarvis Boxing Enterprise became established there, four other promoters in Boston: Billy Ferriabough, Helen Hall, Rip Vallinti and Subway Sam Silverman were all marketing the Metro New England area.

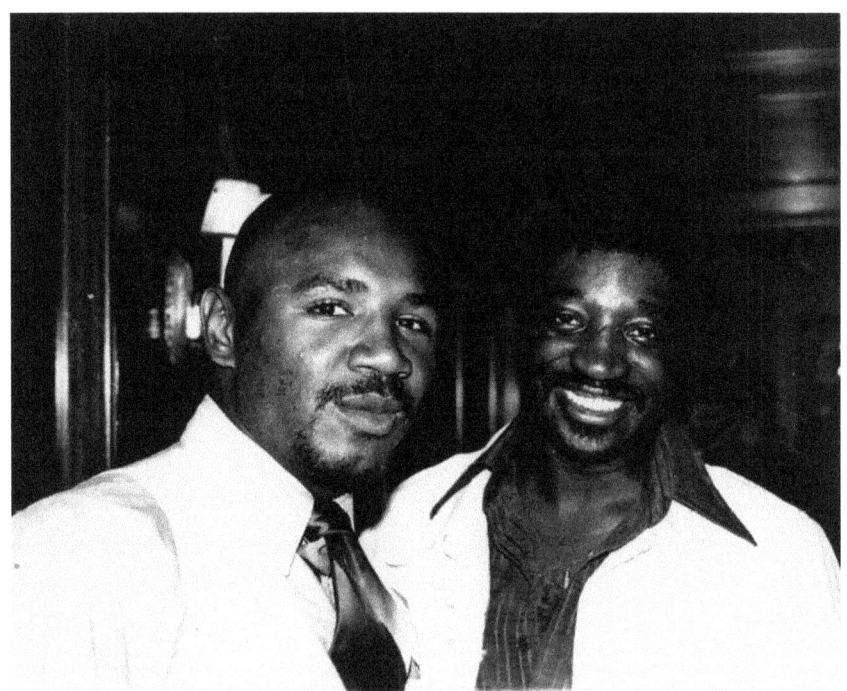

Marvelous Marvin Hagler & Douglas Pendarvis

Doug started working with Marvin to use his right hand as an alternative power punch, making the right hand as good as the left. Marvin started practicing that technique in his mother's mirror, day and night, perfecting his skills as a right hander. That opened up the door for fight-matching abilities in the city of Philadelphia. Doug believed that some of Marvin's best fights started and were fought in Philadelphia, including: Benny Brisko, Willie the Worm

Monroe, Bugaloo Watts, Eugene Cyclone Hart - all the best middleweight top ten fighters – and he won them all.

Doug: believed that the Bugaloo Watts fight was rigged and it was Marvin's first defeat. Marvin took that loss very hard, but he won the rematch in an unquestionable victory.

It turned out that anytime Marvin lost to anyone, if there was a rematch Marvin destroyed his opponent to win a victory. Doug became so close to Marvin that at times he would get into the ring with Marvin as a sparring partner, even though Marvin would take it easy on him.

In observing Marvin, Doug felt that Marvin was getting to much non-productive attention in Brockton; so Doug encouraged Marvin and the Petronelli brothers to go to the Provincetown Inn on the Cape. Doug searched for a boxing training camp in P-town and he met a man named Brooks who had a boxing camp there. Doug cut a deal that Brooks would get the publicity from Marvin's media brand at Brooks' boxing camp. In turn, Marvin could get the training with his team of Pat and Goody Petronelli and keep his sparing partners away from unproductive distractions in his hometown of Brockton, which worked out well for everyone

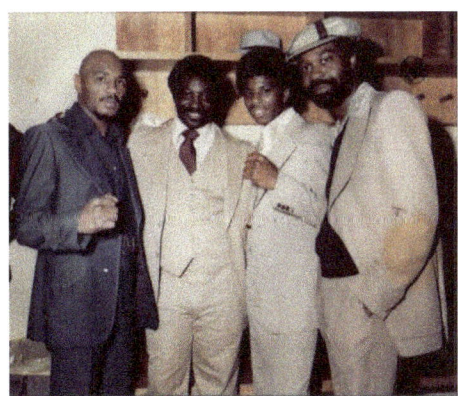

Marvin Hagler, Douglas Pendarvis, Robbie Simms & Haroon Rashid

Then Pendarvis Boxing Enterprise, in partnership with Pat and Goody Petronelli, started promoting small fights in the area like Taunton, Massachusetts at the Rosalind Ball room which was a place that we had many boxing events. We would basically promote their fighters and then Marvin would come too as a guest fighter to sign autographs. Marvin's younger brother Robbie Simms was breaking out as a fighter under the Petronelli and Pendarvis Boxing Enterprise promoted his coming out events along with Mike Cappiello.

Soon after, that came to Boston and Philadelphia with matches and it was then that we got the attention and started working with New York boxing promoter Butch Lewis, he was the promoter handling Michael Spinks and Greg Page fights. We promoted fights in the Catskill Mountains with Butch and he became close friends with Doug and taught him everything that he knew about the boxing game to help us with the boxing network.

From there we started branching off into Atlanta, Georgia with a lightweight professional fighter named Ebo Elder and that is where Doug first met World Heavyweight Champion Evander Holyfield.

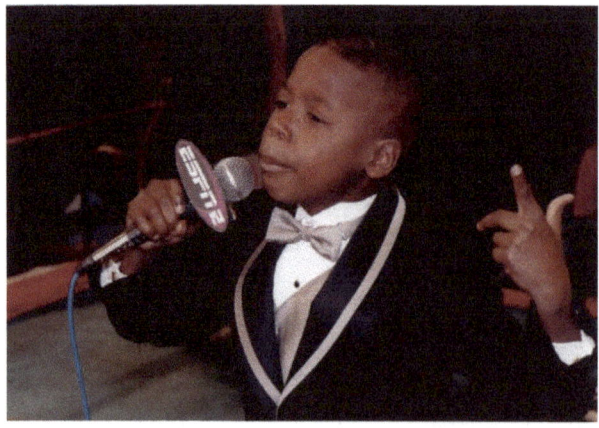

New England Rap Star Little Kenny

At that time Doug was also promoting a young rapper that was called Little Kenny and Evander Holyfield liked that young man so much that would have him perform in his private VIP room at the event. Pendarvis Boxing promoted fights in Worcester, New Hampshire, Portland Maine and all over the Metro New England area.

We also had the privilege to be among some of the Great Hall of Famers in the boxing business like Angelo Dundee, Hector Mancho Camacho, Lou Dova and many more.

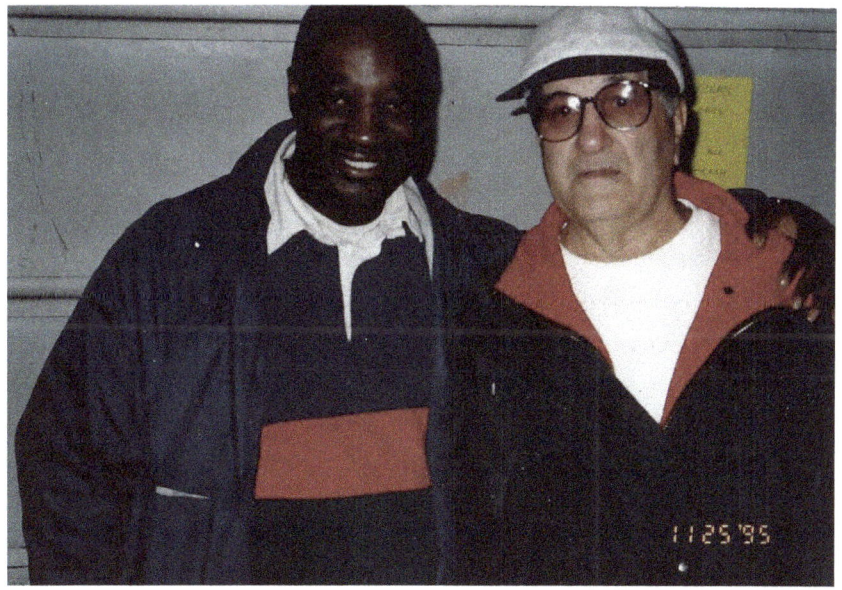

Douglas Pendarvis & boxing Great Marvin Hagler's manager Pat Petronelli

Lou Dova took Doug under his wings and introduced him to all the great ones and Lou was Evander Holyfield's trainer. Whenever Pendarvis Enterprise would have an event New England fighter Richie was able to capitalize on that event in getting other fighters for him to handle in the New England area.

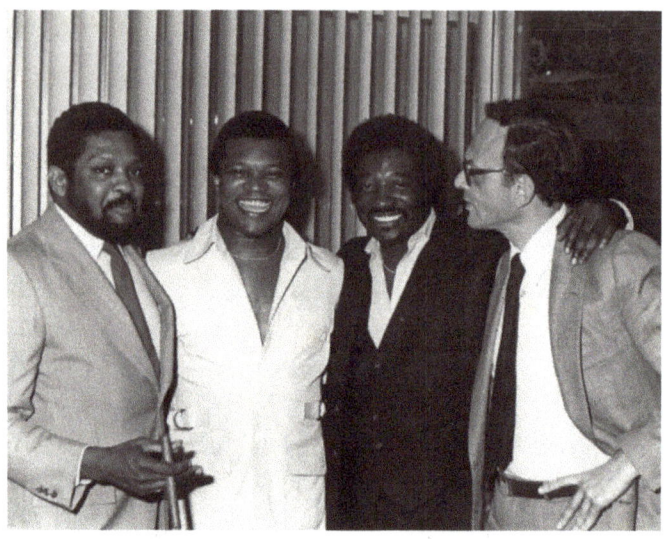

*Butch Lewis, Michael Spinks, Douglas Pendarvis
& the Attorney for World Boxing Council
The New England Knockouts*

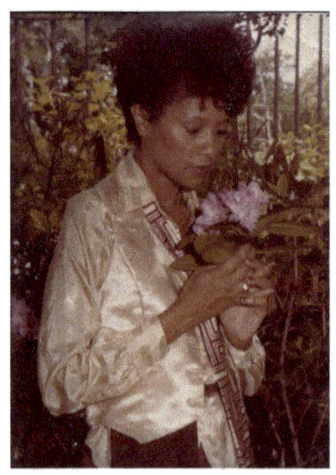

Yvonne Willis - Style & fashion Consultant

In 1971 we create an assembly of beautiful young women called The England Knockouts rounds girls that would enter the rings in between rounds at fights to show the public signs of each round. They were trained and coached how to walk and to have the confidence for stage presence, by a woman that was an expert in doing that while helping the Pendarvis Boxing Enterprise accomplishing our goals. Her name was Yvonne Willis Rose who was a beautiful woman that I had learned to love and respect, and that I had a perfect professional relationship with. We were also neighbors that lived in the same area just blocks away from the now Malcolm X Park, and the Crispus Attucks Drive and housing complexes. Yvonne had a reputation of being precise and professional in her skill set and had events that she was managing or engaged with all over Boston. I had all the confidence, knowing that if Yvonne was working with me we would be fine with our presentations.

After being around her I developed an appetite to have a smart, charismatic and attractive type of woman in my inner circle for the appreciation of equal respect for leadership.

My theory, since then, has been that if two different personalities, male and female put their backs together and form their views there is a 360-degree observation and most likely it will give them an edge for success, if they can stay focused.

The rounds girls, as they were called, were being guided in the way that Yvonne was showing them how to be a positive alert representative and to stay focused, particularly because they would be in sexy bathing suits around all types of men that would have the tendency's to occasionally say too much or go too far. The women were so sexy and beautiful that one time we did an exhibition fight with Muhammad Ali and Peter Fuller and Ali was so taken back as to how beautiful one of the rounds girls was that he literally took her off the floor after the fight into his hotel room, and of course we went with them. Since we were the only ones that could enter into his suite, we had a great time that night. We all took pictures and he signed autographs with everyone who was with us; the girls were ecstatic that they could come and get that close to Ali in his suite. He would tell everyone that he was "The Greatest of All Times."

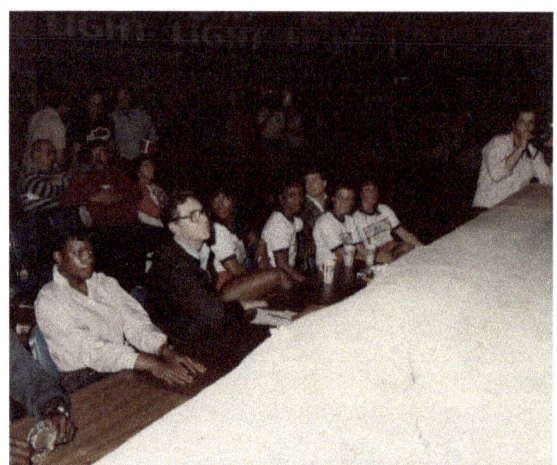

Pendarvis Boxing New England Knockouts, Rounds Girls

Those were great times that we all had and I am sure that everyone had many incredible stories to share about meeting the many celebrities and new lifelong friends that we were privileged to know and encounter along the way.

Douglas Pendarvis, Cynthia Cox & Haroon Rashid

The Muhammad Ali Olympic Training Center was a not for profit 501c 3 corporation that was created by Douglas Pendarvis, Cynthia Cox and Haroon Rashid in 1987 for the express purpose of helping potential Olympic youth candidates to maintain their academic skills while pursuing their dreams to qualify and to be active as Olympian athletes. Our goals were to provide individual tutors to each athlete to insure in their absence from the classroom teaching that they, while training and competing, would not miss their basic education.

We presented this concept to the city of Boston and received approval of the nature of intent; in fact the city of Boston offered, as a donation to the Muhammad Ali Center, an unused closed Boston Public elementary school in the Dorchester area, to renovate and develop into an official location that would house our conceptual concept.

We then attempted to get the concept up and running. But there were far too many hurdles for us to jump and get the project off the ground, in spite of the need for such a concept at that time. Our first hurdle was to get the approval of Muhammad Ali and his family to endorse the conceptual concept.

Doug and I made special trips to Chicago to hand deliver to him at his Mansion on Woodlawn Avenue in Hyde Park Chicago a copy of the schematic plan. We also met with one of his daughters in her suburban home to seek her assistance in making this idea come into fruition, to no avail. Because the legal advisors of Ali felt that they did not want Ali's name tagged onto anything that the legal team of the Ali estate had absolutely no control of. Of course we learned that they had an interest in creating something similar in Louisville, Kentucky, his home city. We did not have a backup alternative at that time and our motivation for pushing up the city level was out of the respect that we had for Muhammad Ali as a social activist/athlete; we all knew of his world services. In addition, the city of Boston would be a perfect fit and magnet for the educational environment in Boston, which we could use to recruit from the metro Boston colleges and university for interns as volunteer tutors.

We had youth volunteers that would come each day to help in any way that they could to get the building ready for renovation, only to be very disappointed that it never caught on and the Ali family did not want Muhammad Ali's name associated with it.

So, to be honest, we were shocked that the idea was so matter of fact rejected, that we lost the desire to pursue the ideas any further. Besides the city was putting pressure on us to deliver the production or they would demolish the building and that is what eventually happened. It was after that action that I decided to leave Boston for Atlanta and pursue my other ambitions that were social activism in the Atlanta Area on the Atlanta black colleges' campus site; thus the idea was aborted.

Ironically, later in Boston, a similar concept was instituted after the sudden death of a Boston Celtics icon, Reggie Lewis, with the establishment of the Reggie Lewis Community Center in Roxbury, directly across the street from the Muslim Mosque, Roxbury Community College, and next door to the Madison Park High school campus, a very attractive and useful center complex with many of the similar concepts of the Muhammad Ali Center.

But we all were very disappointed that our vision could not come into realty at that time.

Meanwhile at Olives Beauty Salon

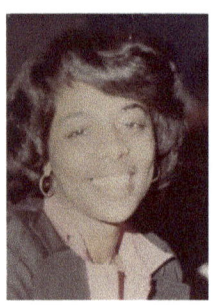

Gwendolyn Palmer

At that time, I was dating a very beautiful and intelligent women name Gwendolyn Palmer, who was a single mom that lived in Cambridge, Mass from Fayetteville, North Carolina. She was an administrator at Northeastern University in Boston. I learned to love Gwen and I asked her to marry me several times, but because of a former experience, I believed that she would not trust or take my offers seriously. Gwen kept rejecting my appeals for marriage, so I allowed my mind to wander and eventually I got attracted to Veronica. Gwen was a great woman; my children loved her. My family loved Gwen and I totally respected her as a woman, but the chemistry of Veronica and I being fellow Artists at that time was the single thing that made me experiment, and eventually I got caught up on Veronica. I often thought what Gwen and I could have done together if things did not go the way that they did. I am sure that we could have been very happy together because she was a good woman.

While working at one of Olive Benson's and my Cousin James Harris' Hair Metric Training Center classes in Boston, I met my future wife Veronica Younger. She was the manager for Olive's Beauty Salon in Atlanta, Georgia. Veronica and I helped Olive, and my cousin James to teach that class. We seemed to click with each other right away and I could not get her out of my mind.

Two months later, after befriending Veronica, I moved to Atlanta and we were married within a year. That marriage created a lot of success for me, and if I had not met and followed my mind, we would not have had my beautiful daughter Rakeemah.

Soon after Veronica and I got together, we made an offer to Olive that she agreed to; and we bought Olive's Beauty Salon in Atlanta from Olive Benson. It was the first hair business that Veronica and I owned. We later changed the name of the salon to Rashid's Hair Care Center. We got a loan and totally redesigned the salon; it was one of the best-looking salons in Atlanta.

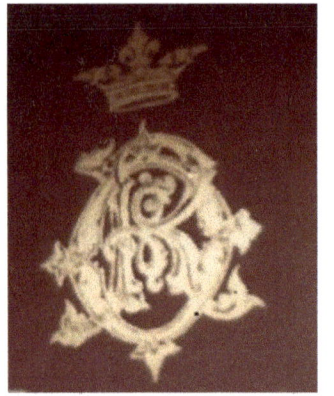

The Rashid's Family Coat of Armor

This image is the Rashid's Coat of Armor that I had designed in the mid eighties for my first Hair & Beauty consulting business in Atlanta. It was a way for me to declare my families Sovereign identity. As I was aware that the Surname that I and most African-Americans was born with had been given to us and my immediate family members in South Carolina during the days of slavery as a legal form of permanent identity for the purpose of a valued property of our former slave owners.

As I then adjudicated myself self identity back in the late seventies, through a court order in the United States Federal Courts in Jacksonville Florida from my former Sir name of Thompson, that to me represented a reminder of slavery suffering and humiliation.

I have since then SOVEREIGNLY declared my liberation from any potential seals, coats of armor or any legal declarations unless that of a willing acceptance regarding a former slave master's children's of any intellectual proprietary identity claims.

However, I have since capitulated and will declare an acceptable and agreeable reparation for the inhuman treatment and sufferings from the descendants of the sealed SOVEREIGN Thompson corporation HUMAN VAULE PRPOERTY RIGHTS and or the United States of America for equal human value property rights.

Chapter Nine

Rashid's Hair Care Center

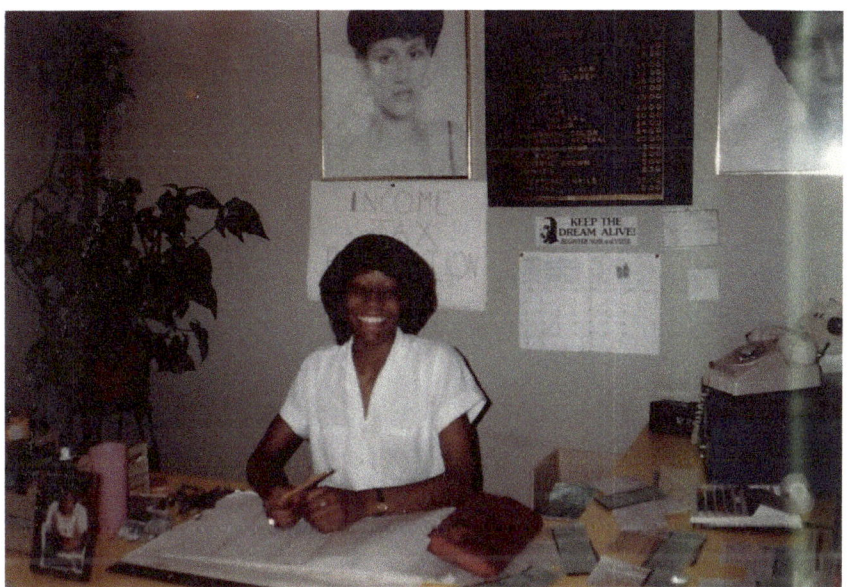

My Daughter Anita as the Receptionist before the renovation of the salon

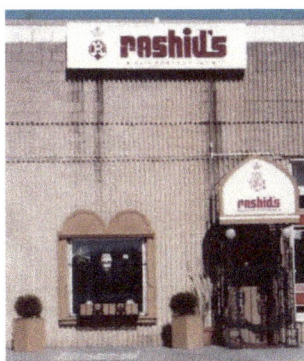
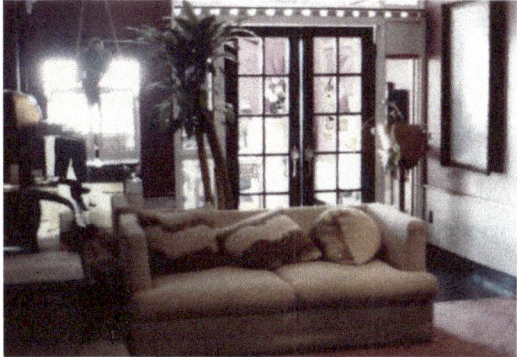

Rashid's Hair Care Center: exterior entrance and inside décor Lounge area.

We did some cutting edge décor in the salon with privatized work stations and a full comfortable reception and private waiting room area, separate hair dryer room area, private employee lounge room, and private shampoo area. Many hair manufacturing companies used the salon for hair product photo shoots. We had the idea that the salon should maintain customer privacy, so we created sections in the salon as well as semi private work stations. It was a great success for the salon in that we received a lot of popularity Atlanta first African American Mayors wife Valerie Jackson or Mrs. Ginger Sullivan, wife of the School of Medicine at Morehouse College: founding dean and director Dr. Louis W. Sullivan among other celebrities and high end professionals in Atlanta.

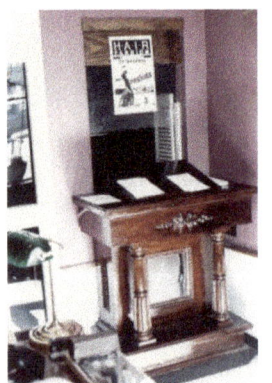
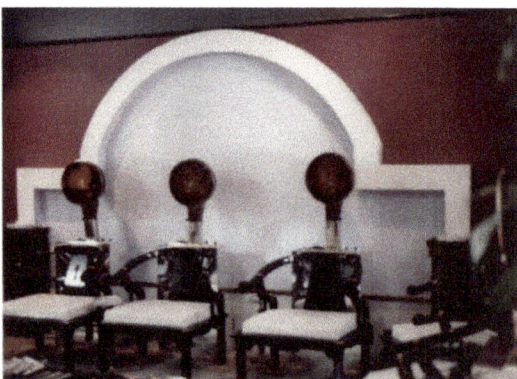

Sign in podium at the entry of the salon, & the hair dryers section

Because Rashid's was a popular cutting edge salon, it was previewed on the cover of several hair care magazines. Rashid's was always busy with students and professionals from the Atlanta University Black Campus Center schools - Morris Brown, Morehouse, Atlanta University, Clark College, Spellman College, and Atlanta Theological Institute. My Daughter Anita was a student at Spellman and she was a receptionist for the salon; that helped drive business from the young students to the salon.

One of the other things that made our business so popular was the fact that both Veronica and I were known in Atlanta and across the country as a husband and wife hair styling team for Johnson Products Company, and we were contracted to teach our skills to hair stylists throughout Atlanta and the country. We made a great team and soon built a strong reputation, nationally and abroad. I, soon after, started getting offerings from companies all over America to represent their product lines.

One such company asked me to be their International representative, and that opportunity took me to several different continents as an advice educator.

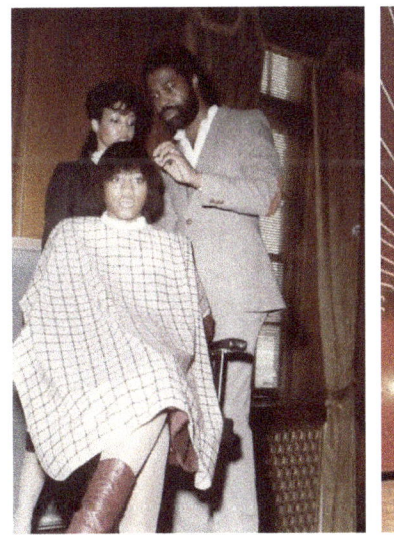
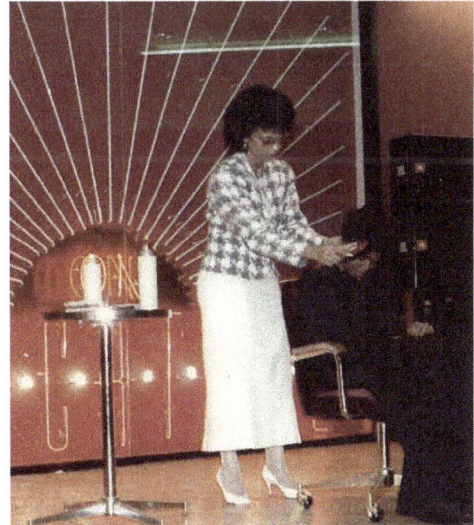

Veronica & Haroon Rashid, Johnson Products Co. Husband Wife Styling Team

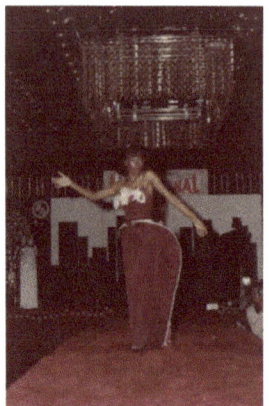 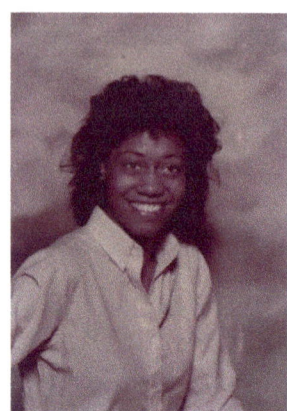

Anita as a Model at the Bronner Brothers Show & as a student at Spellman College

The Rashids, as we were called, were booked to do shows and workshops all over the country. Either Veronica or I and / or, in some cases both of us, were representing their company's interest and, in many cases, for professional hair and beauty associations.

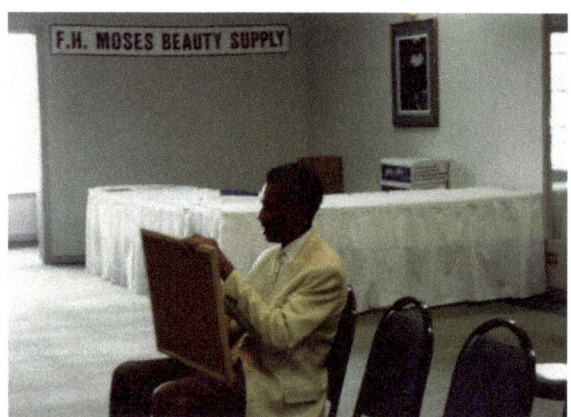

Al Washington CEO of Afam Products Company

One such product and company was the Elentee Vitale Hair Care/Afam Products Company; the President's name was Mr. Al Washington. We were asked by the company to do some exploratory testing on their product line called Vitale products before their marketing was officially introduced into the markets and I later became a feature artist for their company - Afam Vitale Products.

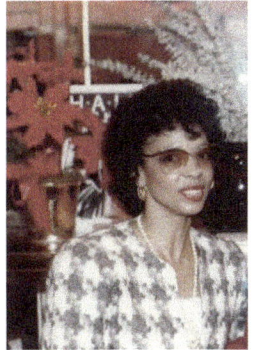
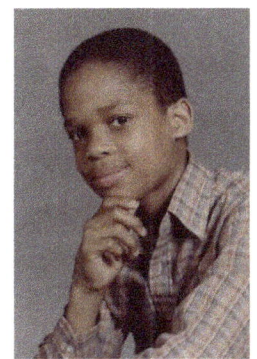

Veronica Younger Rashid   *My Stepson Mark Younger*

Veronica had one child before we met and married. His name was Mark Younger, he was a very smart young man and I was proud to call him my son. Veronica and I, soon after, produced our last child Rakeemah Jamilah Rashid. She was a little angel as a child and Lord knows that I loved that little girl. She eventually, like so many of my children, took after her mother and me to become a hair stylist herself. She loved being in the salon and I knew that she would get involved in the industry one day, and she did.

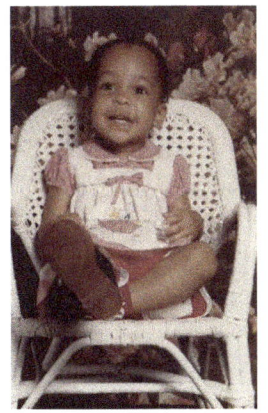
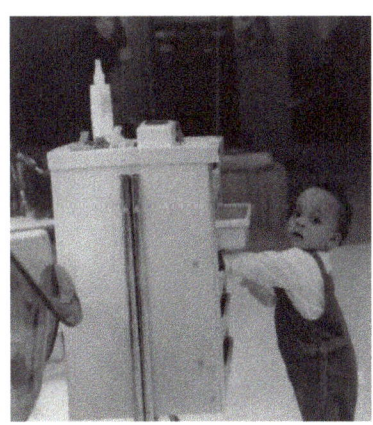

Rakeemah Jamilah Rashid   *Rakeemah practicing for her career*

MY CULTURAL BIRTH RIGHTS

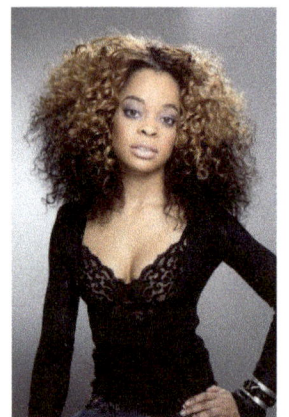
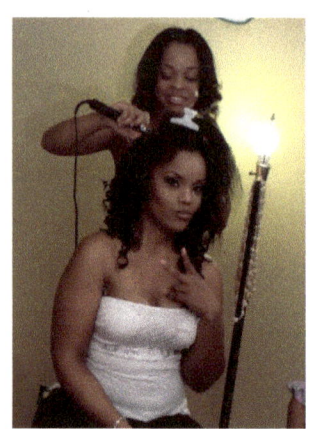

My Daughter Rakeemah all grown up and working as a cosmetologist

It was in Atlanta that I became involved with the television industry. I had a friend from Boston who was in production, at the time cable television was breaking into the cable television broadcasting business, in particular with Ted Turner Broadcasting. The federal government, at that time, made it mandatory that the new network had to offer free cable access programming to the community and if you had a pilot program concept they would allow you to produce your own television production.

My friend showed me how to get involved and learn the necessities to produce my own cable television program. I took up the offer and produced a weekly program called **"Professional Hair Care and the Fashions"**. That program opened a network of information about the hair industry that most people in the industry did not know about.

Each year Bronner Brothers would put on the largest gathering of African American stylists, and celebrities from around the world would come to Atlanta for this show. So I decided to schedule my show at the Bronner Brothers hair shows. I ask Mr. Nathaniel H Bronner Sr., who was the CEO of the show, if he would allow me to tape and broadcast my production centered on celebrity interviews to talk about their input in the industry at his shows, and he agreed.

The first interview was with him and the industry leaders. If you were one of the who's who in the industry, you wanted to be interviewed on the Bronner Brothers hair show, and to be televised on Atlanta Cable Television at that time. One such historical interview was with Dr. Katie Wickham, President of the National Beauty Culturalist League and Alexander Neweia, who was then President of the National Cosmetology Association.

To add to the success, we had the celebrity clients in Atlanta that frequently visited Rashid's. The business was doing well until I started teaching and traveling abroad. I was the International Stylist for a company called M &M Products. The company executives Thurman McKenzie and Cornel McBride; commissioned me to do a three continent tour in, the Caribbean, Africa, and Europe.

Chapter Ten

Three Continent Working Tour

The Caribbean

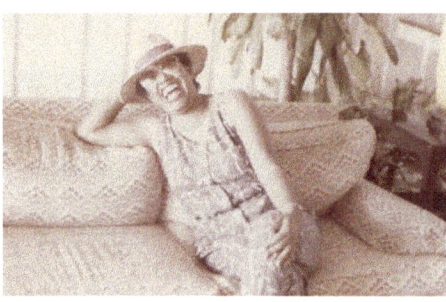

Caribbean representative for M&M Products Mrs. Mary Ellen Reese

When I first went to the Caribbean as an International Celebrity Stylist, it was in Jamaica. I started in Kingston, the capital city, where I was the guest educator for a local beauty supply company. The Caribbean representative for M&M Products was Mrs. Mary Ellen Reese, who became one of my best friends at that time.

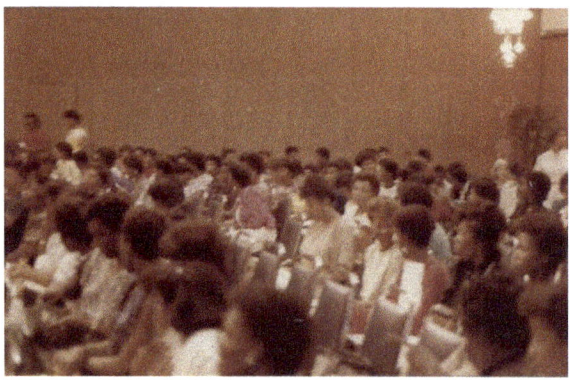

Kingston Jamaica lecture and workshop at the Afro Caribbean Beauty show

While in Jamaica one of the first things that we did was to organize the professionals in the hair and beauty industry to help perfect a professional hair association like the one in America. Overall our lectures, as well as our meet and greet networking tour went very well in assisting in that cause.

Hope Academy Beauty School in Kingston Jamaica

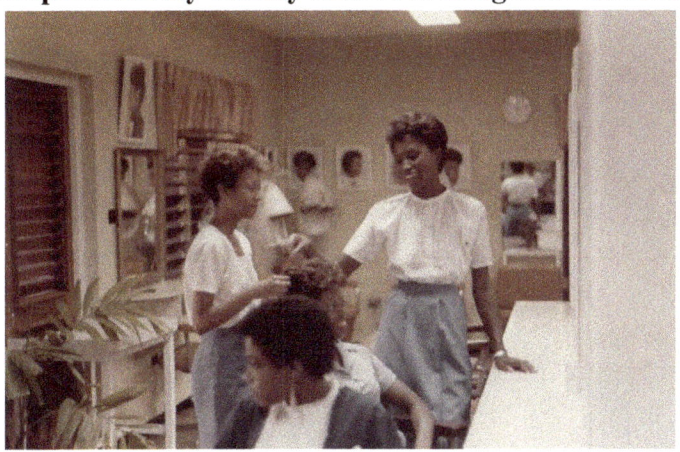

Students at the Hope Academy

The school was a pet project of the First Lady of Jamaica, Mrs. Missy Ceaga. I helped train the staff for the Hope Academy, the beauty school on the Island. I also worked with and trained the Island's hair and beauty association along with the beauty supply companies to produce a trade show on the Island. I was the Featured Artist. I traveled from Kingston to Ochos Rios, Mandeville, Negril, and Montego Bay; and in each city I gave cultural cosmetology and tonsorial arts classes. I made lots of friends there and I returned back to Jamaica at least five times after.

We then went to Bermuda, the home Island of Mary Ellen. Her brother owned a Beauty Salon, a taxi service, and a clothing store. I stayed with her brother and his wife in one of the most beautiful homes on the Island. Bermuda is one of the richest Islands per capita in the Caribbean. I traveled all over the Island teaching in schools and beauty salons.

Barbados Workshop

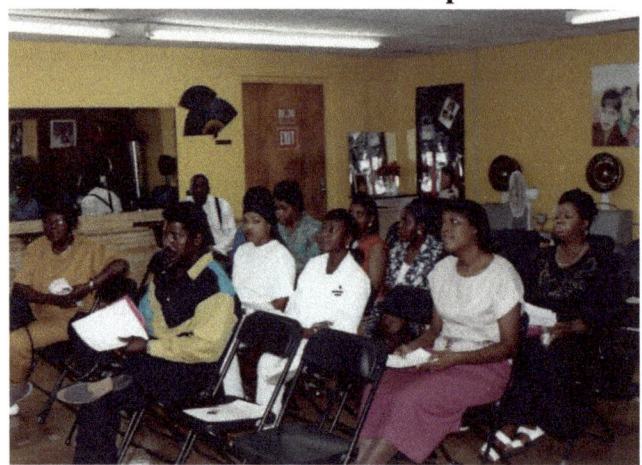

Students at a Workshop in Barbados

I then went to Barbados and stayed at the Hilton hotel, which was right next to an oil refinery. The refinery being so close to the tourist areas of the Island was unsettling for me. We gave hair shows and I taught at all the beauty schools and salons on the Island. One other observation that I had was that the businesses were behind the time in style and décor.

Barbados is a former British colony and the people are hard-working and friendly. The hair distributor that we were working with on the Island also owned a bus service and a construction company; he was one of the wealthiest men on the Island. The Island had a serious tradition of all business shutting down at noon; they would close for an hour or two, and then go right back as though it was a new day. I found that experience in several islands like Curacao, so you would have to wait if you had any intentions of shopping that day. We got along very well with everyone while I was there. I was surprised though that the Island seemed very hilly to me and sociopolitical, very controlling on the locals by the authorities on the citizens. The people seemed very ambitious and dedicated to their work. But it was so strict at the hotels and in tourist areas we stayed in; the citizens were not allowed to be there and fraternize with the tourists unless they were working.

Arriving in the Bahamas

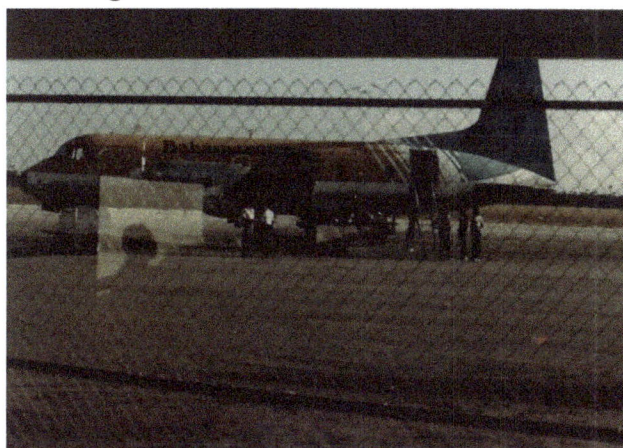

Arriving in the Bahamas to consult the Bahamian Professional Cosmetologist

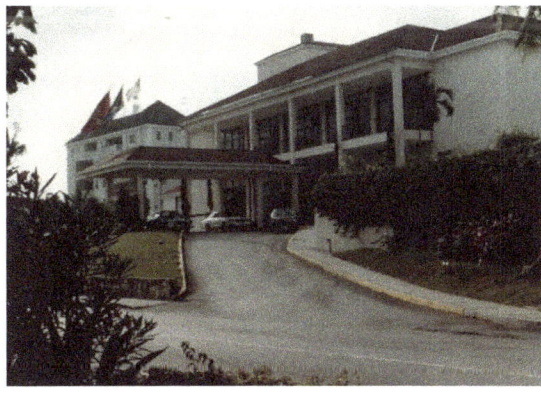

We stayed at the Nassau Bahamas Grand Casino and Hotel

The Island was very much Americanized and, like the entire Island, there were strict restrictions on tourists and the native people socializing at the hotel resorts. But I always managed to avoid the restrictions to meet new people and make friends. Freeport was different from Nassau in that Freeport was laid back and relaxing like most Island cities are, and because of the many casinos, the city of Nassau was a very busy fast active scene. I toured the Island with the distributor, who was a pharmaceutical distributor as well as a hair and beauty supplier. We were teaching in every salon and school on the Island. The people were very festive and friendly.

Curacao: Antilles Island /Trinidad

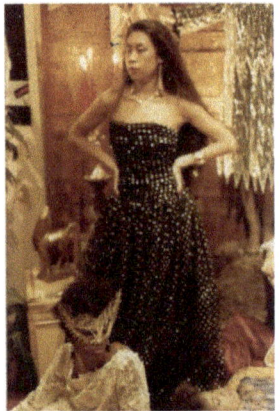

Models at the hair show in Trinidad

We then traveled to Curacao, an Antilles Island. The people are mixed with Dutch, Spanish, French, African and English. They speak a native language called Papiamento, which is a merge of all the languages on the Island.

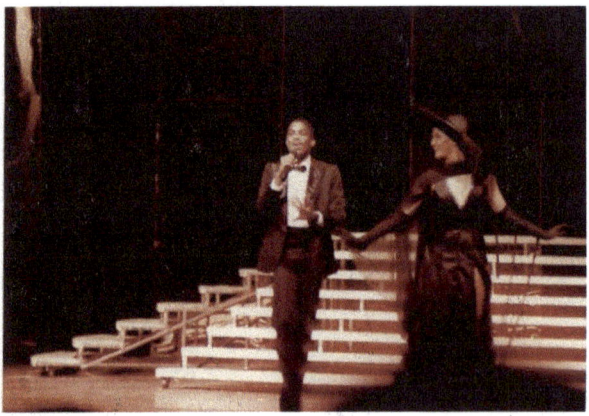

At a Cabaret in Curacao

The distributors are a husband wife team that also, at the time, distributed Frito Lays products throughout the Islands of Trinidad and Curacao. There are casinos on the Island that attract people from Venezuela for weekend fun getaways. You can see the lights from the city of Caracas, Venezuela at night in Curacao. Many people come to Curacao during the Mardi Gras in Trinidad or Rio de Janeiro as an overflow for tourists during the festival. The people are very youthful- looking and friendly. I toured and taught hairdressers throughout the Island.

Chapter Eleven

South African Tour

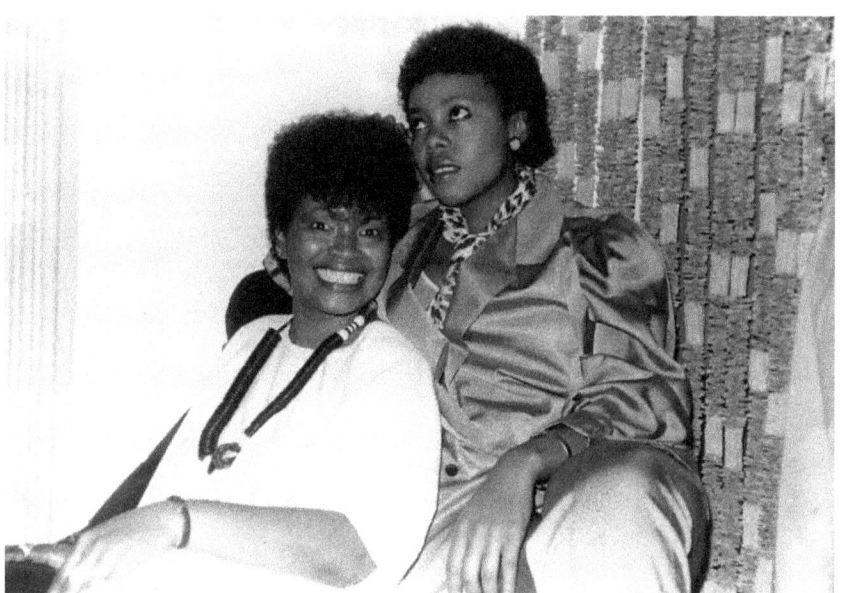

My American business associate on the left and a South African Professional Actress

When I was in South Africa it was during a time when apartheid was being practiced.

I remember talking to one of my peers who was scheduled to go on tour with me. She called me in the middle of the night in Atlanta, scared and uncertain. She spoke of talking to her spouse about not going because South Africa was still at war between the government's, white Afrikaner and its citizens, black Africans. I told her that I had spent my youth protecting the United States of America, in the U S Marines.

Therefore, I was not motivated by fear, only by knowledge. I wanted to know what was really happening over there, and I did not know anybody but Ambassador Andrew Young, who was African American that had been there, so I wanted to see for myself.

We agreed to not look back or try to get too political about the decisions that we would make if our intent was to be pioneers in regards to taking advantage of retrieving real time information about that part of Africa.

As a former marine and African American sociopolitical leader for many years, regarding the invitation to go there, I knew that most of the best information about the world community would be best witnessed on the grounds where the reality of the actions were taking place.

It was more than I thought on so many levels. One of the examples of that in the city of Johannesburg was a serious attempt to modernize the city with skyscraper buildings, modern department stores, and restaurants. The ugly part of the good life in the major cities like Johannesburg was it was created for the white citizens' sovereign use and the so-called colored people were allowed to have special liberty in those major cities. The townships that surrounded every major city were the homeland for the Black Africans. I had the opportunity to observe all of it for myself.

City of Johannesburg

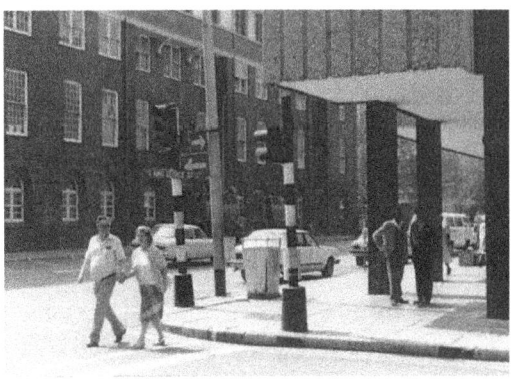

A street in downtown Johannesburg South Africa near the Hotel that I stayed in

South Africa was beautiful and the modern cities like Johannesburg were heavily populated and reminded me of a very modern New York City. The city has tall buildings, a big financial district, a major shopping area, a large restaurant, and a nightclub community. It is a very busy fast pace and Metropolis City, with museums and a top of the line school system that was insultingly privy for the white population.

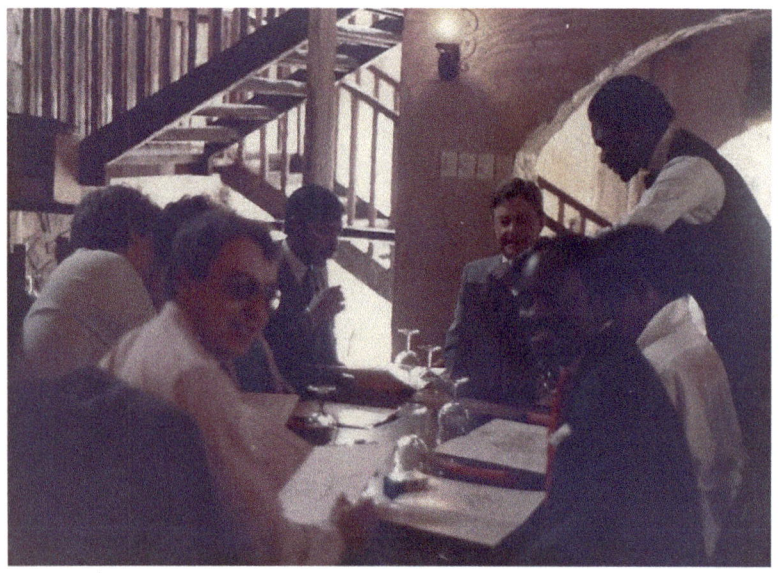

A five Star restaurant in the center of the Johannesburg National Zoo

My first encounter with wild animals in Africa was at a first class restaurant in the center of the city zoo in Johannesburg South Africa. It reminded me of the Tavern on the Green in Central Park, New York.

The cities that I mentioned were populated and enjoyed by white Africanas, and tourists who were allowed to travel in them and see while we were there. Was I surprised when I found out that I was classified as an honorary white citizen, as an African

American visiting South Africa? Because with the control the government had on the Black African and so-called Colored citizens, they were made to stay out of the downtown district after certain hours, unless they had a pass to be there. If I did not have that special honorary classification, I definitely would not have had the privileges that I did. Most of the black people had never seen the inside of some of their beautiful hotels rooms, as I did. That life was so grand for the people that could enjoy it.

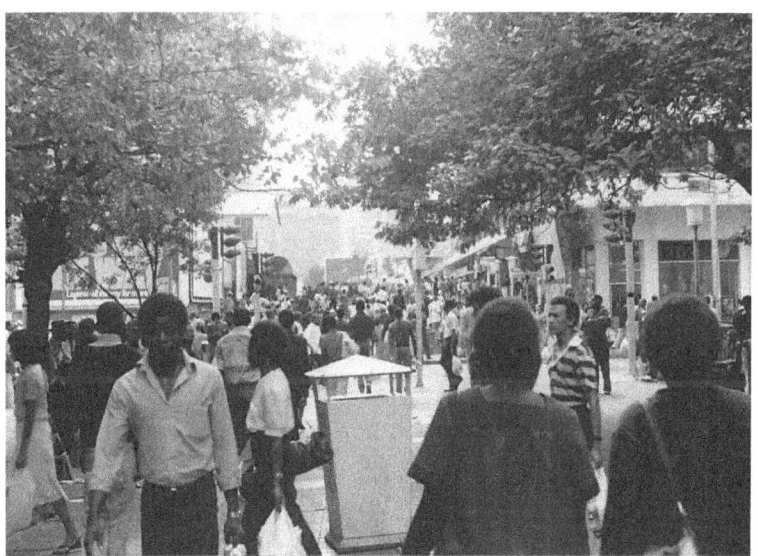

Soweto Township business district

Then there were the black Townships that surrounded those lovely cites like Soweto near Johannesburg, where I was taken on a tour to Nelson and Winnie Mandela's home and Desmond Tutu's home. In Soweto, we were invited to a fast track grade school for the elite blacks; it was called Pace Academy. The school had state of the art equipment and a mostly all white staff that was operating it. It was a colossal difference from the so-called education and

Bantu schools that most South African students were forced to attend, and that they were protesting against.

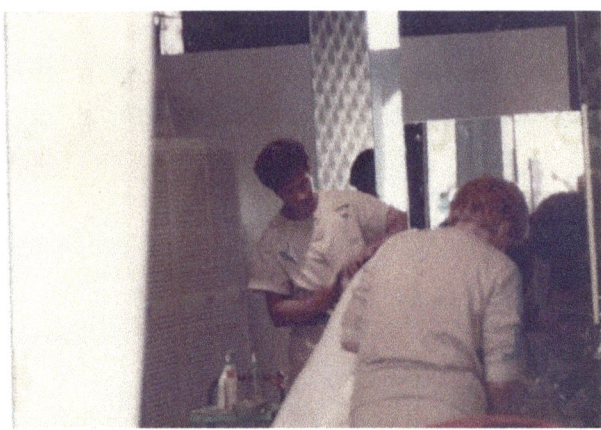

Our first hands on workshop in the popular downtown Johannesburg Hotel

The professional and commercial hair and beauty businesses and South African entrepreneurs were in full attendance of the introduction for the South African M&M Products "Stay Soft Fro" exploratory investment workshop. Part of the introductory was to give hands on workshop of the products.

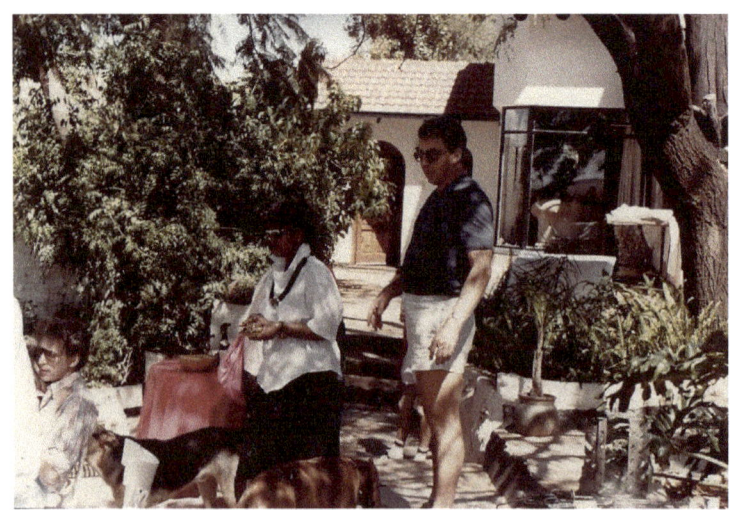

Our USA team at one of the distributors homes for a picnic in Johannesburg

In this scene we were at the personal home of the national distributor for the hair and beauty business that was in one of the suburbs of Johannesburg. It was a send-off picnic for our departure before we left the country.

The City of Durban

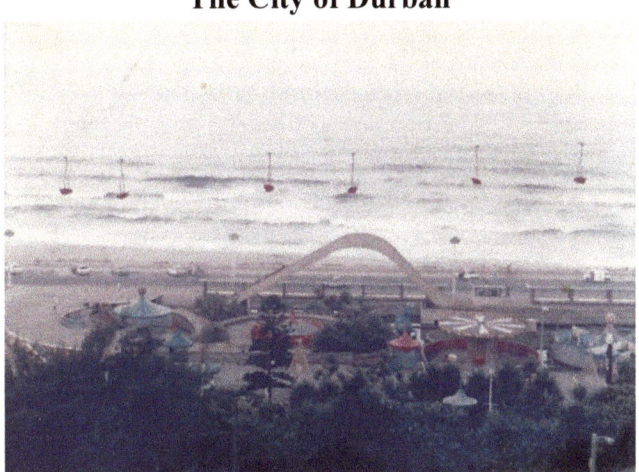

My view from the Casablanca International Hotel in Durban South Africa

Durban sits on the coastline of the Indian Ocean. The city has a very Middle Eastern feeling with shopping bazaars, Ferris wheels, and roller coasters, right on the ocean front. We stayed in the Casablanca International Hotel in Durban South Africa.

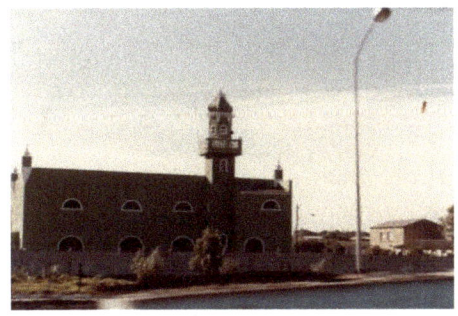

A Muslim Mosque or Masjid in the city of Durban

In Durban I met many Muslims that wanted to talk to me as an African American Muslim, to find out about how Muslims in America manage to practice their Deen or (spirituality) and stay current with fashion and culture. I was told that Wallace Muhammad from Chicago had just left Durban to teach at the Muslim Mosque, so that made them really excited and eager to know about me. I could not answer their questions about fashions and trend because I was not sure that American Muslims had yet put a statement together on fashion. I believe that will come, though, as the community lets go of some of the old style traditions and moderates them to today's trends.

Port Elisabeth was a city that had plenty of the so-called Colored People. It was there that I met a woman who was classified as colored, and we became friends. She taught me the cultural differences between the races. She was a student nurse in a Port Elisabeth hospital, and a model for one of my hair training classes. She told me that most of the colored people were mixed with Indonesian men, and African women.

The men were brought over to work the mines without their women; so many of them married the women that were available. White women were prohibited and there were no other choices, so the men taught the black women their customs and culture, which was Islam. Thus the Islamic influences among these people are very apparent. The colored people there were considered more civilized than the black Africans by the evil minds of Apartheid, and were given a small degree of favor or freedom because of that. Colored people were treated better than blacks because they looked more like the white people, with a lighter skin and straighter grade of hair. This is the same way American mulatto or African Americans that are mixed were treated, especially in the South.

The City of East London

East London is a very busy and old industrial kind of environment that sits on the Indian Ocean. I got a definite British feeling and influence out of the environment with old close homes like in Birmingham, England, or Brooklyn, New York, in America. The people were friendly and very hungry for knowledge. Most of the salons were white owned with black staff. But there were a great number of young up and coming black stylists that were watching my every move.

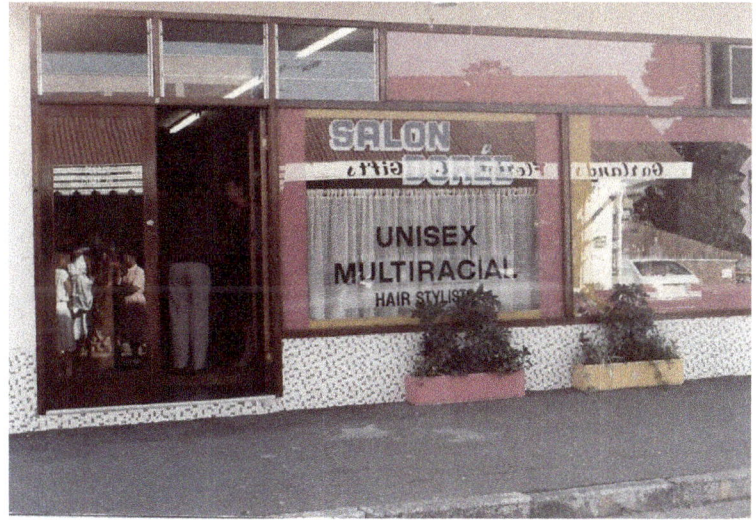

Salon Doree Unisex Multiracial hair salon in South Africa

Working with these young future entrepreneurs, I learned that African culture, and many in the African Diaspora are very gender conscious. Most of the men see doing hair, particularly on women, as a female thing unless you are a homosexual. Like many other environments, I send strong messages to the men that the hair & beauty industry is a good business if you do not allow yourself to become homophobic or too over the top.

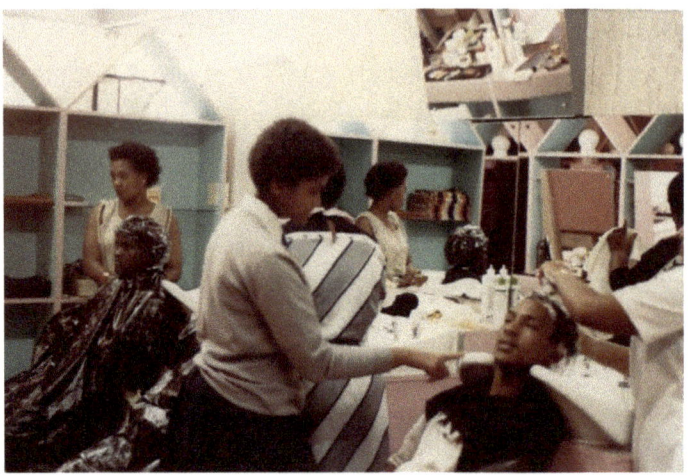

At the Doree salon students following the instructions of Haroon Rashid

In Bloemfontein

Bloemfontein, sits in the middle of the lower southern tip of Africa, it is surrounded by rich farmland. The homes in the city are beautiful, and expensive. It was in Bloemfontein that I met a delegation of African women that told me they wanted us to go back to America, and tell their brothers and sisters that we love them and we are the same, experiencing the same problems. They said we pray for the day that you can come home to Africa, and they can come to America to see their brothers and sisters.

They also managed to take us on a tour of one of the townships near Bloemfontein. There I talked to the common man about youth problems. I tried to explain the deference with civil rights protests, staying in school as the way of the African American black protest, and how many of the African American battles for civil rights were fought on the campuses and streets throughout America.

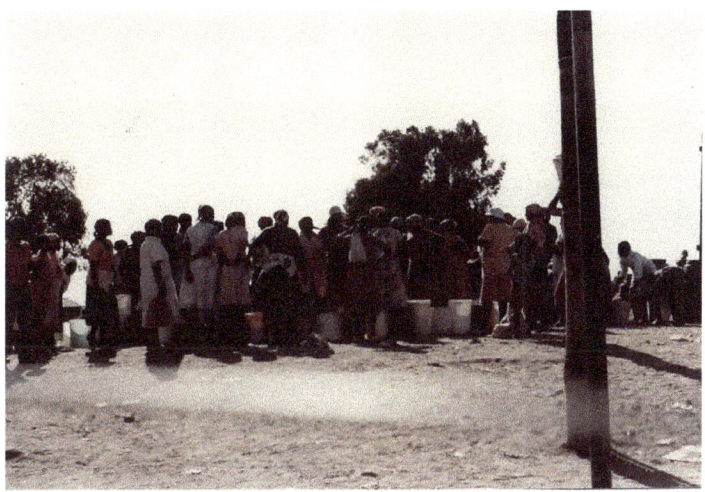
Mothers gathering to discuss their children's safety while they protested Bantu education

I told one male parent that when we were going to school during the protest and we knew that if we decided to throw rocks at police or tanks that we better do it on our way to or from school because our parents did not play that. The Bantu education, as a system of education that white citizens who refer to themselves as and were called Afrikaner, the multiracial as Colored and the blacks as African people. The negative code name for Africans was Kefir. The intellectual level of education was obviously inferior in comparison to the Afrikaner and Colored people, it was called Bantu Education. The African children rebelled against it and that was the start of the protests started by the children. So that man told me that if we told our children to stop throwing rocks and go to school, the children would throw those rocks at us.

Botswana / Sun City were a city like Las Vegas. It sits on the southern tip of Kalahari Desert. It was packed with casinos, cabaret, hotels, nightclubs, and restaurants. Only whites or celebrities could go there, and that is why the natives called this city Sin City. In Sun City, we realized that we had been followed because there were two black men that looked like American black men. They were well-dressed, clean, groomed; and by the time we had gotten to Sun City we knew theses faces were no coincidence. So we assumed they were working for the American government or South African government keeping an eye on us.

Most South African Blacks, at that time, if they lived in the beautiful City of Cape Town they were not allowed to travel to see the top of the world famous Table Mountain, a national monument for South Africans and tourists that were privy to view two major Oceans, the Indian and the Atlantic Ocean merge together.

The irony of it is that, I, as an African American citizen with that insulting passport, was able to experience that phenomenon.

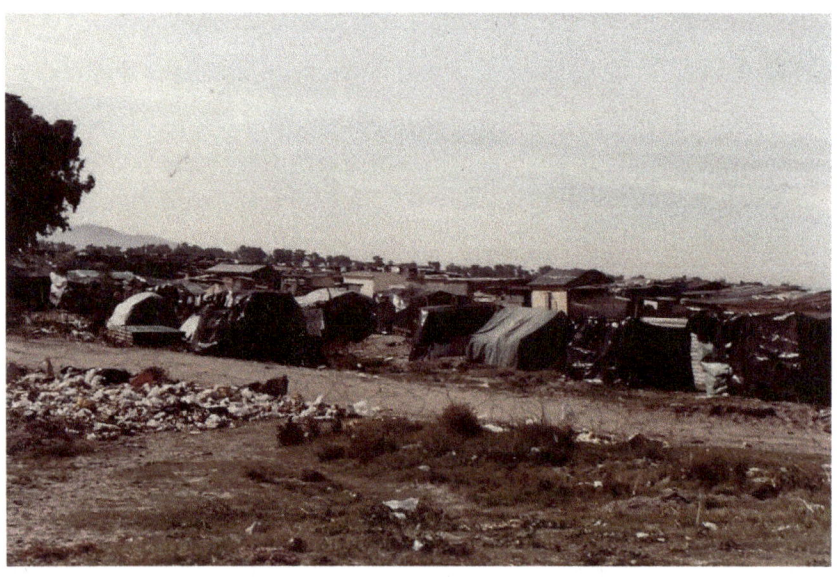

At the Crossroads near Cape Town, there were massive rows of shacks; some were built of cardboard as walls, etc. They looked like the poor shabby towns that are in Mississippi, or worse. But then there were these black independent Home lands: Transkei, the homeland that Nelson Mandela was born in; or Ciskei, Bophuthatswana, Swazi Land; these areas that I visited were massive with many developed cities.

Transkei Section of South Africa

The University of Umtata

I went to Umtata, the capital city in the Transkei, where there was a school being completed, called the University of Umtata. The campus was modern and well-attended. The thing that stayed with me the most is that there were so many Americans as staff members teaching on that campus, it sort of put in perspective why I was there, and that was to teach my people all I knew. Once I got to that way of thinking, I saw people bringing their life stories to me, I saw people following us from work shop to work shop, hungry to see the Americans and ask all the questions they could about everything. I must admit that I was prepared through all of my experience in America, to give and gain knowledge there.

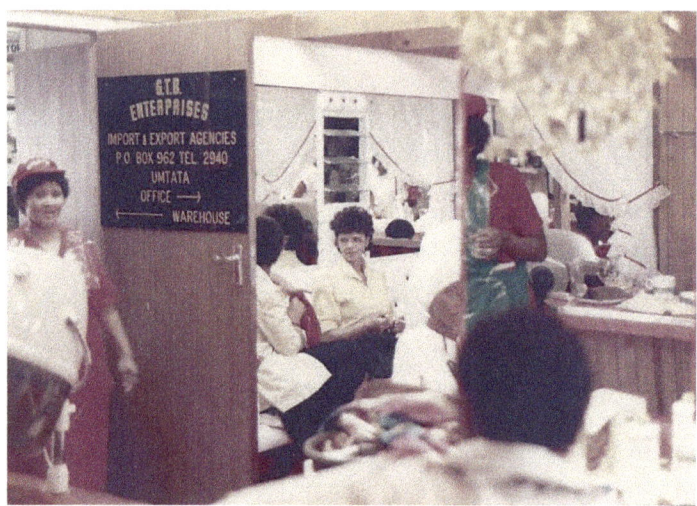

GTB Enterprise an import export Agency Company in the city of Umtata

One incident stays with me more than any other. As we were driving through the Transkei, our car caravan was stopped by men that looked and acted like military security. It turned out that these men were the security of Chief Mangosuthu Buthelezi, the President of the Inkatha Republic Party and the Chief Minister of KwaZulu tribe and it turned out that his son in-law Uhmsci was a tour representative for the sponsors of our trip. We were told that we were invited by the chief for an outing since we were traveling through his territory. The leaders of our team did not want to stop because it was a political concern for them, and it also would throw us off our schedule. We were told that we had to go because; the tradition was that when a head of State, or leader invited you they begin the ritual of slaughter of fresh stock of lamb for cooking. It is considered an insult not to show up. So we went. I for one was happy that we were going, because this would be an opportunity to ask questions if I could and hear from the chief how his people think. It was a great experience. We were told to tell Andrew Young and other leaders in America that their townships matter and that they will not be deprived of quality life under a government that will not recognize them. I was told by the chief that they would rather do for self than beg for the things that they were being denied.

As a former member of the Nation of Islam, I was familiar with that type of manifesto. However, I did see the difference in that in America the racial demographics are not the same. So, I was in agreement with Mr. Mandela and the ANC: one man, one vote position, which was the just and humane equal rights agenda that should be the rule of the land. However, I knew that my reason for being there was to get a hands on knowledge and understanding of what was really happing in South Africa that so few African Americans had the privy to see for themselves before me; so that upon my return to the States I could address it intelligently.

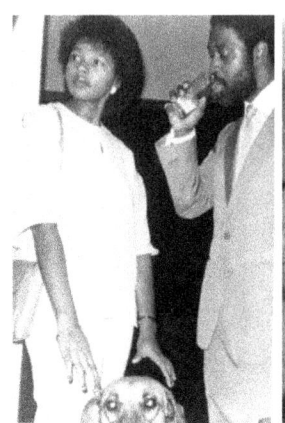

Royal Princes with the Inkata People

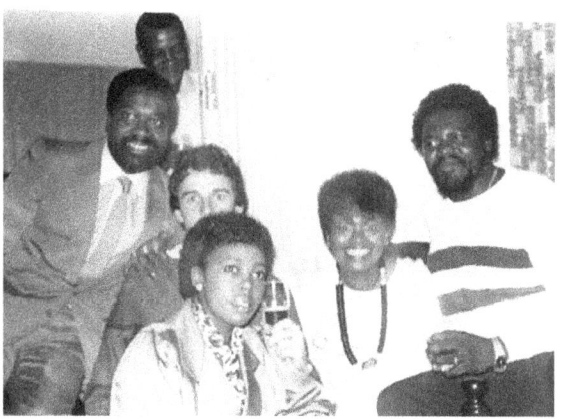

Me with my American associate second from right & Umtata representatives

I left South Africa being offered the opportunity to be in partnership with a group of investors, to open a chain of salons. As much as I wanted to do that, I was advised not to because of the anti-apartheid position of America, so I did not get involved.

Chapter Twelve

United Kingdom European Tour

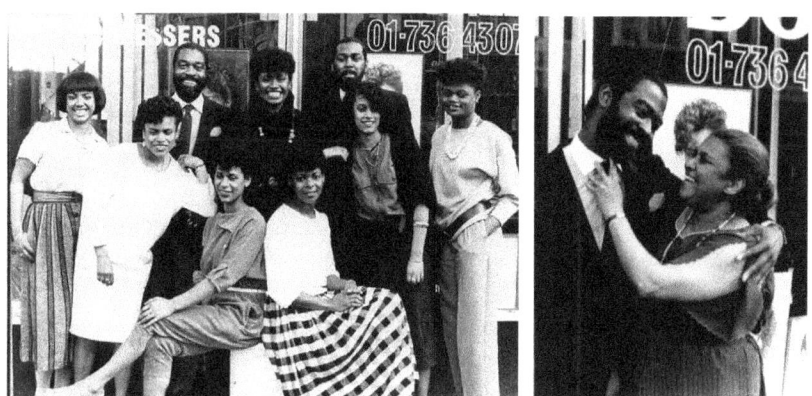

M & M International Team & UK Rep Mr. Ron Baker with models and UK salon owner on the right

London is the major city in England; it is an old but well-kept city. Most of the people of African descent are from the Caribbean or Africa, they are called Afro Caribbeans. There is a large hair and beauty market in London. Most of the stylists are very diverse in that white stylists do black hair as well as black stylists do white. Schools are not that important in England because there is a serious apprenticeship program in place. There was an American representative for M&M International LTD., Mr. Ron Baker, who I was working for in London. He took me throughout the United Kingdom, while giving classes along the way.

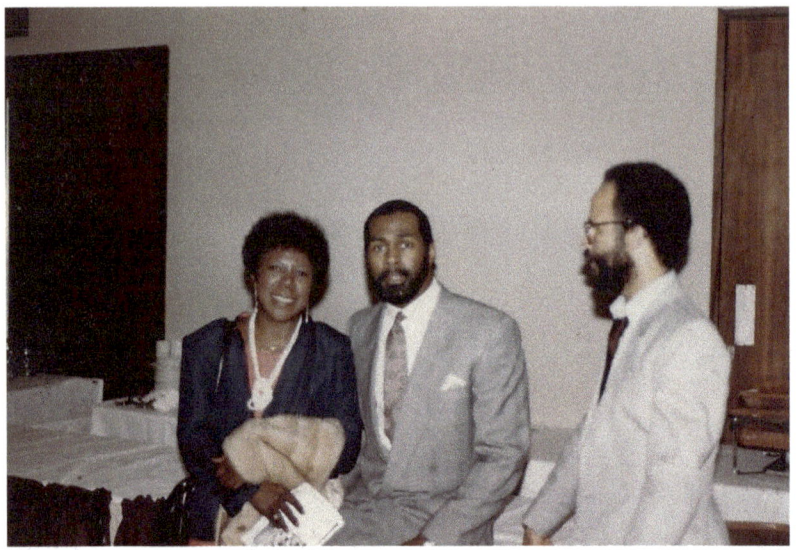
M&M International representative in the middle, Mr. Ron Baker

I met many friends in London and I lived well there. In the Caribbean, the dollar was sometimes as much as ten to one. In Africa, it was two to one, so I was surprised to find when I got to England that the dollar was forty-five cents to the United Kingdom's pound (dollar). I was published in the London news as a visiting hair artist on a three continent tour from America.

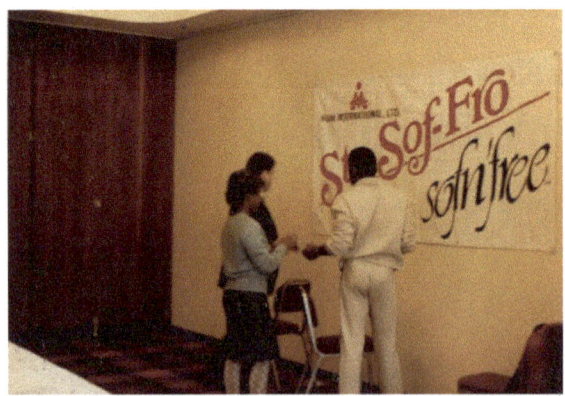
Presentation preparation in downtown London hotel

We taught at the department store salons and trained staff how to work with products and techniques. We traveled to Birmingham, which is more of a working class city with lots of industry. There were a lot of salons in Birmingham; it is a city that reminds you of Philadelphia. I traveled all over the city visiting salons. Americans do not come to Birmingham that often, so we got a lot of attention. I encountered my first racial incident on the tour, when some young white man felt he should tell me that I better be careful in the town because they don't like blacks from America that come to their clubs getting white women all hot and bothered. I can remember telling him that if he did not get out of my face as fast as he could I would beat the British out of his ass. I told him I was not one of your black boys from Birmingham, I am from America and where I come from we don't play that shit. He apologized and said he had too much to drink. He offered me one and explained why he came to me like that. It was, in his words, because whenever Americans came in town, the women would always run to them and most men in the city just don't like it. We agreed to understand each other and he got of my face.

We then went on to Manchester, which is a small hilly urban city; I gave classes at beauty schools and large salons, and then we went back to London.

I know that I was part of a great team of consultants that promoted advance hair and beauty care techniques, as well as programs and organizations that still exist, or are still in practice throughout Africa, Europe, and the Caribbean.

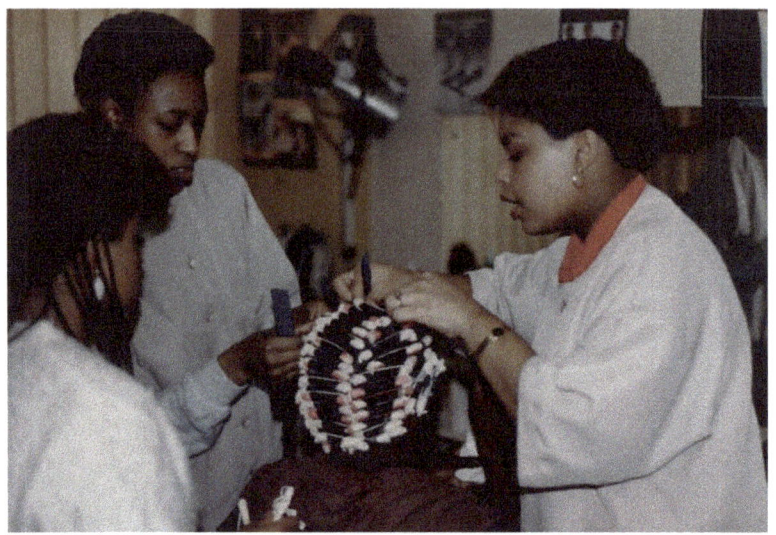

Student's in advance training class

That was a time when the wet curl products were very popular in America and many of the international countries in Europe that had sizeable populations of people of African descent to market the products. So it was in London, England and throughout the United Kingdom that we traveled and taught them how to use the products and how to make a profitable income in doing so. One of the things that I found interesting in the UK was that there were a large percentage of biracial services and salons. Clients felt comfortable with anyone who had the skill set for the services or who might have the money to pay for the skills by whoever their racial factor may have been.

We gave workshops in the major department stores' beauty salons in London where most of the tourists would go while in the city for services.

When we finished the touring and working all over England it came time to come wrap things up and to prepare to go back home in Atlanta, bringing with me a wealth of experience and new contacts that would become very useful later, on my return to London.

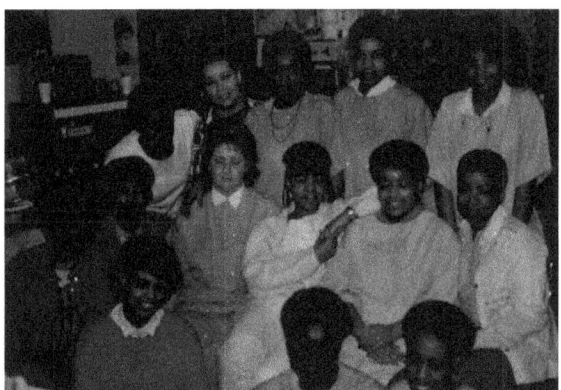

One of the many salon workshops that we did throughout the United Kingdom

All that time, traveling, as good as it was, and spending too much time away from my business and family, regretfully ruined my marriage and my business. Traveling through Europe, while on my three continent educational tour, I met friends in London that invited me to come there and try to make a go of it in England, since things were falling apart in the States. So I packed my tools and moved to London, England.

London was good to me, I met a lot of friends from all over the world. When I first moved there, I lived in an area that is called Stratham with my friend, until I was able to find an apartment in the Elephant Castle area. The Beauty School that I taught at was the Afro Caribbean School of Hair and Beauty in Brixton.

I also became acquainted with the business of freelance hair styling; through that service I met a lot of Britain's stars and celebrities. One of them was an elderly woman from America, called Lady Bea. She said she was married to one of the gentlemen in the royal family, and that is why she was commissioned as the house entertainment on the Queen Elizabeth II Royal cruise boats. Whenever she would go on a cruise, I would stay at her house and watch her property for her. Going to gatherings with Lady Bea, I was privileged to be seen in a prestigious circle of British performers, fashion designers/stylists, as well as hair stylists and makeup artists.

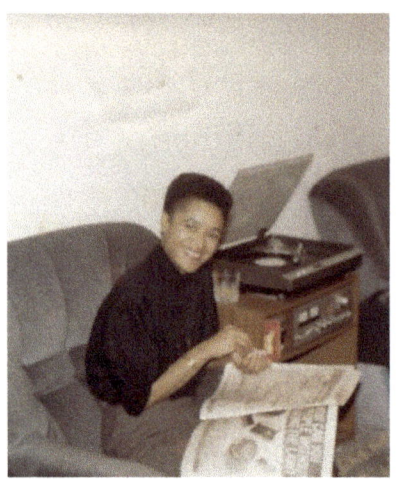 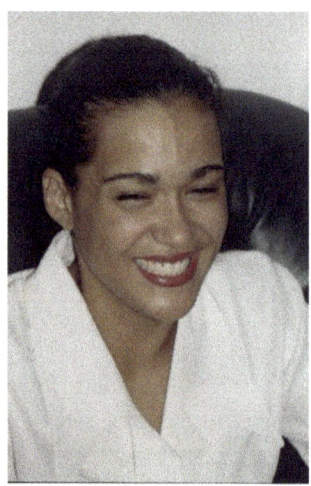

British Fashion Designer and friend in London, Ms. Juliet Callarvlo and her sister.

I also had an opportunity to network the fashion industries, whereby I was one of the hair stylists at the British fall winter Fashion release, on the Kings Row Palace ground. There I met a young designer, and artist that showed me the artistic sides of England. Juliet lived in West Kensington, which, after meeting her, I found myself going to more than anywhere else. She was more than a friend; she was my confidant, someone to help me through my pains of separation and divorce. She did a marvelous job and I will always love her for that.

The first year was filled with excitement, it was good therapy for me at the time because I had just gone through a tough separation and the change was needed. The thing that reminds me of the thrill of London was when I met this African Nigerian man and Caucasian French woman who turned out to be under his command.

We met through a friend of mine. I was surprised to discover that he was a Left Lieutenant in the secret force. It was strange to me because I liked them both as running partners. With them I found myself in all kinds of strange places. I became a regular at the Nigerian Embassy; I can remember us driving in this Citron car that was totally wired with telic- communication devices; the car was wired to the police band radio system. I saw a lot from those experiences.

But when I found out that they were there to warn me, I started feeling blessed, so I decided to go along for the ride. I was told that Americans were on high alert because President Regan had just bombed Libya, and Americans in Europe were targets for retaliation. The one thing that caused so many concerns and brought attention to me, I believe, was the fact that my name is a Muslim name, and because I was a former Minister in the Nation of Islam. We know, from the history of Malcolm X, that the federal government has secret files on people that were members of the government's unapproved or sanctioned organizations. I felt someone had pulled my file and I was on a terrorist watch list, so it was time to go home or back to America.

Chapter Thirteen

Back To America

At the time, I was in communication with a man whom I had done business with before I left for England. He owned a hair chemical company and was in need of someone to run his ethnic division; so I recommended a friend that somehow did not work out for him. He offered me an opportunity to come back to the States and direct a division of his hair chemical company in Elk Grove Village Illinois; so I took it on. The one thing I got out of working for Denna Corporation was that I began to realize that I was a practitioner/artist and not an administrator, so the job did not work out for me. I found myself wanting to do what I was comfortable with, which was doing hair.

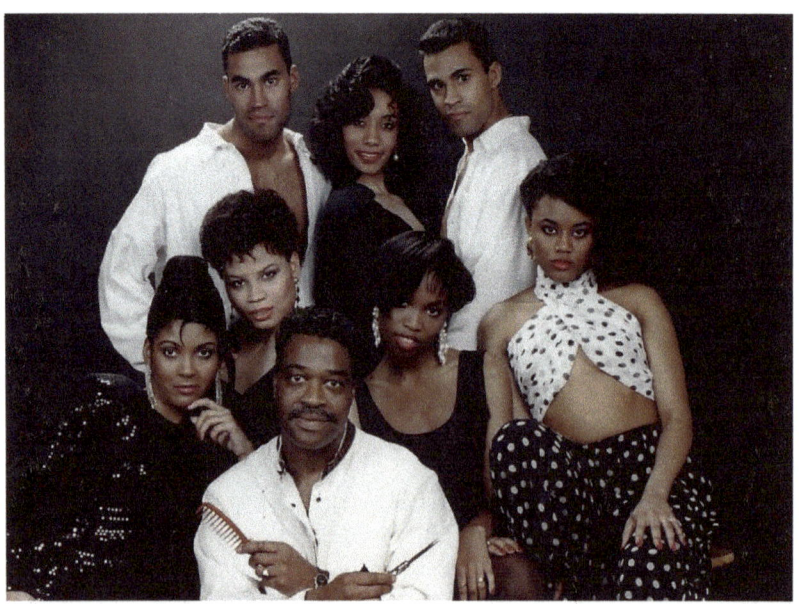

One of many Photo Shoots with different professional photo agents and photographers

In 1987, coming back to Illinois was a joy; on one hand being around my children again, also being around an associate of mine that owned a Beauty salon. She wanted me to work in her place as a stylist. I accepted and in a short time was doing the hair of the City of Chicago Mayor Harold Washington's girlfriend Ms. Mary Ellen Smith at Shur Le Salon in Bolingbrook IL. That network provided me a lot of opportunities and fun, I also began to travel and teach as a beauty consultant, again in the domestic beauty market.

The first company that I worked for when I got back was Deena Corporation in Elk Grove Village; I was the Director of the Ethnic Division. From there I worked for Shur Le Distributorship in Bolingbrook, - Johnson Products - Chicago, Elent'e Viatle Corporation – Chicago, McBride Lab- Atlanta, Carson Products - Savannah Georgia, Supreme Products - Chicago, Revlon - New York, Roux Lab - Jacksonville Florida, L'Oréal -New York, Clairol - New York, and M & M Products – Atlanta, Georgia. My commercial credits include ad campaigns for Fashion Fair, Isoplus, Duke Men's Products, Shades of You Hosiery, and Ebone Cosmetics. My editorial coverage was Rapp Pages, Working Mother, Essence, Ebony, Bride's Today, Shoptalk, Upscale, EM, Jet, and Black Elegance.

The Miss Black America Pageant, Hair Styles Director

Coming back to America from Europe was a very rewarding experience for me, in that I felt I was bringing back some new European cultures that I knew were unique during that time. The first job I had been at a chemical company by the name of Dena Corporation, where I was their Global ambassador. Things went well there but I really wanted to do some mainstream salon services again, so when my friend that I knew, who lived near the plant in Elk Grove Village ask me to come to partner with her business, Shurle's Salon in Bolingbrook, I accepted the invitation.

It was at Shurle's Salon that I was asked by Ms. Jo Green, the producer of the Miss Black Illinois & Miss Black Chicago pageant, which was part of the Miss Black America pageant, if I would be the official hairstylist for the productions. I agreed and that was the beginning of a very interesting connection in American history.

For four years I was the official hair stylist of the Miss Black America Beauty pageant in Indianapolis Indiana, until Mike Tyson was accused and convicted of raping one of the contestants, Ms. Desire Washington. After that the, pageant could not get the respect of the public's support to keep it going; but my sons, and my hair crew had a great time over those years traveling to different locations for those pageants.

Working in the pageant I felt honored to help those young beautiful women feel good about their chances to be crowned Miss Black America and to, in some cases, be their guardian from the public when we were out on location doing photo shoots for the pageant's marketing presentation.

I remember the day that Mike Tyson came to visit the girls. He looked as though he was a child in a candy store as he watched those beautiful young women lined up in bathing suits in the lobby of the hotel that we all stayed in. Later that day Mike invited a group of the girls to a music concert featuring Johnny Gill. History was made after that venture and it was not a good one for Mike or the Miss Black America pageant. I walked away from that experience with a very close friendship with Cynthia and was a part of maintaining her personal and public image. Cynthia also was a third degree black belt martial artist instructor at the time of her entry into the pageant; in fact, part of her talent exhibition was a marital art demonstration. I learned to love Cynthia because she was a very beautiful woman with a fierce character of confidence.

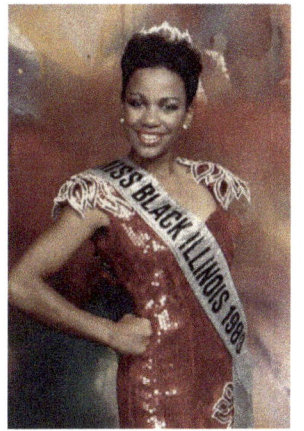 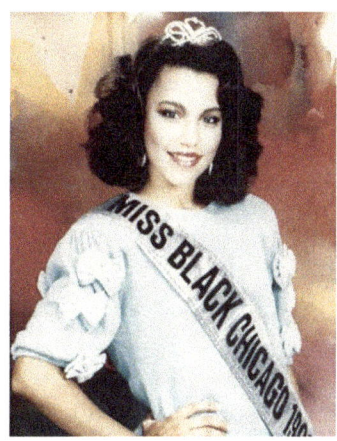

1989 Miss Black America's Pageant Queens: Miss Black Illinois Ms. Cynthia Thompson & Miss Black Chicago Ms. Melanie Martin

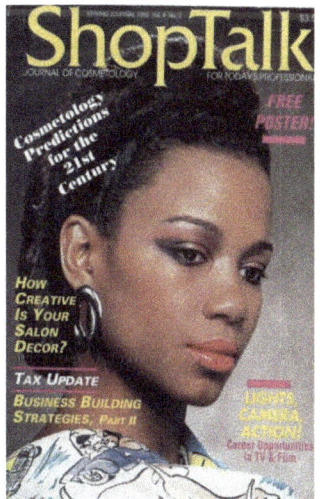 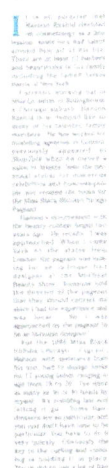 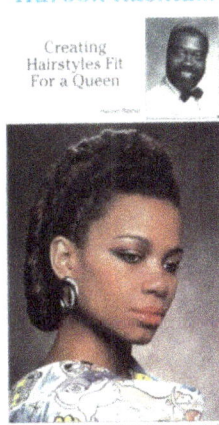

Cover for Shoptalk Magazine and a story on my hair and image consultant services

MY CULTURAL BIRTH RIGHTS

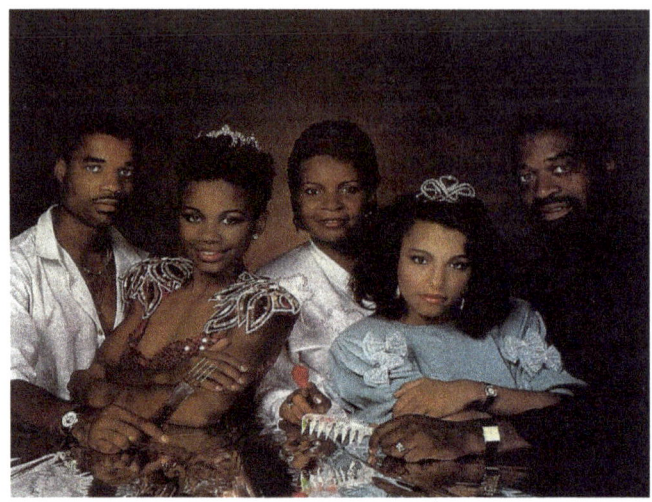

Haroon Rashid on the far right his son Aaron Rashid on the left Hair designers for the Miss Black America Pageant; in the middle is Lavinda Wilson Makeup artist with 1989 Miss Black America & Miss Black Illinois Cynthia Thompson and Melanie Martin left to right. Crown Queens.

While living, and working in the suburbs of Chicago, one thing that bothered me the most about Chicago was the response of the people after the death of Harold Washington. The African American community started fighting among themselves to the points that no one of color felt entitled to govern the city. That bothered me for a long time, until one day while taking my friend Juliet from London on a tour we stopped at the Du Sable Museum. Somehow I made a connection with his life and legacy, and have been talking to others about this man ever since.

To compare his great accomplishments in the city, being educated in France, he was so intelligent; being of French European descent from his father and African Haitian decent from his mother; and marrying and having children by a Native American woman, set the tone for a multi-cultural tolerant man, Leader, Businessman, and Founder of the city of Chicago. I realized then and now that the only race in the city that Mr. Du

Sable founded is the Human race and that legacy of diversity, sovereignty and human rights should be the theme and motto of Chicago.

I finally moved back to Chicago to work in one of the most elegant salons in the city; it was called Van Cleef Salon. I was very proud to work in that place, it was formerly a church that had been modernized and was owned and operated by a man that I will always admire, Michael Flowers (Rhani). He is a man that has great work habits and is a hard working dedicated professional.

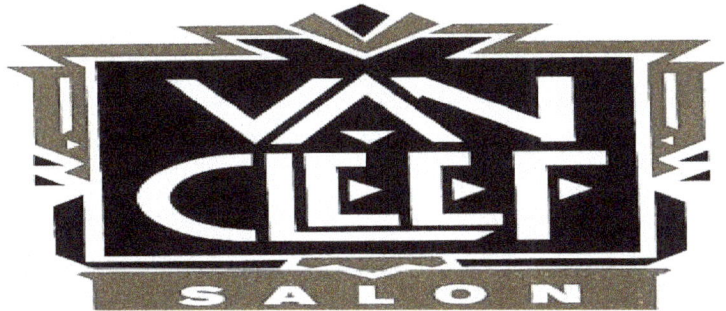

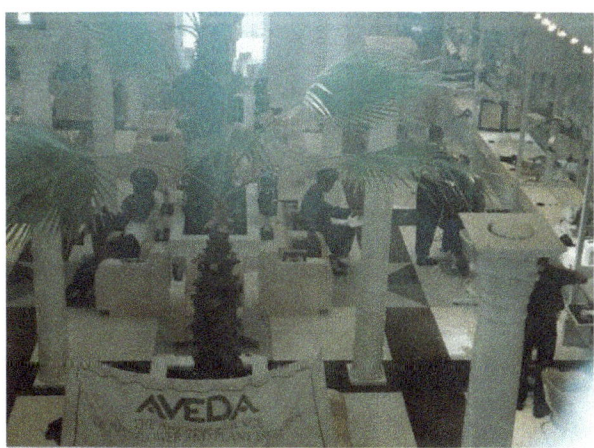

Upper level veiw inside the historical salon that 1st African American First Lady of the United States and her family were coming for services in Chicago - Van Cleef Salon

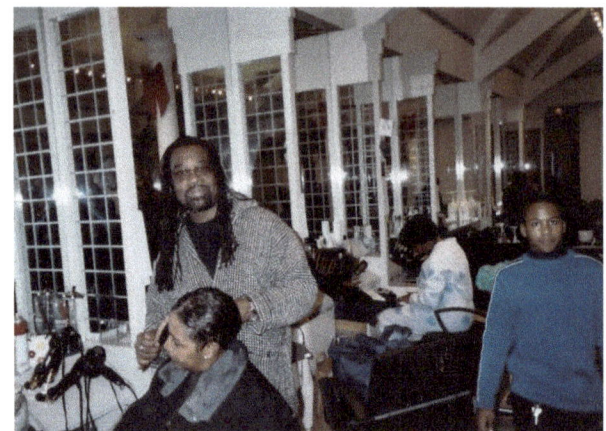
Happy days at Van Cleef Salon

While at Van Cleef Salon I also became a member of the Chicago Cosmetology Board, and was an advance cosmetology educator in Chicago. At Van Cleef I began to build my elite clientele in Chicago: Joan Johnson the CEO of Johnson products; Alison Payne, WGN news; Jonathan Rogers, President of Discovery Channel; Muriel Claire, News reporter - WGN news, Pete Myers - Chicago Bulls, John Mod - Radio broadcaster (V103); Sonja Gant, TV anchor, morning show (WGN news); and Don Lemon, CNN News broadcaster.

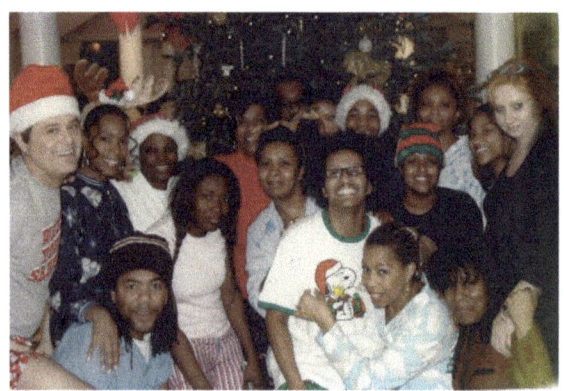
Van Cleef Staff Xmas Celebration

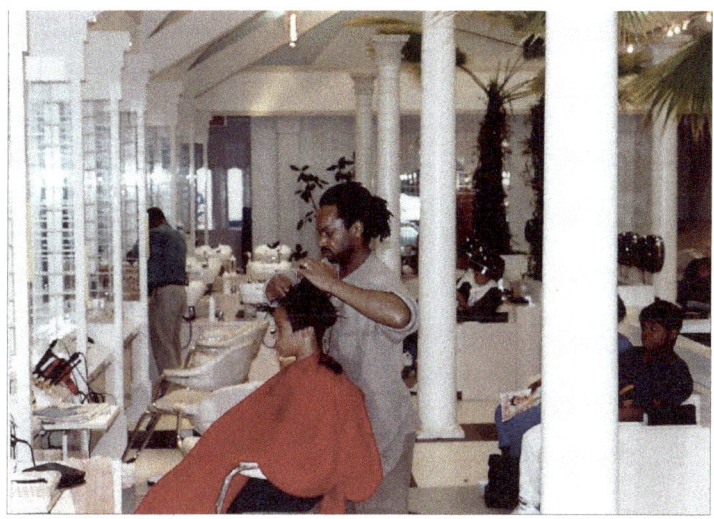

The inside of Van Cleef Salon with a view next to my work station

I did not know what it was that still bothered me about Chicago, until one day while I was working in the salon cutting a man's hair when I heard a loud sound, and felt a warm feeling on the back of my leg. Everybody was screaming and when I tried to move I realized that I had been shot. I had been through some rough situations before coming to Chicago, but never this completely violated. At first, naturally I was scared, but then when I put together what had happened to me I got angry, and bitter. I was first angry at the thought someone cowardly took their insecurities out on me without dialogue because, to this day, no one has come forward and explained to me why they would do such a cowardly thing to me. But then, a more sinister thing happened, the media gave their interpretation of a jealous lover dispute. I watched some of my so-called loyal clients and some fellow employees, and opposed to showing concern about my welfare as a victim, they seemed to agree with the criminal's rational. That act of inhumanity by all that was involved put a scar on my heart because my comfortable beautiful environment had been destroyed.

Not everybody was like that; Rhani and his family showed me love. I remember one day one of Rhani's clients came to me, she was a TV Celebrity. She took me to the back room and held me; and then she told me she knew the pain that I was experiencing because she too had been a victim of the same kind of violence. She was shot in the head and left for dead, but of course she survived and she makes it a point to reach out to fellow victims. She said because no one knows how it feels to go through that kind of violation, and drama but a victim. I will always have nothing but respect and love for the compassion given to me by these special people.

My spirit for Chicago was being challenged, and then I met a young lady name Jada Goodlett. It was Jada who convinced me that if I would go to the Million Man March that she wanted to go and would help plan the trip with me. I agreed but told her that I would go with my guys and she would have to go separately so that we did not get distracted from our purpose. She agreed and made the journey in support of us. I really respected and loved her for that.

For me, that trip was more than an historical event; it was a sign of unity among black men to America and the world. It also was a spirit that the men and women who attended it empowered themselves to take on the responsibility of leaderships for change in their lives. It was so great being among that body of people; words will never explain the pride that I felt that day as a black man, when I watched men with tears of joy and sorrow in their eyes while we hugged each other before departing from Washington D.C. at the famous Washington Mall.

The Million Man March

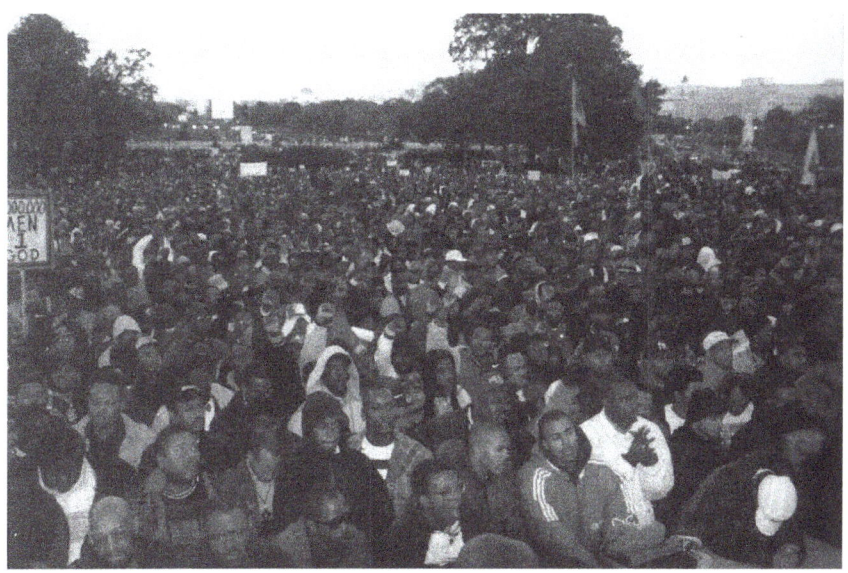

Haroon Rashid, in the center 4 rows up was 1 in a million at the Million Man March

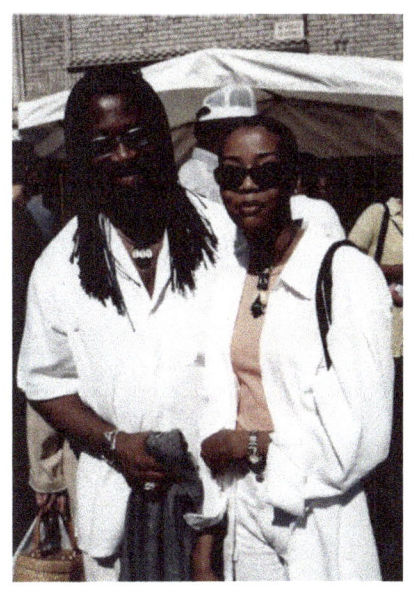

Jada, My Fountain of Youth

She was an ambitious, daring, and culturally exciting young person. I had such a need at that time for a good change; I fell in love with her. I met her doing her hair. We started to talk with each other and ten years later we were still talking to each other and seeing each other every day. So again, it was there at Van Cleef Salon that I went on the famous Million Man March, as well as meeting my fountain of youth Jada Goodlett. Going on that March was such a great experience. One of the staff members gave my son Hakeem, the desk manager at Van Cleef Steve and myself each a Million Man March tee shirt as a gesture of support for our drive to Washington D.C.

Jada moved to New York after that to attend the Fashion Institute of Technology. I felt the need to get away to be with her; I missed her so much. I also felt the need to get away from Chicago where my spirit had been damaged and I also wanted to be closer to my family and loved ones in Boston, and New York.

Chapter Fourteen

When I Moved To New York

While living in New York Jada helped keep me on the fashion trend, because she was a student at F.I.T, and New York is so culturally diverse that I began to see a difference in Chicago style. To me, it was almost like being in London again with the art and fashion industry; she became, as Juliet was my confidant, guide, and loved one. My first job in New York was at Naomi Sims Salon on 57th Street & 6th Ave., right across the street from the Motown Café, where I would go to lunch sometimes and watch the Motown review performers.

It was a quaint and pretty salon, and since my cousin James Harris designed and opened the salon for the fashion Model Naomi Sims, and one of our longtime friends from Boston, Rudy Townsel managed it, that even though James was not working in the salon I felt welcomed.

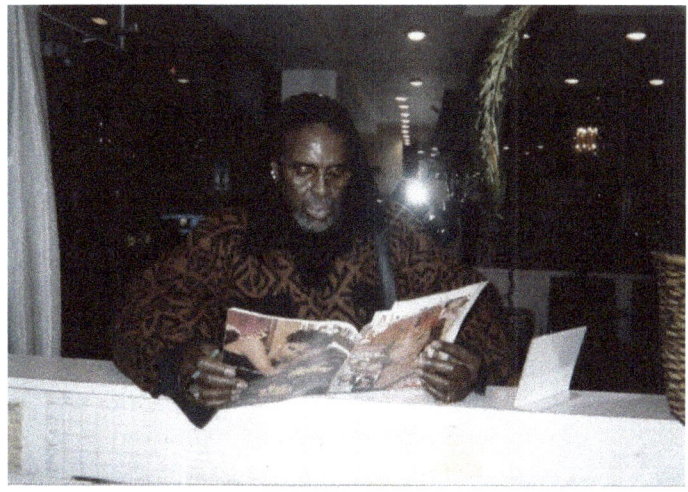

Naomi Simms salon manger Rudy Townsel

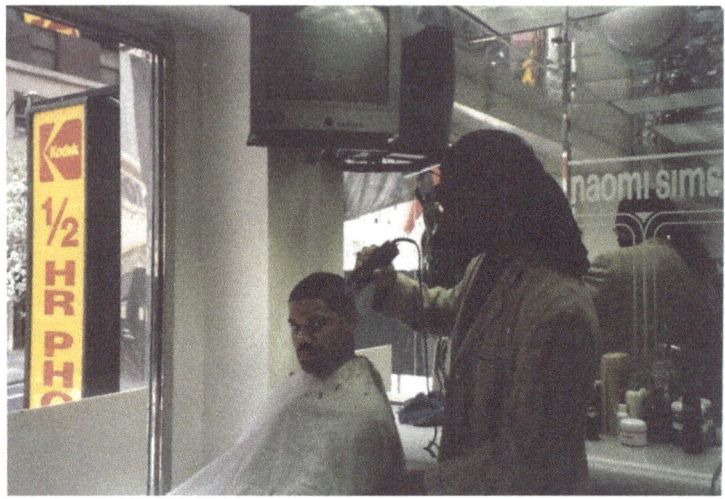
Cutting my Son Hakeem's hair at Naomi Simms Salon

Based on my previous salon experience and high end clientele in Chicago, I knew that I would have a hard time developing the type of business that I felt capable of in New York at the Naomi Simms salon. That being said, I started looking around for other opportunities that I felt would be in my favor.

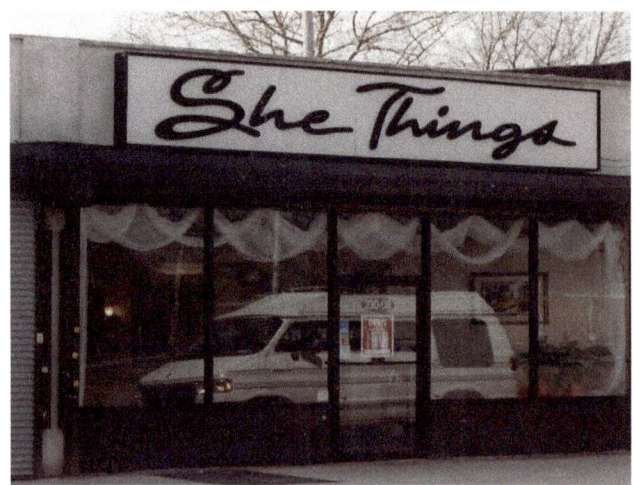
Outer exterior entrance of the She Things Salon in Queens New York

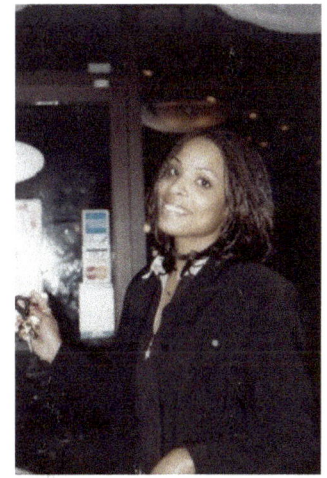 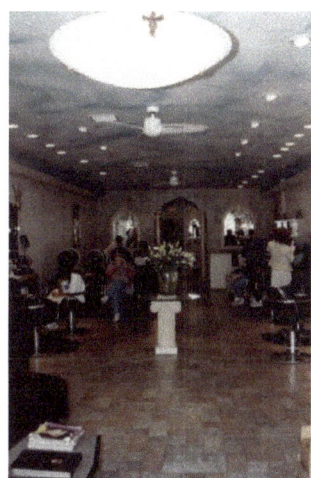

Spinderella: of Salt-N-Pepa, on the inside of her salon at "She Things"

I was still traveling back and forth from New York to Chicago every other weekend when I found out that Deidra Roper (Spinderella), of the hip hop group Salt-N-Pepa had opened up a salon called She Thing in Queens, and she needed a styles director. So with as many ideas that I had at the time for my vision of the new salon trends, I felt the need to be in a position to do it; so I took the job as the Styles Director at She Things.

The one thing that I found troublesome about She Thing was its location:

A - It was in the Boroughs of Queens. B - It was located on an industrial frontage road facing the expressway.

It was unlike the salons that I was accustomed to in Manhattan, and that I believed the upscale clientele she was attracting to her was used too. We talked about the idea of a shuttle service to escort the clientele to her spa salon but I believed that she and some of the staff were beginning to settle for the isolated location, as a matter of fact; and I just did not see it that way.

Deidra did not have a hand on type position in the salon; she left those responsibilities to her sister who was the salon manager, and I believed like most new ventures it was perceived that the business would develop and take off with time. I was always taught that in an upstart business, the number one rule for success is the location, regardless to who or how much you put into it. However, I tried to make a go of it in suggesting incorporating the concepts of a more spa like salon; but things did not work out as I thought they would for me in Queens, so I left and finally found a place that I thought was a better fit for me in uptown Manhattan.

The Gazelle Day Spa

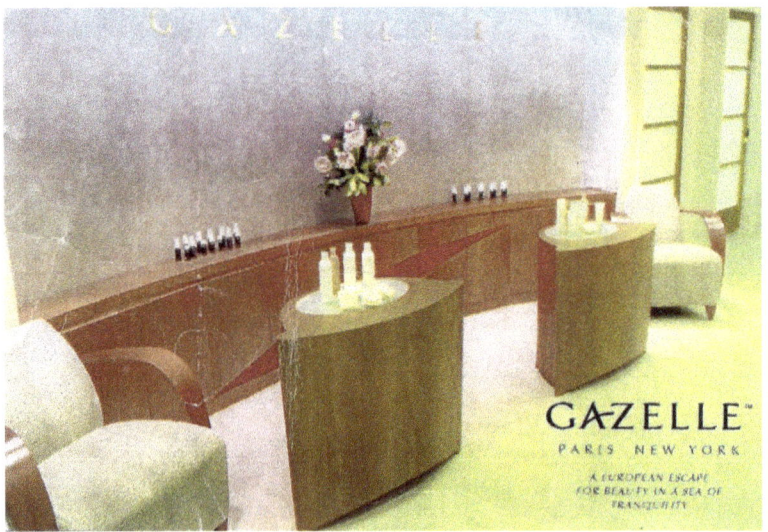

The Gazelle Day Spa interior

The Gazelle Day Spa was in class by itself; a modern décor, professionally run first class environment; the actual salon was a private room within the spa. We had two-hair specialists and we specialized in hair care treatments; it was there that I learn about the usage of natural herbs, oil, and tinctures.

It was a full day spa, owned and operated by Ms. Patricia French an African American woman that had lived in Paris, France for years and had created a product line that was marketed for the international market in Africa and Europe for women of color called Gazelle cosmetics.

She brought her products to New York City and created a flagship Spa to promote and distribute them. It was the first of its kind that was meant to attracting the high-end clients of color by catering to total spa services. Gazelle catered to most of the celebrities in New York or international tourists searching for the services that we offered. It offered full whirlpool Saunas, Steam rooms, Massage and Facials, Make up and Manicure/Pedicure rooms. It had a full lounge with personal Gazelle labels on champagne and wines. Individual serving of foods and beverages: each client was given gowns and toiletries for showers with individual wall lockers for changes. We offered special Herbal hair and body treatments. It was there that I also met many of New York's celebrities and leaders.

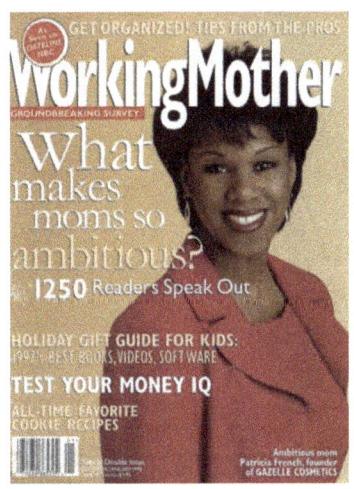

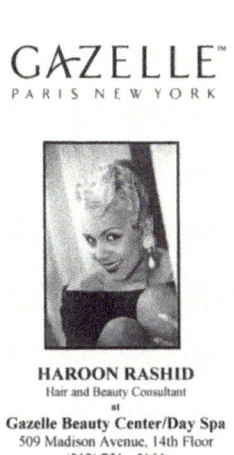

HAROON RASHID
Hair and Beauty Consultant
at
Gazelle Beauty Center/Day Spa
509 Madison Avenue, 14th Floor
(212) 751 - 5144

Ms. Patricia French, Founder of Gazelle Cosmetics & Gazelle Beauty Center & Day Spa in Midtown Manhattan

The Crown & Glory Salon

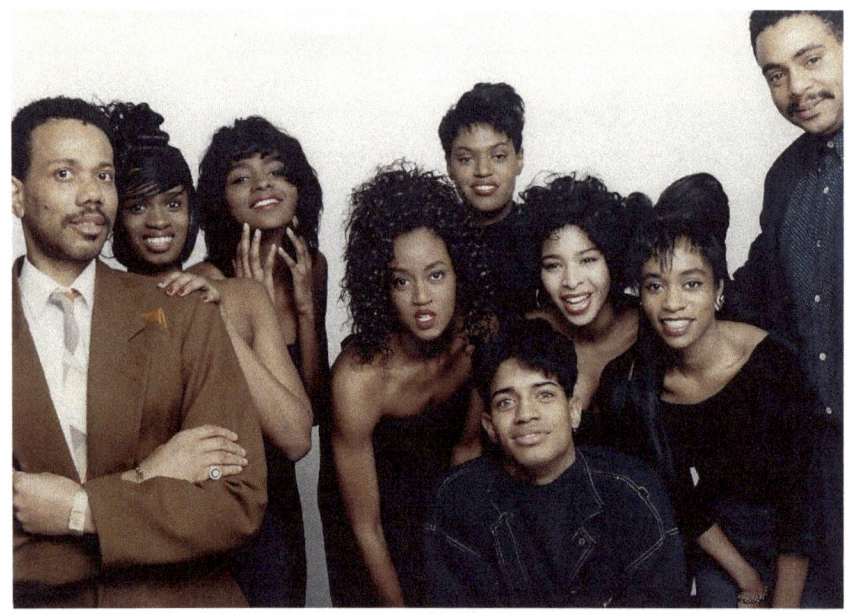

On the left is Richard Green owner of the Crown and Glory Salon in upper Manhattan and staff at a Photo Shoot

I was also working in a salon in midtown Manhattan Called Crown and Glory; this salon belongs to a good friend of mine, Richard Green. In his salon everyone had an agent, and was doing some kind of commercial work. My agent Ken Barboza had three of us working in Richard's salon; it was a fun place to be. One of the best assignments that I had with Ken was working at the New York Fashion release called "Fashion on Seventh" doing the hair of the leading top models in the country. The Mahogany Door also was a place that the top hair stylists, makeup artists, models, celebrities and actors came to for services.

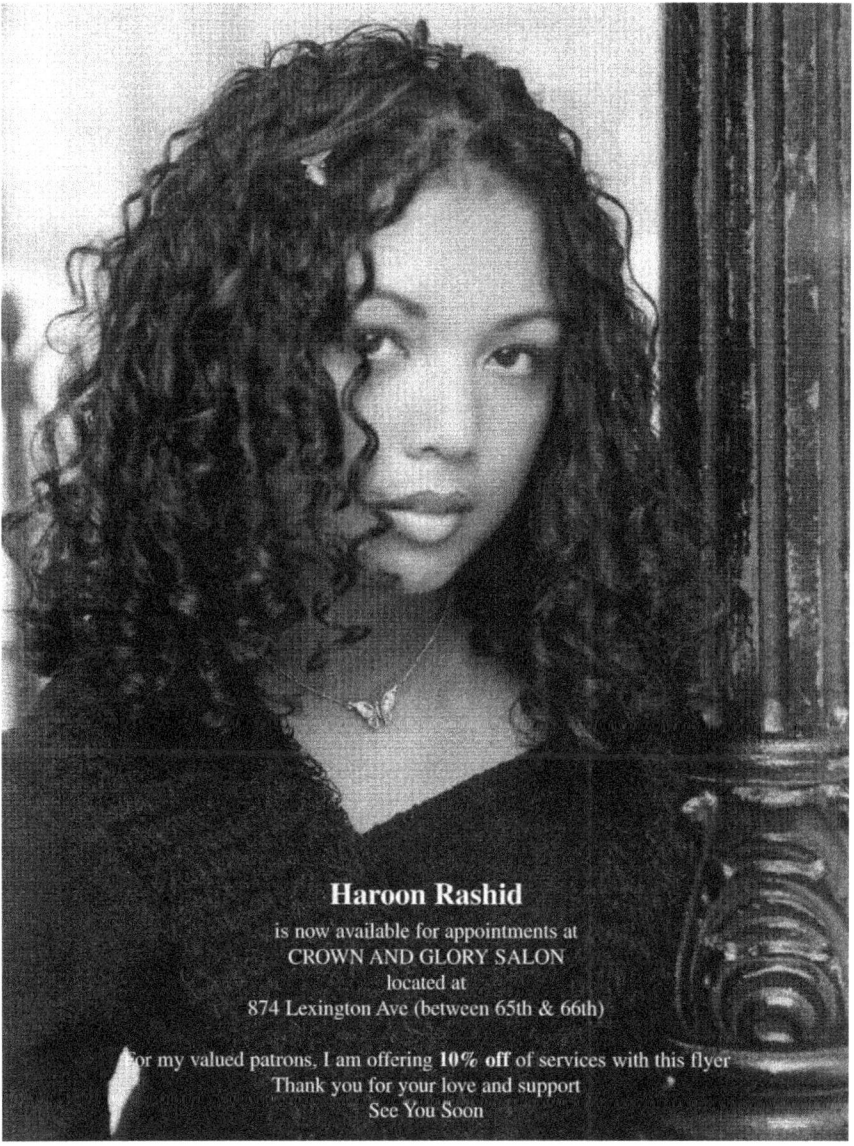

Crown and Glory marketing advertisement for me

But when my cousin James opened his Salon in Harlem, the Mahogany Door, I felt the need to support my family and move on. I was still going back and forth to Crown and Glory, part time, as I had clients that preferred the midtown versus uptown Manhattan location and I was still working with Ken Barboza's agency from that salon. It was mostly because Richard and I were good friends and I did not feel comfortable leaving him in a negative way, which worked out fine, until it became too complicated to manage the two clienteles back and forth. That is when I decided to make the total move to the Mahogany Door Salon in Harlem.

The Mahogany Door

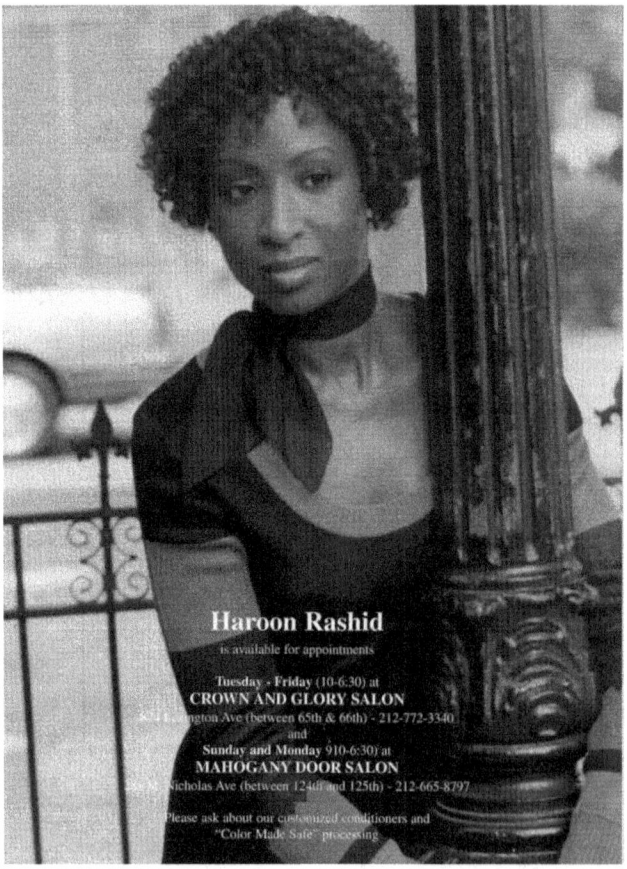

Crown and Glory & the Mahogany Door marketing advertisement

At any given time, the top stylists in New York might come to work at Mahogany Door for a day, week, or a month, just to be exposed to the environment, and techniques of James Harris in his salon. The clients that Mahogany Door was attracting were the elite entertainers of New York. From the Apollo Theater in Harlem to the Broadway theaters in Midtown Manhattan the salon was attracting actors, musicians and sports stars. Recording executives from Motown International, Kadar records and many more frequently visited the salon. Ms. Audrey Smaltz, Executive Director of the Ground Crew fashion consultants not only was a client of James Harris and the Mahogany Door, but she hired out many of the Mahogany Door staff for the New York City Fashion on Seven international seasonal Fashion Trend release events.

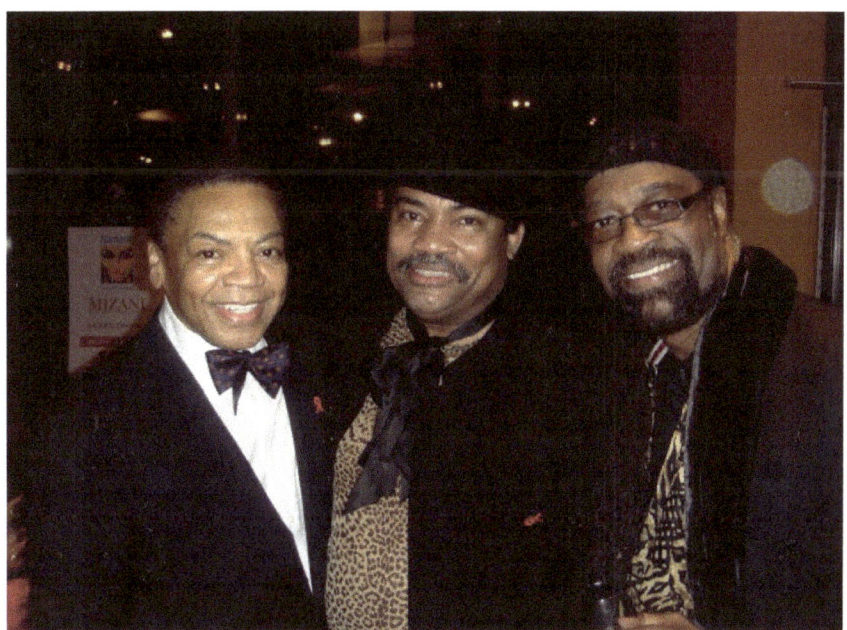

Oprah Winfrey makeup artist Mr. Reggie Wells, Mr. James Harris & Haroon Rashid

MY CULTURAL BIRTH RIGHTS

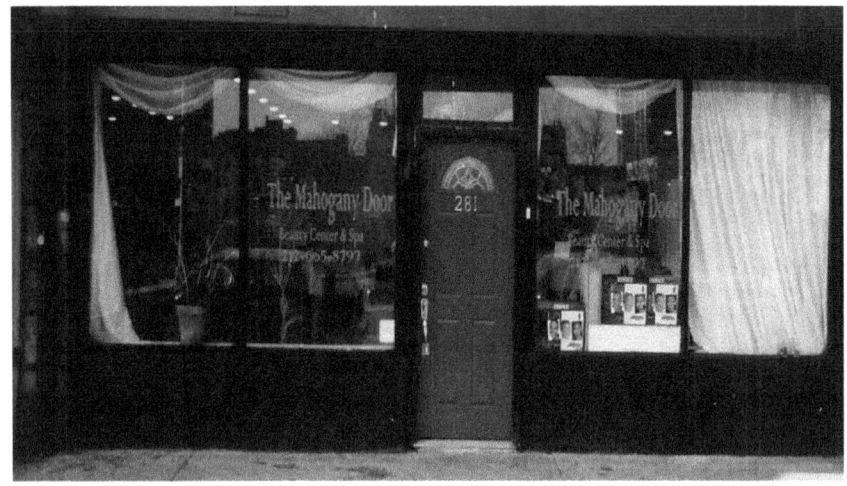

Mahogany Door was the pride of Harlem on 124 Street and Saint Nicholas Avenue.

James Harris, the owner, had the ambition to create an upscale salon in the heart of Harlem that would give the sense of pride to people of color in Harlem. I was always a fan of Harlem and the history of the Harlem Renascence that was financed by the late Great Madam C.J. Walker. She was the single person that made the beauty industry global with her hair and fashion shows in Harlem. Not to overlook the roots of the Apollo Theater that is indebted to her known works with the likes of Langston Hughes, whom she had financed, and many more in the spirit of African American edutainment. It seemed easy to feel the energy of ancestral cultural roots in the Harlem community.

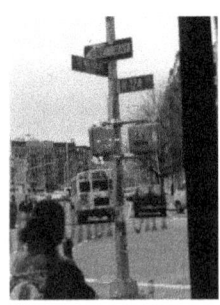
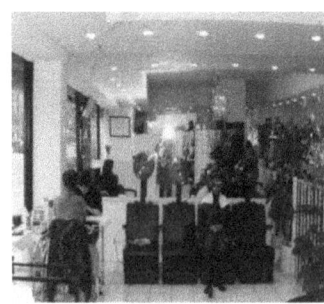

124th Street at ST. Nicholas & Inside the Mahogany Door salon

The interior of the salon was well lit with full length mirrored walls throughout the salon. There were chandeliers in every ceiling throughout the salon and, like the Gazelle day spa, there was Champaign and beverages served to the clients. The Mahogany Door was also the salon that was frequently contracted to do or provide operators to do professional photo shoots. Regardless, if they were for magazines or hair and beauty marketing industries, we were very busy in the salon or on assignments on location.

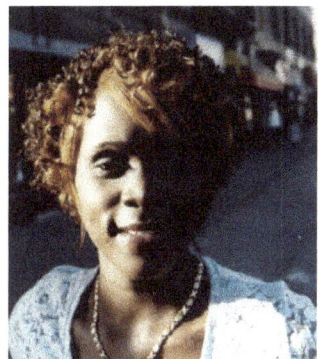 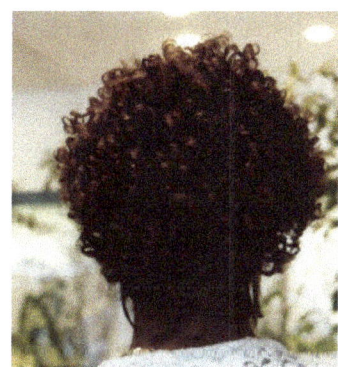

Photo Shoot on Texture Curls for Black Hair & Beauty Magazine at the Mahogany Door Salon

This was a photo shoot for multi-texture multi-color soft curls hair styles for women of color, which was very popular at the time in New York. I had built a reputation for those type services and I had a large clientele that was in demand of the styles.

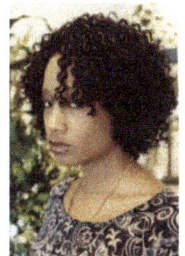 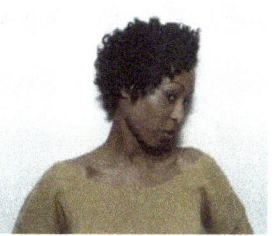

Photo Shoot on Texture Curls for Black Hair & Beauty Magazine at the Mahogany Door Salon

In the late nineties, we were experimenting with soft texture looks on natural hair, especially among the female actors who had found our services to be helpful because of the many hair changes that their hair was required to make adjustments to. We were also contracted to do casting productions for multi-diverse clients of all persuasions.

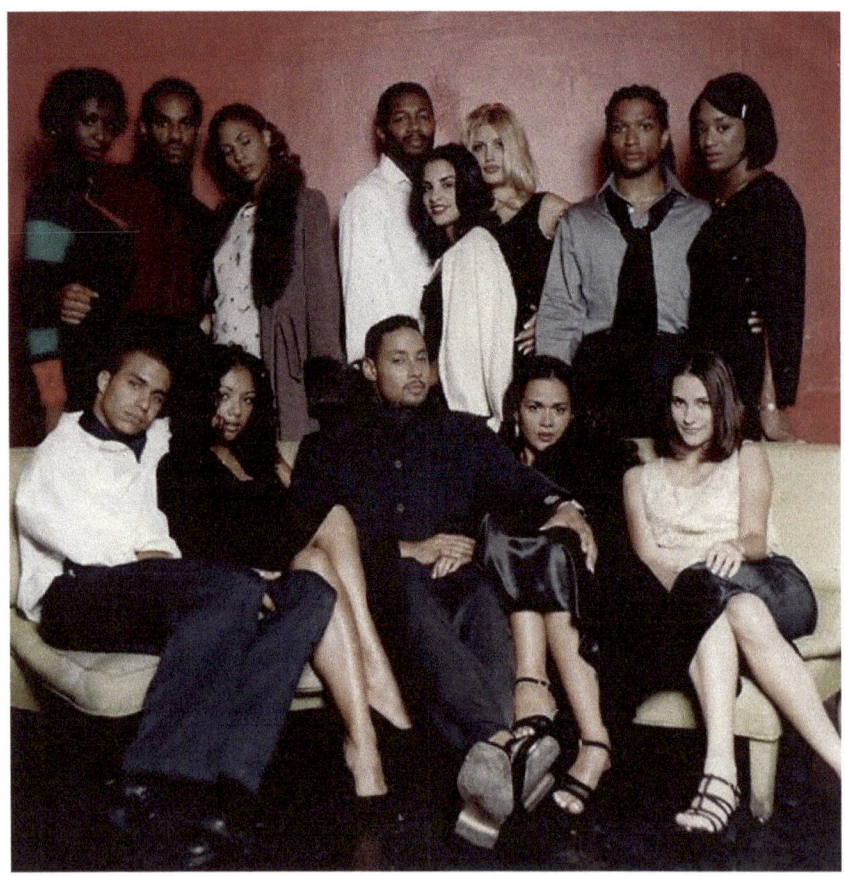

Hair Photo Shoot group shot was taken while at the Mahogany Door

This photo shot was taken in a Brooklyn New York at a night club for commercial advertisement uses.

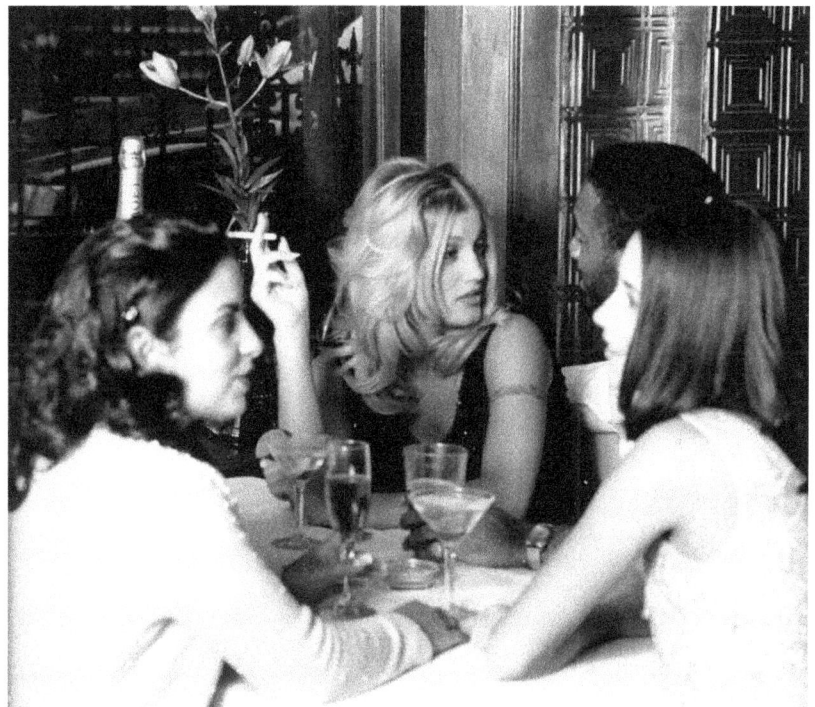

Hair Photo Shoot group shot while at the Mahogany Door

1998 the Mahogany Door Salon produced a fashion show called "A **Night in Harlem**" it brought the stars out to Harlem and was the talk of upper Manhattan. From musical great Roy Ayers as the musical entertainment to Audrey Smaltz as the fashion show narrator.

Immediately after the show, all was well until my sons and daughter opened Visionaries, Day Spa in Chicago. They asked me to come back to Chicago, and help them run it. At that time, I did not want to go back to Chicago. I was enjoying New York way too much, but I thought it was the right thing to do, so I went back. I told Jada that I was going back to Chicago and after I got things set up I would send for her to join me. She really did not want to come back to Chicago; in fact, when I got situated and it was time for her to come be with me, I had to go get her and reason with her against her desires to come back to Chicago.

Chapter Fifteen

The Visionaries Day Spa In Chicago

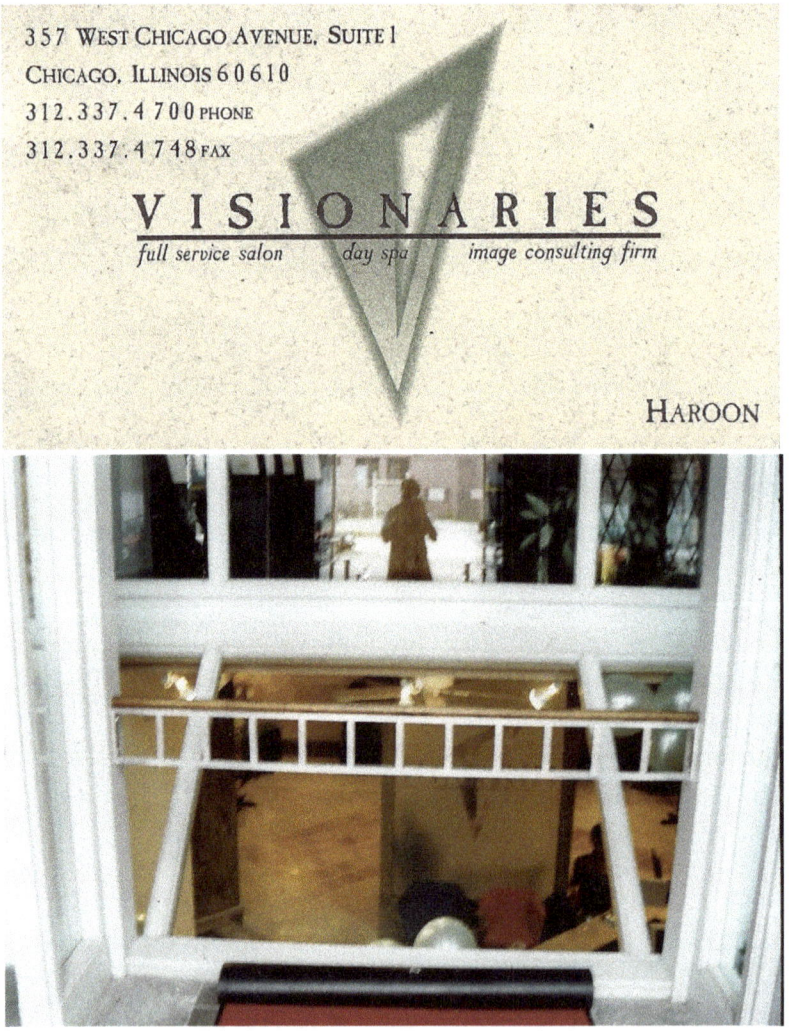

Visionary Day Spa upper view entrance into the salon

When I came back to Chicago I came with a critical eye on style, fashion and social cultural divide in Chicago. I did not know that this dissatisfaction would lead me one day to what I discovered the missing legacy and well-kept secret of Mr. Jean Baptiste Pointe DuSable. From that moment I made the connection of greatness in this man, and the more I saw how much potential the City of Chicago could have, especially for people of African descent, under right guidance. I felt God gave me a new spirit to renew the life, history, and legacy of my ancestor and mentor, as well as give me a new sense of purpose.

At first, Jada and I hated coming back to Chicago and leaving the flavor of New York. We decided that we were going to find a way to bring some of the diverse spirit of New York to Chicago. That attitude kept us going back and forth to New York and looking for a network in Chicago to build on.

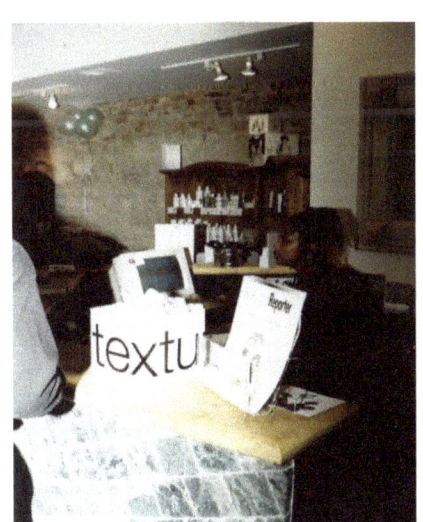 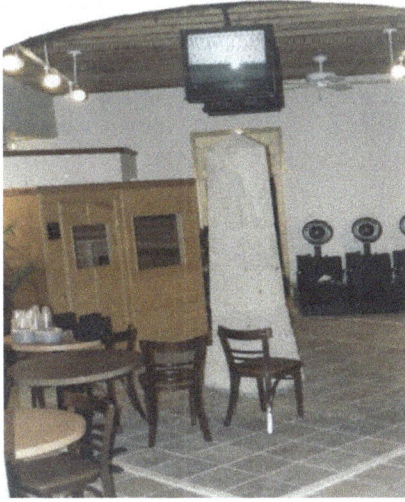

Visionary Spa front desk area and rear Sauna Massage room and lounge

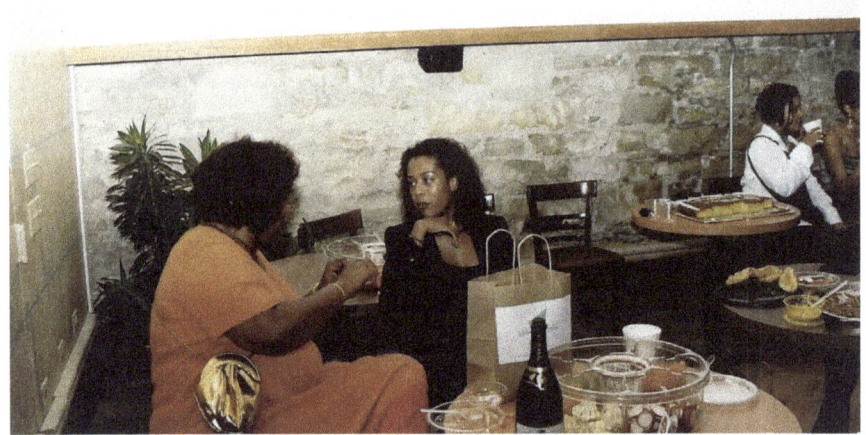

Jada networking at Visionary Spa in the lounge area

We soon settled in and started looking for ways to make sense of our return back to the city of Chicago that I left to live in New York, because of the spirit of violence and the tolerance by Chicagoans to normalize that behavior.

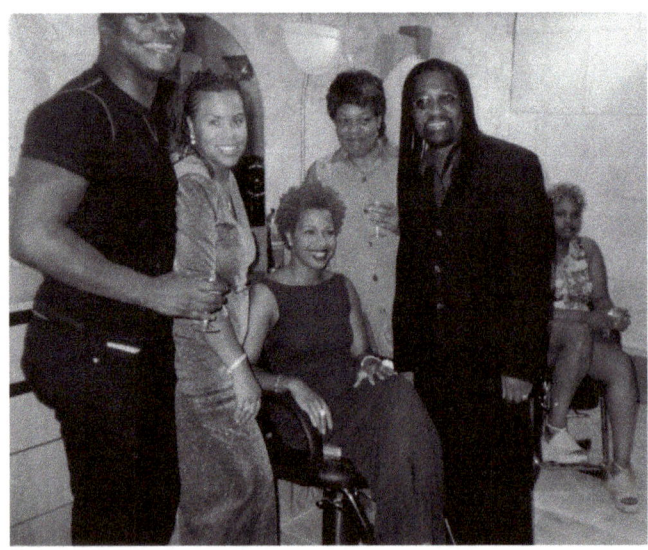

The Grand opening of the Visionary Salon celebration with my colleagues and friends Christopher Canty, Bonnie Deshong, Gayland Rose, Menoria Taylor & Haroon Rashid

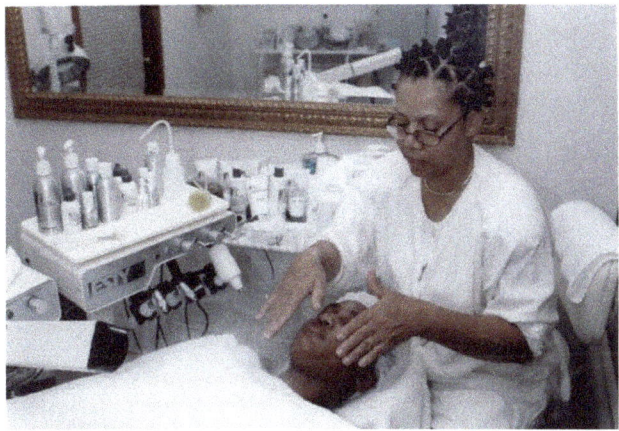

Visionary Day Spa Facial room and Esthetician Sheila Rashid

My former wife Sheila Rashid went to cosmetology school and studied to become a licensed esthetician and she was excellent in her services. Visionary was truly a family affair; my oldest son, Aaron Rashid, and my daughter, Darya Rashid, both were hair consultants; my youngest son Hakeem Rashid was the salon manager. We were well-respected, and again we were building a new reputation as the salon and people to go to in Chicago for full salon services. When it opened, the Day Spa was the only one of color in the near downtown Gold Coast area.

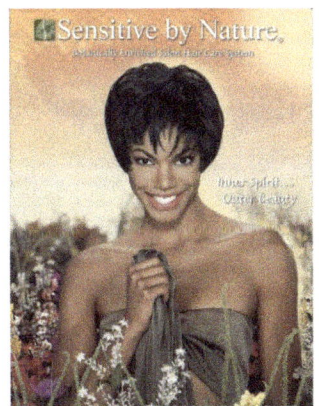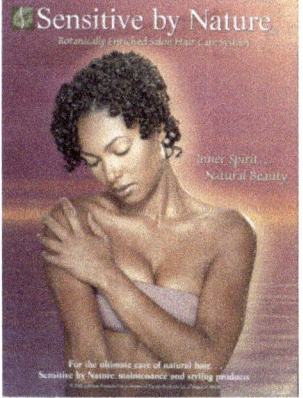

Johnson/Carson Product Company Sensitive by Nature Photo Shoot

While working as a styling consultant for Johnson / Carson Product Company, I was part of a launch for a new product line and concept call Sensitive by Nature. It was a very good line of products; I was asked to do the hair for the commercial print advertisement headshots. Of course after negotiating for the best fee, I agreed.

The job was done at the corporate headquarters in Savannah, Georgia. While working on the shoot, I got a call from my sister in Jacksonville, Florida she informed me that my grandmother was in the hospital in a critical condition; and if I wanted to see her before her termination I should come to visit her then. So I broke away from the shoot and went to visit my grandmother.

I stayed for two days; she appeared to be stable; even though she said to me she wanted to go home, she kept saying I am ready to go home. Sandra told her when you get better you will go home, so my sister suggested I should have time to finish the shoot then come back; she would keep me in touch. Two days later while we were finishing the photo shoot I got the call from my sister Sandra letting me know that she had passed. I felt guilty and hurt because I left, rather than stay. My mother told me that I should not, because she believed Mother as we called her, held on to life to see me before she passed. Being the person my grandmother was, I later realized when she said she was ready to go home she was talking about the kingdom of heaven with God and Christ Jesus. I felt comfort in that understanding because I knew she loved the Lord so much and there could have been no better place for her.

Once Sensitive by Nature was launched I became a part of the styling team. We traveled throughout the country introducing the line to hairstylists and distributors.

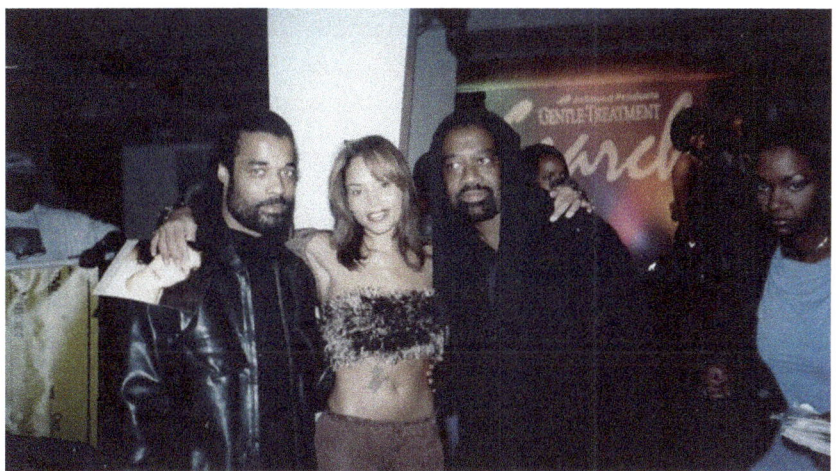

Aaron Rashid, model and Haroon Rashid

At the Midwestern trade show in Chicago, I asked the Sales Director for Carson products what I would have to do if I wanted to be a distributor of the line. She informed me I would need to purchase a minimum order and they would extend a line of credit for the rest, based on orders that I could generate.

I said cool. I decided to start a For Profit and a Not for Profit corporation. I convinced Jada to partner with me and I then called on my network of people and sons Reynard, Aaron, etc. to get involved; we all agreed to go for it. We launched a company; Reynard asked me to use the name for the Distributing business that was called Salon Development Group and we became the Midwestern Distributors of the line, as well as an advance educational resource to hair stylists. In 1999 I found a newly constructed two-bedroom condominium for Jada and myself to move into and use as a Corp office and warehouse of merchandise. It was near the University of Illinois campus in a very quiet neighborhood. Soon after, we bought inventory and started our business.

One of the other opportunities that came to us at that time was that we were asked by the Efalock Professional Tools Company to be their Distributor, which turned out to be a very exciting new line item for us.

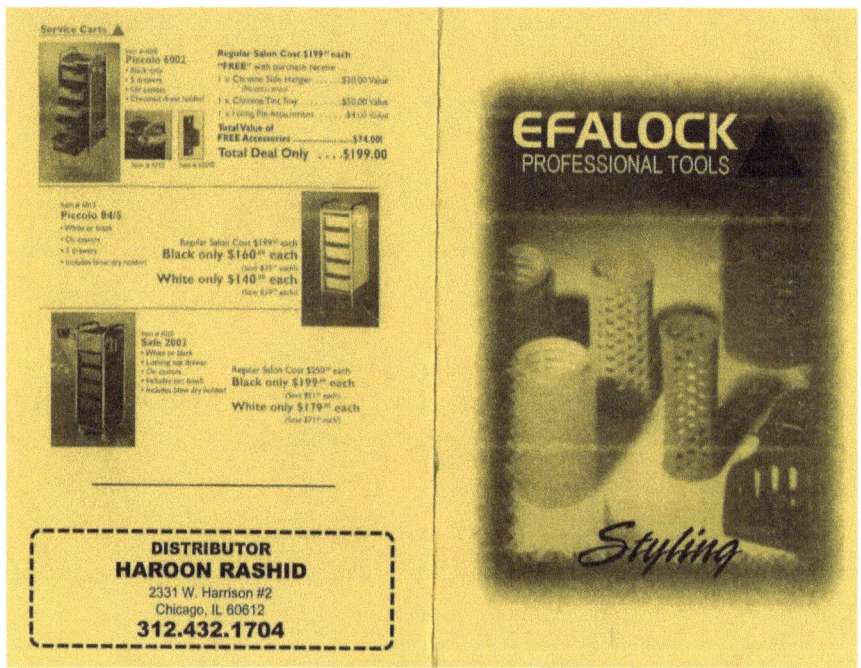

Efalock Professional Tools Company Midwest Distributor

Carson's Product Company repositioned the sales of (SBN) to the mass general market. The line that we purchased was no longer a professional line and our sales team could not move the products at the rate of profit we needed to sustain. We found ourselves competing with mass beauty suppliers and drug store jobbers, mostly Asian wholesalers in the Midwest. We, soon after that, had to sell our inventory and take the loss. That transaction nearly destroyed us individually and set us all back from the business.

NEW YEAR'S EVE 2000
BEGINNING OF THE MILLENNIUM FACTOR

I, like everyone I knew, believed that New Year 2000 was a very special date and that something crazy was going to happen. The love of my life at that time: her Mother and Dad came over to celebrate with us. We looked, listened and checked the media for a sign of something and we pleasantly celebrated that nothing did happen. To be honest, I was shocked because I was taught so much about that time it was hard to believe it went so smoothly.

In 2000 two disturbing things did happen to me:

1. While my woman and I were traveling back and forth to New York visiting her friends, she met someone that she became attracted to and we separated for a while.

2. The other thing was Jada lost her mother, whom I loved like a mother; and I got back together with her for support. Then came September 11, 2001, America was attacked by a radical group of Arabs in New York - the World Trade Center, and Washington D.C. at the U.S. Pentagon. I began to see the fear that I had on New Year's Eve 2000 play out one year later, and I was hurt and petrified over the tragedy.

The World Trade Center bombing changed our desires to travel as frequently to New York as we did before. After that violation, the spirit, freedom and aggressiveness changed in New York more than ever, we decided to work at making Chicago our permanent home. We put all of our energy into building our business ideas and we made tremendous success.

Two years later as she quoted on a TV program called "Bridezilla" Jada met the man of her life and married him. I still respect her for what she has contributed in my life when we were friends. Even though I can say in hindsight I should have married her when I had the chance. I know that the mission I am on may not have been this clear if she had not shaken my world and made me aware of my feelings, and later stood by me through my trials in building the DuSable awareness when I brought it to her. That really helped me in my success. I'm totally grateful to Jada for that.

THE INCREDIBLE RIDE

After my split from that sad situation, I began to believe that relationships never change for me; I think that one of the reasons for that was because I began to feel a need to be in one where someone would be giving me attention that, to be honest, I may not have deserved.

I felt dependent to have someone to live the remainder of my life out with, as I realized I was getting older and losing a lover and friend of ten years. So I found myself looking for the characteristics in women that I felt would be of value to me in a lifelong relationship: like being a parent, having religious respect, having marriage or commitment experience.

One day, while working on a client's hair at Visionaries Day Spa I met that women and through our good conversations and great chemistry we became friends. She was absolutely beautiful to me, and I liked everything about her and I had just come to realize that our relations with our perspective mates were on the brink of destruction. We found comfort in talking things out with each other, she became my confidant and I hers. In all fairness I got distracted from my previous relationship with my new friend who started showing me I could have her if I really wanted her and instead of me putting all my eggs in one basket and making it work with my former friend like I have done so many times in the past, I started cheating with my new friend because I began feeling sorry for myself.

Things moved real fast between us after our separate break ups; unwisely we replaced our respective partners for each other without taking the critical time out to heal from those previous relationships.

Even though I knew that kind of behavior rarely works, I was so attracted to her character and beauty that I felt challenged to pursue her and take the risk; to me it was worth the try at that time. She had a twin sister and they were Geminis, not that astrology means anything to me, but by being a Gemini myself I was intrigued with dating someone like her to see how it would feel and how much chemistry we really had in common.

I met members of her family; they were all good religious people. The one thing I noticed was that most of her family members were close associates with her ex-husband and his family, as they all either grew up in or were associated with the same church. The values among them were conservative Christian views and her former husband was an assistant pastor at the same church she loved going to. Me being a believer of Islam and as liberal as I am in nondenominational religion, I knew that I would never be accepted in the church that she attended or among the guarded like circle of family and friends. Even though I knew that it was not intentional I sometimes felt critique like I was just a temporary outsider among them.

In my heart, I knew that any person that had been in a relationship with one person for eleven years and had no real dating experience until meeting me would be challenging and risky. I also knew there would come a time that she would want to know how it feels to simply date and see what it is that she was denied by being in a committed relationship for so many of her vital years. I further knew that there would come a time that the obvious age difference and religious difference would come to a head; but to be honest, she was worth the risk for me at that time in my life.

In spite of that, she and I decided to move in with each other downtown Chicago one block from City Hall. We moved in a building that I lived in before I left Chicago to live in New York before meeting her. We traveled together and experienced different environments together. We visited my family in Boston and while there we went to Martha's Vineyard on the Cape. Later she, her daughter, her young cousin and I all went on vacation in New York City; it was her first trip to New York. The kids had a ball and I enjoyed exposing her to the East Coast cities and she really liked it; in fact she said she would like for us to live in New York when her daughter was off to college.

When we first started going out with each other, we attended as many events and night clubs that we could, pending her getting a child minder for her daughter. I felt it was important for us to get out to places that she was not used to going to, like night clubs, concerts, festivals, movies, plays, theaters etc. So every weekend I would try to do something to wine and dine her in different ways - restaurants and events throughout Chicago - I really enjoyed doing that with her.

She had a beautiful eight- year-old daughter that I got a chance to know, by helping her get to school each day for the first school semester that we lived together. This was her first year going to Chicago public schools and it was unlike the suburban school she was accustomed to, prior to moving into Chicago. She was afraid at first to put her in the Chicago Public Schools. She felt, like most people, that the Suburban School systems were better, and they were! She felt that her daughter was doing well out there and that the Chicago Public School system had a bad reputation. She feared that she might not do as well in the Chicago schools, so she entertained the idea of keeping her in the suburban school and driving her to and from the suburbs each day on her way to and after she got off work.

In talking to her, I convinced her to look into the Chicago school system, for the schools that had a good record of achievements. I suggested that she should apply to them for her. I knew that Chicago had some good schools because I was working with the Chicago Public schools sponsoring DuSable literacy essay competitions in the systems. I have been to great schools and seen brilliant children with good teachers and administrators.

She investigated it and found that I was right and that her daughter would have to take a test to get in the good schools; she did and scored high enough that she was selected into Hawthorne Scholastic Academy in Lakeview Chicago.

She was used to driving her daughter to a Pre School center on her way to work. The Suburban School and Pre School was close enough to where she lived at that time, which made it easy for her to manage. The Public School buses in Chicago that picked up and dropped off children at her school did not pick up at our home location downtown Chicago, and there was no pre School system available that we knew about, so I volunteered to help get her to school on time. So her daughter and I would travel on the public train every morning; being it was her first time riding a train, she loved it. Rain, snow, cold or otherwise, she was always eager to take the ride on the train and not miss a day. At eight-years-old she was an exceptionally smart ambitious child who loved to read and cook. I became attached to her.

After a year of living together I decided to do the right thing, I asked her to marry me so that she, whom I thought was a highly moral conscious person and her family, would respect our relationship and me.

I was unprepared for her answer; she said no and that she was not ready to commit to marriage again. She said she was afraid to go back into a marriage contract for fear that if it does not work she would have to go through the pain of divorce again. I understood, but I was shocked like most men that have been rejected from such an important decision as marriage; your ego steps up and you find yourself asking *what is going on*? After all, for me this was the second time that I experienced that rejection.

It turns out in her telling me that she felt I was not committed to her enough and that I was waiting for the right chance to leave her for a better choice. It was not true at all, I had already made that transition and when she realized she was making a mistake about my intent it was too late for she had already began experimenting with another man. Once that happened it was like Eve in the Garden of Eden after eating the apple, she began to see all my shortcomings, including the age differences that started following the suggestion of her sister and friends to explore other men that might have more to offer than I. They suggested that she experiment and told her that she did not have to be loyal to me. I got to tell you that suspicion is an evil thing, it is considered one of the original "Seven Sins" and it will definitely destroy what is right or good in people.

There are words in a song by the R&B artist, Leala James, which I will recommend to any person when you see something like this happening to them; the title was called My Joy! The lyric is "You better learn to love yourself first".

Trust me, if you do not, you will find yourself on one incredible journey and if you have short patience you should walk away because you will be tested of what you are made of.

I was beginning to feel that I was not supposed to match well with the Chicago women because of back to back rejections and somehow there seemed to always be, as in the case of most of my relationships, there is always a third party that helps in their decision making. I had the displeasure to listen as she would defend the honor and character of this new person as a highly educated great man, I felt she was implying as she spoke to me that he compared to me, and my associates were people who were beneath her and her new man. I was just a hair stylist, that went to a beauty school and I was no comparison to them; in fact she in anger told me I was nobody compared to her new choice.

Her words were, at the least, condescending and demeaning. She tried and made me feel that his accomplishment was her new version as a measure of a man for her. As though, after all that I had done since she met me, in her mind was nothing compared to the other person's deep rich pedigree for his and perhaps her future. I was hurt, but I forgave her soon after, because deep in my heart I still loved her and I knew that her inexperience in relationships was the major factor in her decision-making. These following statements are meant to be food for thought to those that might read them of lessons learned.

THE GAME OF CHEATING

I share these words as food for thought; in the game of cheating there are three players.

1. **The Primary Person**, this is the person in the game that permits the game to begin and takes the risk of winning or losing.

2. **The Perpetrator**, this is the outsider of the relationship that is permitted by the primary to play the game, this

person generally has the least to lose and is most likely to win.

3. **The Victim,** this is the one person that is most likely to get hurt and lose in the game. In this game someone will lose, someone will win and someone will get hurt.

Generally, the perpetrator has the advantage because they are most likely to have information of everyone because the primary generally reveals all the shortcomings and negative information about the victim's lifestyle and a great deal about their own to justify why they are cheating in the first place. The victim is the only one that is kept in the dark; they rarely even know the name of the perpetrator, not to mention their lifestyle, they are at a terrible disadvantage. The primary also reveals all the things that they are looking for to the perpetrator to give them a jump-start into the game. All the perpetrator has to do is listen and act accordingly and they most likely will win in the game of cheating. Cheating is an ugly game; someone has to win and someone has to lose, shame on the winners. The sad part of this theory is I know it well because I have been a player in all the roles in my life. I am not proud of that at all.

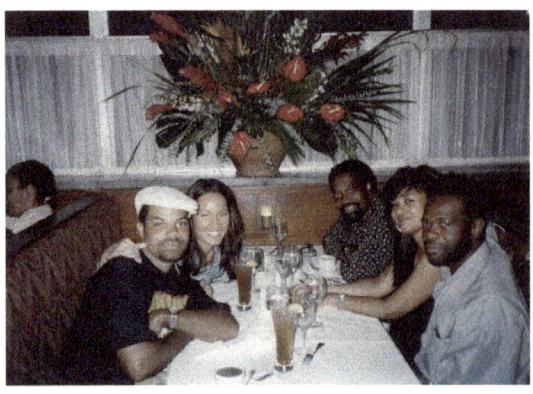

Hakeem Rashid, Tanya Rashid on the left, Oji Young - his friend from Philly & Haroon Rashid at Bea Smiths Restaurant in Manhattan

THE PRISON, PRISONER & PRISON GUARD

Oji is probably the best friend that I have had over the years, he is from Barbados, and he has a lot of different ways of viewing issues; and we seem to advise each other on our point of view in regards to personal drama.

One day as I was explaining my point of views of why I was on lockdown mode about my feelings and I would not give in. He told me a profound story. The story is about a man that guards his women or relationships like a prison guard would a prisoner.

1. The prison: He said in society when a person does something wrong and is judged and convicted, civilized society will lock that person up for a time in prison. It is a place that most people do not want to go, because the main thing that prison does is strip a person of their freedom, dignity, liberties and civil rights; again definitely not a popular plan, vacation trip, or place to go.

2. The prisoner: Feels guilty or innocent as charged, once they are locked up. They feel confined, victimized, angry and controlled, not a good way to live on a daily basis.

3. The prison guard: Even though the guard believes they are doing their duty, watching over the prisoner; but in order to do that work, the guard must go in the prison and be locked down with the prisoner in a place that is meant for criminals, not free men and women. They must surrender eight or more hours of their day in prison with criminals and willingly give up their

freedom to do their work for their happiness. In other words, when we lock someone up physically or mentally you have to be willing to be there as their guard in your prison to serve your Justice. That is not a job for everyone, certainly not for me.

HOLDING ON

Another lesson was given to me from my cousin James Harris; James is an international Hair Fashion Stylist. In one of his lectures to hairstylists he made a brilliant analogy that I adopted; it is about the lesson of letting go to gain. He said if you begin to take all the things that you want to keep; like money as an example, on your person, you fill all your pockets, you put things between your knees, under your arm pits, your arms, under your chin, your teeth, elbows, legs, crotch, in your buttocks, between your toes, fingers, on top of your head, sooner or later you will run out of places to hold things. In order to get anything else that you are attracted to you have to start letting things go in order to receive.

I am very clear that my purpose for being in Chicago was not for personnel love and relationships but instead to do what God has always wanted me to do, his will in the City of Chicago. That is to work for the dignity of my people, my ancestors and my descendants' legacy. Love and happiness will come; if I do my mission God will lead me to the joy I need, I have no regrets for my reality. I will not give up on Love that is an act of confusion, and evil control over good.

I got distracted as to why I was in Chicago and I had to be brought back to reality and put on the right track.

I am a social activist that is blessed to be living at the beginning of the twenty-first century. I believe the work that I do is critical to my descendants' future and I will not willingly act common about such an important time and my responsibilities therein.

One underlying fact came out of my twisted experience in Chicago; that there is a spirit of continuance, tolerance for violation; and there is a lack of trust, and loyalty among its people. I must tell you I have seen this spirit appear over and over again. Even by people that are supposed to protect you: your family and loved ones. I remember the teachings of Imam Wallace Muhammad when I was in the world community of Islam under his leadership. He said that when some elders get old they don't trust their own youth, so they begin to hide their money or valuables and sometimes forget where they hide them.

It was soon after that experience when Visionaries Day Spa went through a financial crisis and we had to close the Spa. So once again, I went back to my friend Ranni Flowers and returned to work in his Van Cleef Salon.

Chapter Sixteen

Back To Van Cleef Salon

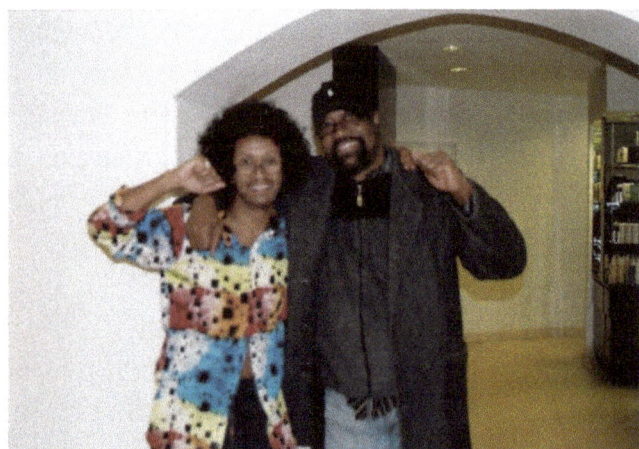

2002: Rahni Flowers owner of Van Cleef Salon and Haroon Rashid back together again

Coming back to Van Cleef *was* very good for me I began to reacquaint myself with many old and new clients. I also started very quickly building a new body of clients and friends. I also would get my eyes open about a very valuable body of information regarding the history of Chicago and its founder Jean Baptiste Pointe DuSable.

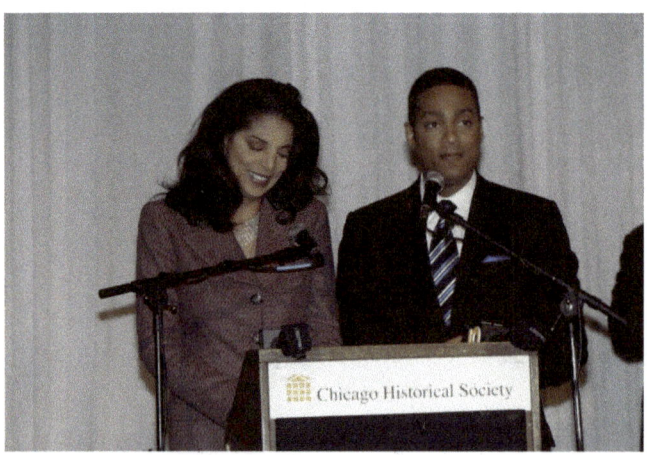

Allison Payne WGN 9 TV News & Don Lemon NBC 5 TV

At Van Cleef Salon, this time I had a lot of TV news anchors, like Alyson Payne, Don Lemon and many other key media and political personalities such as the First Lady Michelle Obama and her family. That opportunity enabled me to pursue into my deep areas of personal interest that I had vowed to address upon coming back to Chicago from New York.

Many of the players of my ambitions were right there coming each week to the salon for hair services. There were social, business and political leaders that I would lobby and seek support from to be a leader in the discussion of progressive change.

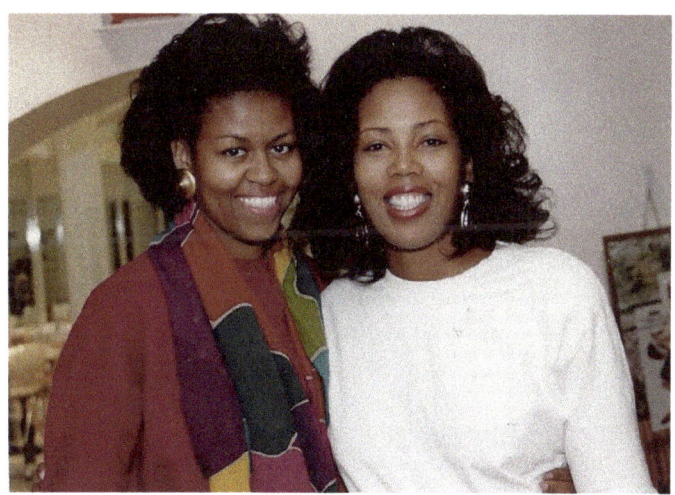
Michelle Obama & her sister in-law Janice Robertson

One of the most important of such clients was Michelle Obama. At the time, she was the wife of then State Senator of the State of Illinois Barack Husain Obama and she was an Executive at the University of Chicago Hospitals. She was getting her hair done by Rahni and I was doing her sister in-law's hair, Janice Robertson. Janice had her own bicycle and sports equipment business in

Wisconsin. In collaborating with Michelle regarding my interest in advancing the discussions on how to commemorate Chicago's founder, and she being a native of Chicago leader, Michelle was able to see right away the value in what I was advocating and agreed to help. After my explaining the mission statement that Friends of DuSable was actively engaging in partnership with the city of Chicago and many leader's city wide she became the key figure in my accomplishments as an activist for equal human rights.

After President Obama was elected as the first African American President of the United States, Michelle and their family became the First Lady and The First Family. The press gave Van Cleef Salon a lot of media coverage as the salon that the First Lady attended. That word out created a great spike in business for Van Cleef as well as popularity as a celebrity salon. The largest professional hair and beauty convention, The American Beauty Show producers made a request that they would like to give a tribute to the Van Cleef Salon at the first major show, after the inauguration for their part in making history. Rahni was uncomfortable in doing the presentation so he asked me if I would help put a team together that would represent the salon, since I had so much more experience in working the shows and in doing presentational workshops.

I asked my good friend and peer, Karen Lemon; we picked a few models and put together a platform production that went off very successfully.

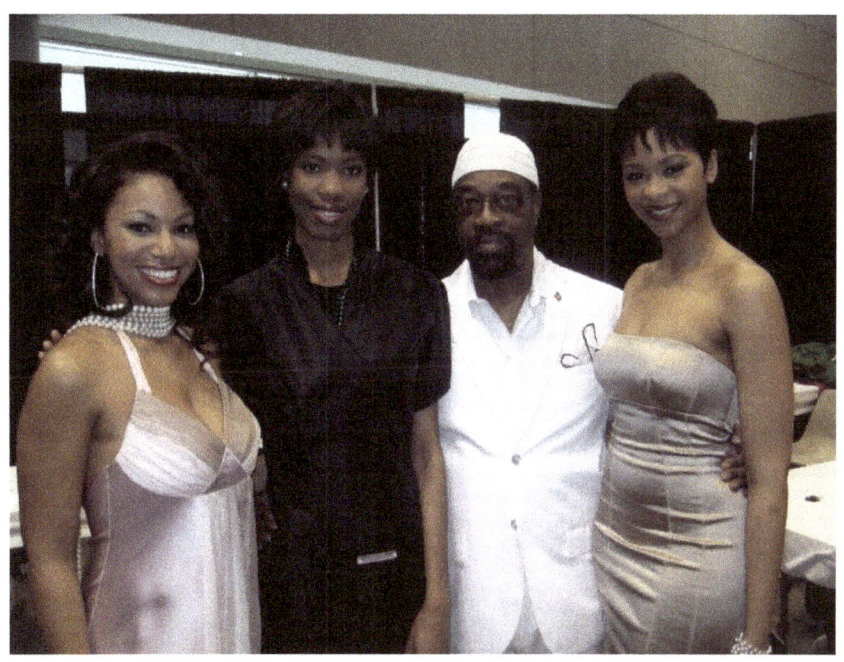

Tribute to Van Cleef Salon for being the Salon that serviced First Lady Michelle Obama

These are the models that we used to demonstrate the type of services that Van Cleef salon was doing, which attracted so many celebrity clients in Chicago. Again there was also that premiere factor to consider about our experience at that time wherein there has never been an African American First Lady before that moment in time. Therefore, Van Cleef salon and its staff was a part of that historical cultural experience. The salon was under the total occupation of the secret service, inside and out. The block that the salon was in, on Huron Street, was under total lockdown on the ground and rooftop when the First Lady would come. Our clients had to, happily, make adjustments with the security to come in and out of the salon when Michelle, her mother and daughters would come for services every week. We were all so proud of her and her family that we treasured every moment we had with them before they finally left for Washington DC. On the last day that Michelle, her mom and daughters left, the salon was so emotional for me, because I was always so instinctively on a security alert mode while in her presence; even though I knew she had the best security in the world around her. I felt an urge to be on my guard to protect her if I had to; so when I watched her getting ready to finally leave, my heart had a rush of pride and remorse for her. She embraced the staff on her way out of the door. I personally will always treasure that heartfelt embrace that she gave me as she was leaving.

Obviously, the press could not get enough of the activities that Michelle and her limited entourage would bring and so every newspaper, television, radio and magazine was covering First Lady Michelle Obama and at some point while she was there and immediately after she left the Van Cleef Salon and Chicago.

At the hair show people from all over the country came to the exhibition room where we held our workshop and discussions, many asking how did it feel to be in that environment during those history-making times. And the hair & beauty magazines did interviews and took pictures of our models and works.

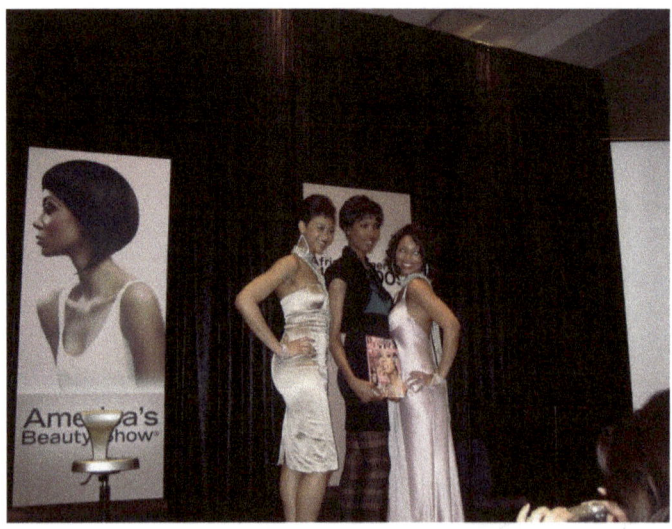

The America's Beauty Show and Black Style Magazine presentation and photo shoot

THE HISTORYMAKERS

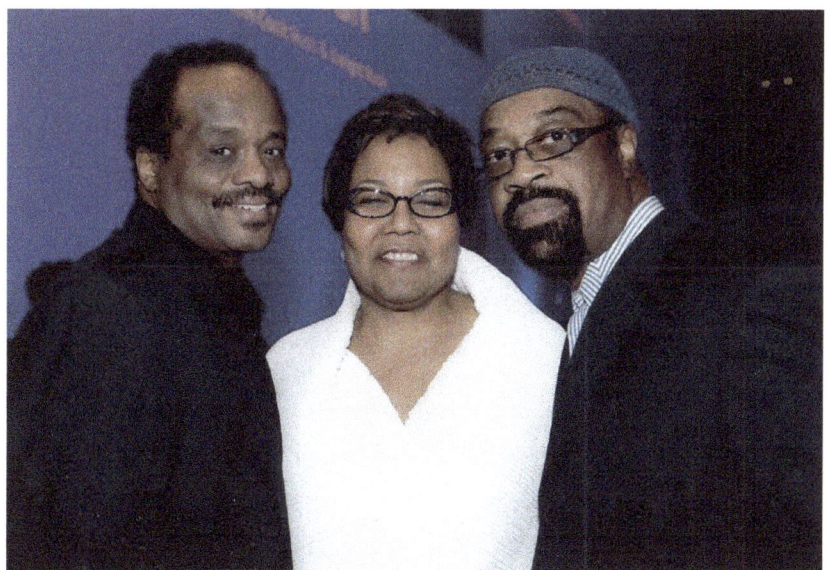

Hairstylist Leigh Jones CEO of HistoryMakers Julieanna Richardson & Haroon Rashid

One of the other proud accomplishments that I was privileged to be a part of at Van Cleef was that I was asked by a client if I would be interested in being the hair stylist for celebrities that would be honored and filmed for broadcasting. It was called, An Evening with The HistoryMakers.

In that capacity I was able to meet and or work with many of African America's premier dignitaries and celebrities. Julianna and I worked together on her productions with Julian Bond, Gwen Ifel, Nancy Wilson, Ruby Dee, Denise Graves, Russell Simmons, Cathy Hughes and Spike Lee

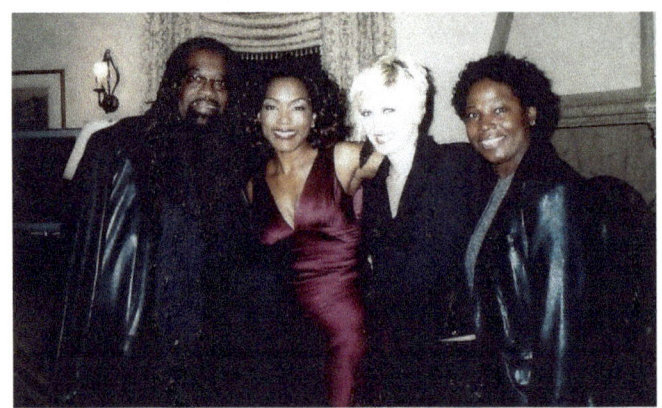

Haroon Rashid's Styling Team for The HistoryMakers with Angela Bassett

The styling team that I was in charge of required a makeup artist and a hair assistant and our job was to maintain a finished look during and in between sets on all personalities that would be aired, unless they brought their own hair and makeup artist for that purpose. I worked with the History Makers events and productions for five years until I did my last production with the fabulous Miss Angela Basset.

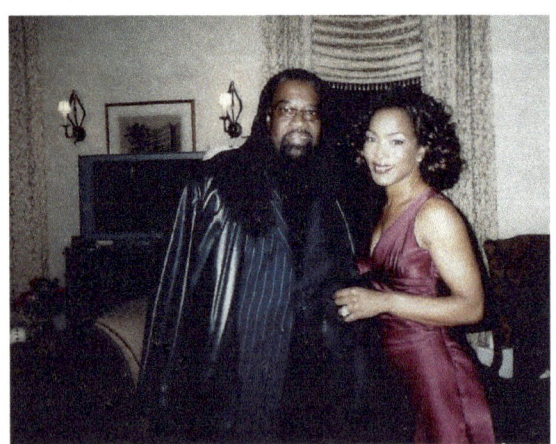

Haroon Rashid and Angela Bassett

I was so honored to work with Angela Bassett because she is one of the actors that bothered to achieve a good higher education. She went to Yale and studied the science of her craft. Most important she is a gifted artist and absolutely beautiful, I looked at her and said to myself right away, *that woman is smart, ambitious, compassionate and beautiful; she is my kind of woman.*

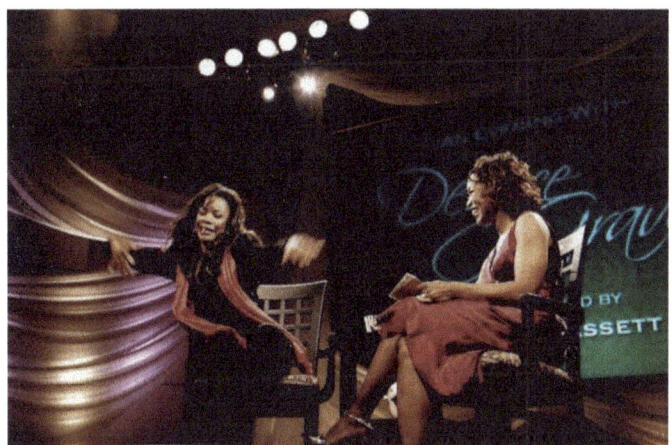

Angela Bassett interviewing Diva Opera singer Miss Denise Graves

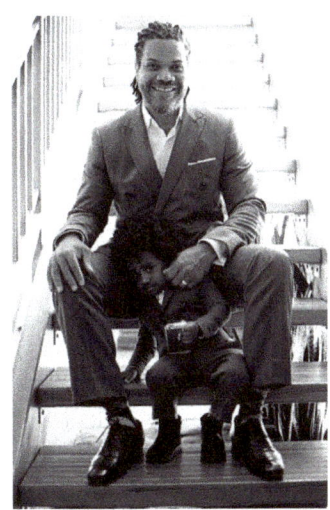
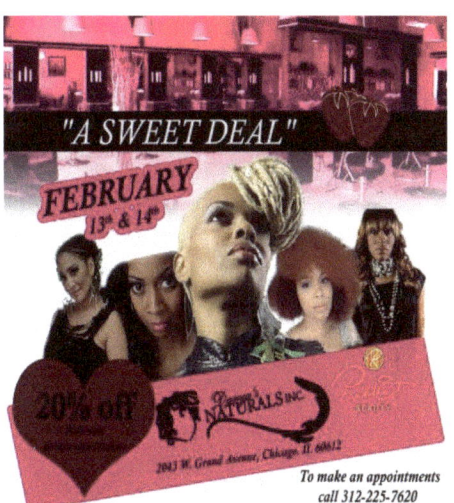

My son Hakeem with his son seven & my daughter Darya with her staff at Darya's Natural hair

One of things that I will proudly say has happened in the new millennium was to see that my daughter Darya and son Hakeem matured in their cultural artistic "Birth Right" as leaders in their own space. Hakeem developed his own men's and boy's custom fit clothing line called <u>Hearts Remained Made to Measure</u> and my daughter Darya as a Salon owner, advance educator and hair product line owner called <u>Darya's Naturals, Inc.</u>

Part Two

THE CHICAGO SPIRIT

Chapter Seventeen
My Manifesto Of Change For The Spirit Of Chicago!

As I have previously mentioned that my life had always been one that I felt born to feel and know that I was a free sovereign man and that I would stand on the side and to identify with those that exercised those same rights.

When I finally learned about the rich history and legacy of DuSable he became a person in character that I wanted to be like and would identify with. I became immersed in his accomplishments and was shocked to witness how unbeknown to so many fellow Americans his legacy was to them. I became fascinated that all the information you would need to know was right within plain sight it was available upon research.

I have personally seen the value for myself and others in particularly people of the African Diaspora develop a great American pride in diversity with a true sense of inclusion entitlement once they discovered that the third largest city in America Chicago was founded by a person that looked like and was one of them.

In the narrative that is now popular in Chicago in which I was fortune to begin leading the discussion that led to Chicago's WTTW TV network using the brand name the film documentary: From "DuSable to Obama" there is a great message for the next generations of future leaders vision of the compatibility of these two great men's valuable lifestyle's whom I believe that both of their glorious roots was Destin to emerge in Chicago.

That is why I included in my historical timeline so thoroughly the services of DuSable that I no history will show what I was instrumental in accomplishing in Chicago with pride for full public discloser. I give this comprehensive information with the intent that if I don't tell this information it might not become transparent or become compromised.

One might come to the conclusion that I have completely immersed myself into the character mode of DuSable in my senior years of social political service and I affirm that is true.

I truly believe there will be a measure of encouragement for some that read within the timeline of my services in Chicago that I proudly and deliberately promoted this very important character in my Chicago history of advocacy and that is why I soon adopted the narrative that "I Am DuSable!" in a mission orientated way.

The Chicago spirit, in particular, is tainted and needs healing from a history of false legacy and negative reactions, as does America. So we have designed a concept that we think can address some of these issues, we call it Spirit of DuSable Healing and Wellness. We believe there is a first step to wellness, and that is healing. We believe a lack of the sense of personal entitlement or knowledge of self brings into play all the negative factors that destroy our natural growth. Many of us will abort our personal success or happiness, not to mention the rest of African Americans because we just cannot believe we deserve it. I believe that Chicago, more than any other major city in America, struggles with a psychosocial disparity, which spawn's apathy particularly to people of African Descent.

Know for sure this is no accident; oh no, this has been a deliberate action on the part of every immigrant cultural society that came to Chicago. The city of Chicago that was hosted by Native Americans, and developed into an immigrant and migrant settlement for so many people, eventually became America's third largest city. Yes, it was a well-kept secret that a man of African descent, Jean Baptiste Pointe DuSable founded Chicago.

Imagine if African Americans, nationally, and people of African descent, globally, would have known they too had a ancestor in American history that was credited and celebrated on the same level as Columbus, Lincoln, Jefferson, Pulaski and other great American pioneers and unlike the stories that were told for centuries that the only accomplishments that the African American accomplished was centered around the experiences of slavery.

Of course, we know that African Americans were not the only people that were brought to America as slaves and given freedom; the Irish, the Asians and other indentured slaves also came to America as property of others.

But the deliberate manufacturing and institutionalizing of the Negro as was done to the so-called Negro on the Caribbean Island was recorded in the Willie Lynch papers. Separating the slaves from all traces of themselves, their culture and of their sovereign land and leaving them totally dependent on the slave masters' wicked version of his culture and names, but void of any sovereign rights in the new land called America. What land is Negro land? Where is it? African people have always refused to accept the so-called Negro as one of their own, until recent years when African Americans have been without a sovereign homeland to claim as their own. Even though the Irish were slaves, when you hear the names McCormick, Daley, O Toole, or Mc Bride you are not surprised to see an Irish person with those names or Lee, Kim or Wang being Asian; but when you hear an African American named Haroon Rashid, Barrack Obama or Wallace Muhammad, well now that seems odd, even to African Americans. That is only because African Americans are the only ones of former slaves that were stripped of so much culture. Even though both classes were given freedom, one is considered a free man and the other lives by a subculture that is secretly considered a freed man, whereby one that had a slavery history can be integrated into society unnoticed; and the other has signs of the disgrace still branded to his implanted cultural experience, the names of his former slave masters.

The word Negro, where did it come from and why is it still being used by a few???? Even though it is now politically correct to say African Americans, a term that was started by progressive blacks to liberate themselves from slavery terms put on the African American race through the institution of shame and disgrace of slavery conditions.

African American was adapted in the mid-seventies; however, even today some African Americans and others of the twentieth century still refer to the former slave children as Negroes.

THE ORIGIN OF THE N-WORD

In the book "The Story of The Moors in Spain" by Stanley Poole, which was first, published in 1886, in the introduction written by Dr. John G. Jackson reads the following on the subject.

In ancient times, Africans in general were called Ethiopians; in medieval times most Africans were called Negroes. The Greeks named the Ethiopians. The word Ethiopia means burnt face, "from the Greek names ethios + face. This description referred to the dark complexion of these Africans, which the Greeks attributed to sunburn. In the literature on Africa, Africans are commonly identified in two groups: one progressive, the other backward. The progressive people are called Hamites, Kushites, Moors, etc., whereas the backward ones are called Negroes. Negro comes from the Latin word Niger, meaning black. Hamites, Kushites and Moors were also called black, but they have been inducted into the white race.

The word Negro; was manufactured by the Atlantic Slave Trade; or to put it another way, there are many species of small fish in the ocean; when put into cans they are called sardines. There are no free fish called sardines; they got that name only after being enslaved. A fish became a sardine when imprisoned in a can, and Africans become Negroes when they are put in chains. According to American law, anybody with an African ancestry, however remote, is a Negro.

To follow this logic, since the human race originated in Africa, everyone in the world is a Negro. Therefore, a word as vague as this, does not mean anything.

So the African American being branded as a Negro was not expected to be a progressive thinking person and was believed to depend on others to survive in the new America. Even after so-called freedom, there were no names to reclaim their culture, or homeland to go to. Like the Ford Automobile the so–called Negro is a product of, and was made in America.

Some believe that, without a linage of a sovereign American citizenship status, there is no justification for free sovereign rights like reparation for African Americans. There are some that believe their giving of freedom to the former slave and allowing education and amending civil rights was a debt paid in full.

What would take this debate to a world court to decide? Most Americans would be shocked to know that America was once under the protection of the Moroccan Nation and that their government gave America its first Sovereign rights in international waters under the Moroccan flag when America was being treated like a negro in its beginning stages by the global community after breaking away from British, Spanish and the French sovereignty and declaring itself to established its independence as the United States. This legal status was so important to America that it accepted the offer from Morocco for those rights. That being said let me tell you the story of an African American that in his day was considered as a sovereign citizen in what is now the third largest city in America. This man owned, in his day, what is commonly called and known as the Gold Coast of Chicago; also called the magnificent Mile, from Chicago Avenue to Chicago River

North/South and from Lake Michigan to State Street East/west and this man just happened to be of African descent.

I would like to talk about a few of our ancestors that I admire and that we can learn a lot from and who have paved the way for African American Empowerment, Entitlement and Reparation. Little is spoken of the free blacks in America that came to this country as immigrants and never experienced slavery, owned land and was sovereign citizens in America. This is the story of one.

SOVEREIGNTY

There are two common terms that I believe every African American must ask themselves in the twenty-first century, *do these definitions apply to me?*

#1 sovereign:
1. DOMINANT, predominant, paramount, preponderant, preponderating, supreme, transcendent, surpassing; absolute, ultimate.

2. FREE independent, autonomous, autarchic, autarkic highest, loftiest, chief, principal, foremost; governing, ruling; commanding, directing.

#2 sovereignty:
FREEDOM: independence, autonomy, autarky, autarchy, supremacy, ascendancy, command, sway, control, dominion, power and authority.

It is believed by some that Jean Baptiste Pointe DuSable was a sovereign citizen in Chicago and he operated under the sovereignty on the land that he purchased from the Native Americans, the original landowners in Chicago.

He exercised all the characters that made up a sovereign citizen and according to history, he was respected as such by all that came to the region. He experienced something that history seem to be unknowing or willing to talk about, the history of American pioneers of African descent that had full Equal Human Rights in lands of this Nation. Clearly driven by the affects of twentieth century overt racism, it has been Civil Rights, as opposed to Human Rights that have been fought for and accepted by the made in America so-called Negro.

So the question is still asked at the gate of the twenty-first century, is the African American a creditable Sovereign citizen with Sovereign rights and do African Americans really have full Sovereignty under the law in America.

Chapter Eighteen

Free Blacks In America

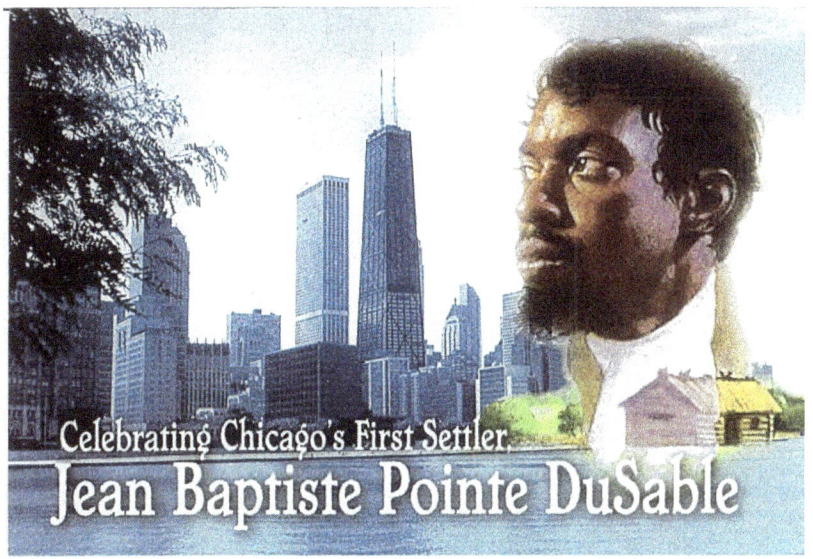
Celebrating Chicago's First Settler Jean Baptiste Pointe DuSable

Jean Baptiste Pointe DuSable was a famous frontier trader, fur trapper, farmer, international scout, businessman, and authenticated father of the nation's third largest city in America- Chicago. Historical records do not agree as to the origin of this great man. But I would like you to consider the theory that he was looked at, in his time, as a Moor; we will talk about the importance of that later. However, history insists that DuSable was born a free black, around 1745, in St. Marc, Saint Dominique (Haiti). He was the son of a French mariner and an African-born slave mother. His father took him to France to be educated, and afterwards, he worked as a seaman on his father's ships.

He was a powerfully built man, well-educated and cultured. He had a love for European art and, at one time, owned twenty-three Old World art treasures. He spoke French, English, Spanish and several Indian dialects. At the age of twenty, DuSable was injured on a voyage to New Orleans. Upon reaching the shores of New Orleans, he learned the Spanish government had taken over. The French Jesuits, a Catholic order, protected Du Sable from being enslaved until he was well enough to make his way up the Mississippi River. He later settled in Peoria, Illinois.

In the early 1770's, DuSable built a cabin and eventually owned more than 800 acres of land in Peoria. He enjoyed a special relationship with Illinois territorial Indians. He took a Potawatomi Indian (Kittihawa), Catherine, as his common-law wife and fathered a daughter, Susanne, and a son, Jean.

There is a parallel of the African American labor and the South African Colored people whereby many of the African American freed men and women and runaway slaves turned to the Native Americans for support, and mates, as did the Indonesian labors in South Africa turn to the Africans for the same. Some years later, he left Peoria and made his way north until he reached the Great Lakes area. The promise of greatness of the "Chicago" area, and which DuSable decided to settle, had been passed over by others before him. None had the foresight to look beyond its barren, damp, marsh condition, nor did they have fortitude to make "nothing" into one of the greatest locations in the Western Hemisphere.

In 1779, starting from scratch, DuSable built the first permanent home on the north bank of the Chicago River, where the present day Tribune Tower stands. His land extended onto the present Wrigley Building sight and beyond, on the Chicago River front. It was a well-constructed house consisting of five rooms and equipped with all the modern conveniences of the times. Later, despite the disadvantages, DuSable established a thriving trading post in a short time; he became well-known as far away as Wisconsin, Detroit and Canada. The trading post consisted of a mill; bake house, dairy, smokehouse, workshop, poultry house, horse stable, barn and several other smaller buildings. His post was the main supply station for white trappers, traders, woodsmen and the Indians. The Chicago portage boomed. It became the key route for merchant trading, and DuSable sent wheat, breads, meats, and furs to trading posts in Detroit and Canada.

DuSable became a man of considerable wealth and means. He also owned a substantial quantity of field and carpentry tools, which indicated that he must have hired men for fieldwork and building assignments. In addition, he owned an appreciable quantity of livestock, poultry, and hogs.

In 1784 DuSable brought his wife and children to Chicago. And, as DuSable was a devout Catholic, he waited for the first Catholic priest to come in the area to marry him in a Catholic ceremony to his wife Catherine. In 1796, their granddaughter became the first born in the city of Chicago. On May 7, 1800, DuSable sold his entire wealth for a mere $1,200 and moved to Missouri, where he continued as a farmer and trader until his death. On August 28, 1818 DuSable died and he was buried in a Catholic cemetery in St. Charles, Missouri.

In 1968 the State of Illinois recognized Jean Baptiste Pointe DuSable as being the founder of Chicago.

Chapter Nineteen

The Spirt Of Dusable

Serene Entitlement & Empowerment Foundation
Friends of DuSable

The Friends of DuSable was founded by Haroon Rashid in 1999 to establish formal recognition for Jean Baptiste Pointe DuSable. The organization's main objective is to preserve an annual commemoration for DuSable, the founder of modern Chicago, as an integral part of the celebration of the Chicago's incorporation date on March 4th each year. In order to properly commemorate DuSable, we needed to increase awareness of DuSable's contributions throughout all of the city's communities.

The purpose of the commemoration was to reinforce the common thread that tied early Chicago to present day Chicago diversity. DuSable's legacy reflected diversity at its best and provided a gleaming example of what Chicago could be, given the knowledge of its roots.

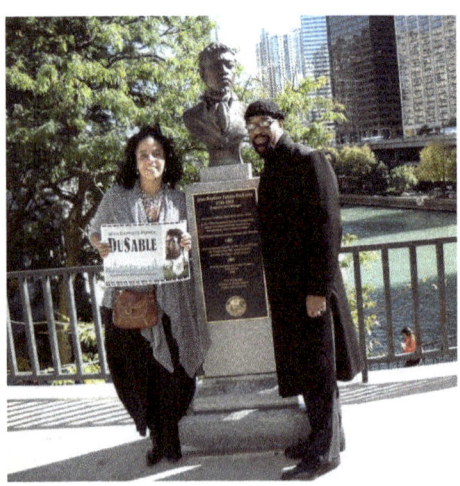

The original pioneers for Friends of DuSable: Maria Jossey Owens & Haroon Rashid

Let me tell you my story of how I and why I became so consumed with this man's life and how it has become an important part of my legacy that I proudly leave for my descendants to learn from: December 1999 while talking to one of my clients, Maria Jossey, about Jean Baptiste Pointe DuSable, the first non-native settler and immigrant in Chicago. I was telling her how I first heard of DuSable from one of my elite hair clients, Mary Ella Smith, who was the fiancée of Chicago's Mayor Harold Washington. As I was the one that styled her hair for both of Mayor Washington's inaugurations, she once revealed to me that Mayor Harold Washington had great knowledge and pride of DuSable and as a former student of DuSable High school that he had campaigned for the Mayor of Chicago under the banner and in the spirit of DuSable; and that in fact he, Mayor Washington, considered himself metaphorically speaking as the rebirth of DuSable's legacy and he had great plans before his untimely sudden death November 25, 1987 to commemorate DuSable's legacy in a global way.

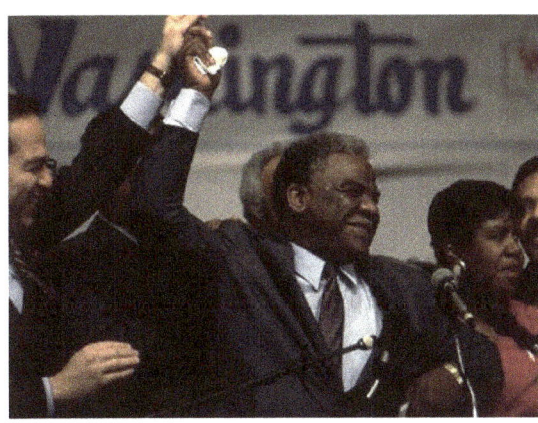

Chicago Mayor Harold Washington and his fiancée Mary Ella Smith April 29, 1987 at his second Mayoral Inauguration

Maria and I discussed how it was a shame that there was no real available public information about this man's incredible legacy. We decided to put a plan in action that would do just that. We felt the best way to disseminate information of him at that time was to have a parade in his honor. I went to My Second Ward alderman Madeline Haithcock in the ward that I lived in and ask her if she could help me establish a parade for DuSable, she advised me to write my plan and give it to other council members and see what the Mayor's Office of special events felt about it; and she would help as much as she could, so I did that. Another client of mine Alicia Ferriabough whose dad I knew from my youth in Boston was a student at Northwestern University Law School, in Chicago. She told me of a program that the school had to help organizations create bi- laws and become registered with the State as a non-profit using the students as an assignment. I went to the Director of the program, Professor Dr. Thomas Morsch. We were assigned a liaison person, Ms. Paula Wells, who worked with the students and us until we created the Serene Entitlement and Empowerment Foundation 501-C (3) by laws. We gave it the name (S.E.E.F.) because our original plan was to address the forgotten heroes from the African American experience. DuSable was just one of the many stories that, once properly told to many, instills the true sense of inclusion and patronage as a race of our ancestor's contributions in the development of the United States and helps to level the cultural divide of others.

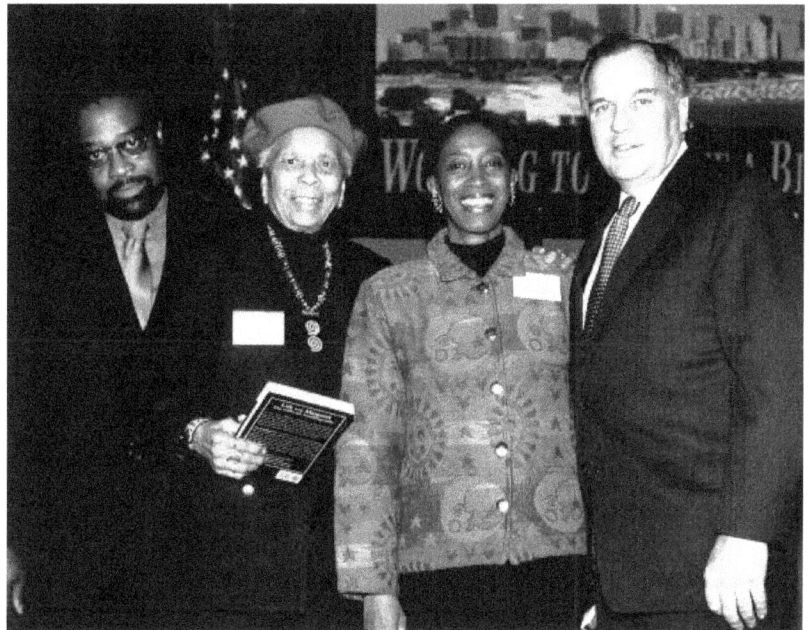
Haroon Rashid, Dr. Margaret Burroughs, Dr. Jean Pierre & Mayor Richard M. Daley

The Mayor's Office of Special Events, upon our request to have a parade to honor DuSable, assigned a person that worked with our efforts to see if the citizens of Chicago would participate. For a year, we were allowed to conduct monthly DuSable collaboration meetings at the Chicago Cultural Center.

It was after one of those meetings that Dr. Margaret Burroughs, Founder of the DuSable Museum, agreed with our efforts; and she said that she would help and recommended that we change our name to Friends of DuSable, which we gladly did. It was then that we created and made public our Core of Initiatives.

1999 CORE OF INITATIVES
OBJECTIVE FUTURE INITIATIVES

DuSable Day Commemoration Ordinance

An ordinance was drafted and submitted to the City of Chicago Commission on Human Relations, the ordinance was awaiting approval by the City Council's Human Relations Committee. The ordinance called for the City of Chicago to incorporate a citywide day of commemoration of Jean Baptiste Pointe DuSable on March 4th, the day Chicago was incorporated. The ordinance, introduced by former Alderman Leonard DeVille, had 19 aldermanic co-sponsors.

To bring awareness of this mission, the Friends of DuSable and the Commission on Human Relations held a rally, "DuSable Now", on June 22, 2002. the speakers included: Haroon Rashid, Founder of Friends of DuSable; Former Alderman Leonard Deville (21st Ward); Alderman Burt Natarus (2nd Ward); Commissioner Clarence Wood, Commission on Human Relations; Russell Lewis, Director of Collections and Research: for Chicago Historical Society; Bessie Neal, President, of the DuSable League; Commissioner Mary Dempsey, Chicago Public Library; Dr. Burroughs, Founder, of the DuSable Museum, and Commissioner of Chicago Park District; Antoinette Wright, DuSable Museum; Jesse White, Illinois Secretary of State/Jesse White Tumblers; Bishop Perry, Titular Bishop of Lead, Clausel Rosembert, Consul General, to the Haitian Consul; John Low, Former Attorney for the Potawatomi Indian Tribe; Arnold Romeo, Director of the African Council of the Commission on Human Relations. The Master of Ceremonies was John Davis of CBS 2; the featured performers were the American Indian Center Drum and Dance Group, Chicago Opera

Theatre, Ben Sexton as "DuSable", Jesse White Tumblers, and Tamboula Haitian Drum and Dance Group.

Chicago Dinners

During Unity Month this past September, the Human Relations Foundation in conjunction with the Commission on Human Relations and Friends of DuSable hosted two "Chicago Dinners". The Chicago Dinners were implemented a decade prior in order to promote dialogue about issues of race in the Chicago land area.

The Unity Month Chicago Dinners, held at the DuSable Museum and the American Indian Center, brought together the African American and Native American communities. Both parties expressed an interest in continuing the dialogue, and presenting the issues discussed to the various cultures in Chicago.

Publication

The development of two Elementary level text books was underway. The "Big Bo ok" would cater to children in Kindergarten through 2nd grade. A second publication would be written for children in the $3^{rd} - 4^{th}$ and 5th grade. These publications were distributed in museums and school systems throughout Chicago, the State of Illinois, the greater US, Haiti, and France.

Speakers Bureau

The Speakers Bureau was formed to continue our outreach to the greater Chicago area. Our primary focus was educational institutions, schools, museums and libraries. In order to maximize our efforts, we would build upon our relationships with Chicago Public Schools, Chicago Catholic Schools, Chicago Public Library,

Chicago Historical Society, DuSable Museum, and Bronzeville Children's Museum, and the American Indian Center.

Newsletter

Our newsletter, that was launched March 2004, served as a central resource for current information on all the DuSable oriented initiatives. The initiatives: DuSable Park Steering Committee, DuSable Park Coalition, DuSable High School Administration and Alumni Groups, The DuSable League, DuSable Museum, The African Scientific Research Group and more, all of which we had close relationships.

Consuls Generals

The French Consul, Haitian Consul and most recently the South African Consul endorsed the DuSable Initiative. We worked to incorporate it into the DuSable Commemoration celebrations. In the spirit of diversity, we planned to build relationships with all 43 foreign Consulates based in Chicago.

Research

Efforts were in place to secure funding to conduct further research on Jean Baptiste Pointe DuSable's history. We collaborated with the historic DuSable League, the African Scientific Group, the French and Haitian Consulates, the Catholic Church, as well as the Native American community, to trace DuSable's roots and identify his living descendants. DuSable's travels took him to Haiti, France, Canada, Louisiana, Missouri, Wisconsin, Michigan and Illinois. There was a wealth of information at the various Historical Societies, Libraries and Museums in the aforementioned regions.

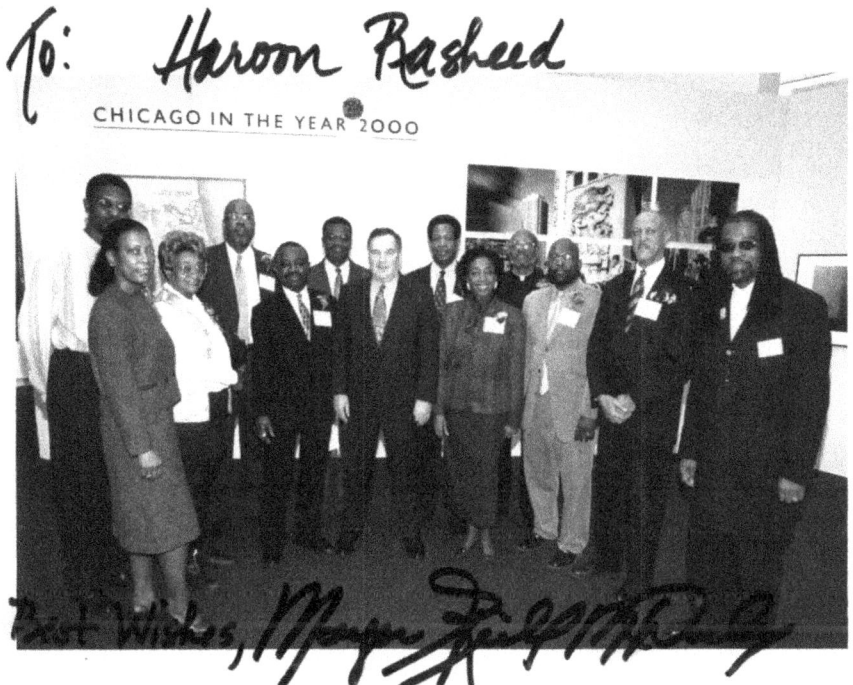

2000 Chicago Commission on Human Relation African Advisory Council on African Affairs members with Mayor Richard M. Daley

My confidant Maria suggested that since the untold story of Jean Baptiste Pointe DuSable is about the first human relation experience in Chicago, I should ask the Commission on Human Relations to help us in our efforts to bring recognition to DuSable in Chicago. So I contacted Commissioner Clarence Wood who assigned the deputy commissioner to talk with me, he suggested that I apply to be a member of the commission on Human Relations African Advisory Council to make this a council agenda. Upon Maria's encouragement and help with the application I did that and was voted in by City Council as new member and approved by Mayor Richard M. Daley. The City of Chicago: Commission on Human Relations Advisory Council of African Affairs in the year of 2000.

As a council member I pushed the DuSable recognition agenda to the members and they unanimously agreed to make it a line item. We drafted an ordinance and sent it to the Commission on Human Relations board for a Vote to be approved. The commission then approved and made the draft a Commission on Human Relations ordinance. The ordinance was then sent to City Council for a vote, to have a day to honor DuSable.

To our surprise half of the alderman or council members, manly African Americans, voted for the ordinance; the remainder did not. The bill remained unfinished for six more years before going into effect.

CITY OF CHICAGO
COMMISSION ON HUMAN RELATIONS

presents this

Certificate of Appreciation

to

Haroon Rashid

for serving as a member of the Advisory Council on African Affairs, and making contributions to help improve the lives of the African community in our city, which positively affects the livelihood of all Chicagoans.

Rahm Emanuel
Mayor

Mona Noriega
Chairman and Commissioner

Arnold J. Romeo, Director
Council on African Affairs

2011 Final Acknowledgment of Services Recognition from the City of Chicago

2011 Final Acknowledgment of Services Recognition from the City of Chicago Commission on Human Relations Advisory Council on African Affairs

DuSable Founders Day Commemoration Essay Competition

In 2001, the DuSable Commemoration promoted the writing of the famous, comprehensive "Essay Competition" for 3rd, 4th & 5th graders enrolled in Chicago area public and Catholic schools. That same year, we merged an ongoing partnership with the Chicago Department of Cultural Affairs, Mayor's Office of Special Events, City of Chicago Commission of Human Relations: Advisory Council on African Affairs and the Chicago History Museum for the City of Chicago Annual Birthday Celebration/ DuSable Commemoration Day on March 4th. We then decided to celebrate Jean Baptiste Pointe DuSable the Man and his legacy without the ordinance and we chose the City of Chicago official Birthday as the day to do it. The way to do that was decided by having children's essays in Public and Catholic schools on how to celebrate DuSable, having programs in public Libraries and city colleges.

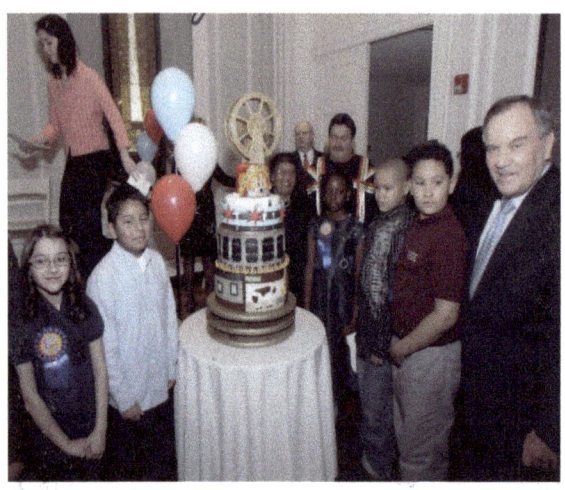

Mayor Richard M. Daley with DuSable Essay Winner during the Chicago Birthday Celebration

Public Announcement

FRIENDS OF DUSABLE 10TH ANNUAL DUSABLE COMMEMORATION ESSAY COMPETITION

Chicago History Museum, 1601 N. Clark Street
Sunday, March 4, 2012   12:00pm-5:00pm
Program Begins at 2:30pm

Chicago is increasingly being poised on the world stage as a city to be noticed. We are once again pleased to present the 10th Annual DuSable Commemoration Essay Competition in conjunction with the City of Chicago 175th Birthday celebration. The competition is presented by Friends of DuSable NFP. Please take a look at this year's prompts. They will be CELEBRATING IMMIGRANTS FOR 175 YEARS, as 2012 is the 175th birthday year of Chicago, IL.

Friends of DuSable NFP, along with the Chicago History Museum, Bronzeville Children Museum, the Chicago Loop Alliance & former Chicago Commission on Human Relations

African Advisory Council are proud to partner in co-producing this stellar event.

In these uncertain economic times we again are continually challenged as to how we were to put this event together. Our resolve was to press forward, knowing we not only owed it to our students, but to the entire city as well. It is equally important to stay committed to our focus which remains single minded "To promote and maintain the legacy of our city's first non-native resident, Jean Baptiste Pointe DuSable".

During this event, we will also be honoring the winners of the 2012 DuSable Commemoration Essay Competition. The winners are 3rd 4th & 5th grade students from Chicago Public & Catholic Schools. Come and witness the students that will be selected to read their essays, along with their teachers, parents and guest in a private DuSable Commemoration display room as they are all recognized and receive Apple ipad2 and other awards for their accomplishments. There will be refreshments and photo opts for them and our guests.

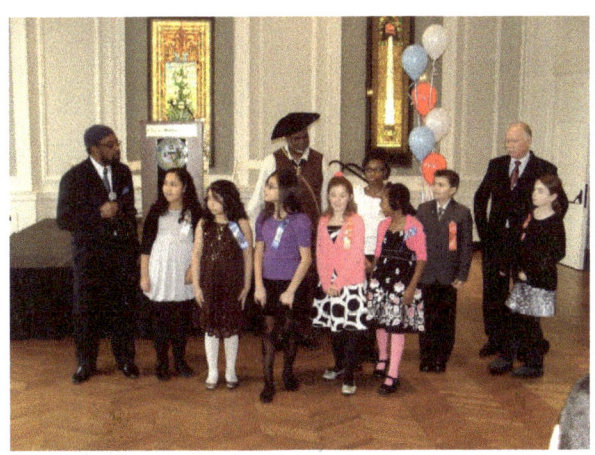

Haroon Rashid, DuSable actor, Chicago History Museum Executive Vice President Russell Lewis & Chicago citywide DuSable Essay winners

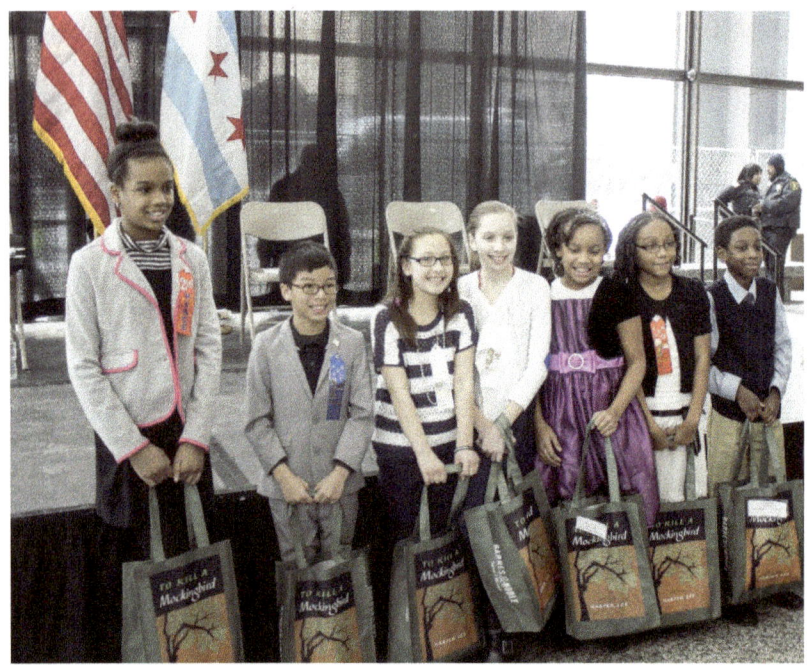

March 4, 2014 DuSable Commemoration Day Essay winners after receiving their essay award prizes

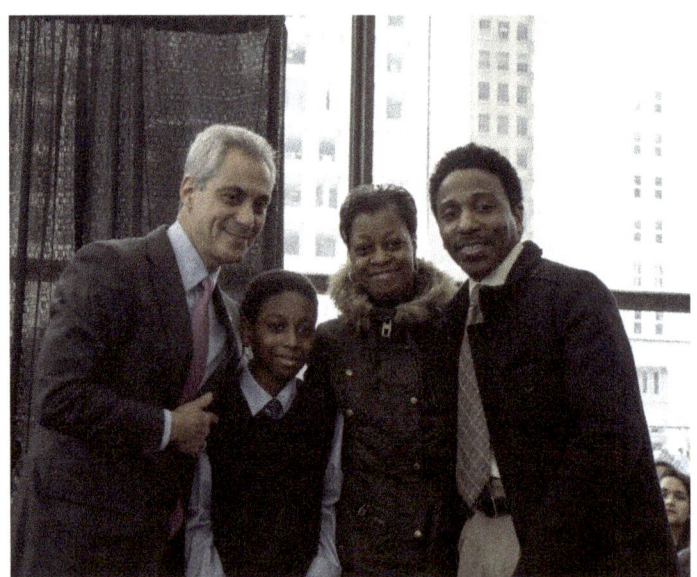

March 4, 2014 Mayor Rahm Emanuel in celebration with 1st place DuSable Essay Winner & his family

2001 "A Fight for DuSable" Pro-boxing/fundraiser

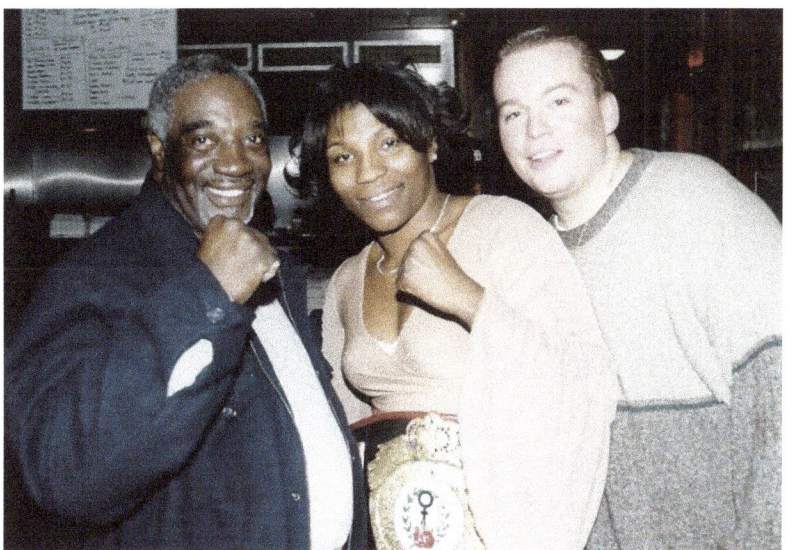

April 20, 2001 Douglas Pendarvis, Latisha Johnson and Little Paki

Friends of DuSable decided to bring awareness to the city of Chicago of our efforts to commemorate Jean Baptiste Pointe DuSable by using some of the skills that my brother Doug and I had as boxing promoters, by creating our first outreach event that was called *A Fight for DuSable* boxing fundraising event at the Chicago Hilton Hotel.

DuSable Now! Information Rally

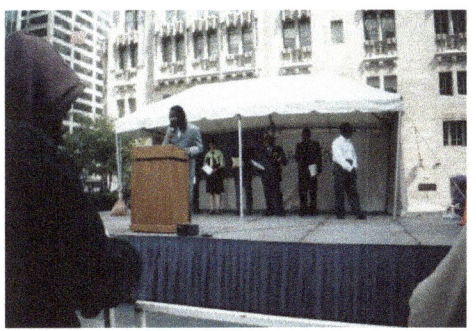

Speakers at the at the DuSable Now Rally

In 2002, FOD launched an information rally entitled DuSable Now to encourage conversation of the erection of a statue or likeliness of DuSable at his home site in Pioneer Court (near the junction of the Chicago River and Upper Michigan Avenue. This is a couple of examples of the media coverage of the efforts and the events.

Written by Annan Boodram
New York Times: July 2002: It's time to give du Sable his due.

That's what supporters of Jean Baptiste Pointe du Sable said Saturday (June 22) as they rallied along the Chicago River near where the Haitian-born immigrant built a home and trading post after he became the first settler to arrive in what would become Chicago.

Records do not agree on the precise spelling of his name and it may be found variously as Pointe de Sable, Au Sable, Point Sable, Sabre and Pointe deSaible. Du Sable, who appears to have been a man of good taste and refinement, was a husbandman, a carpenter, a cooper, a miller, and probably a distiller.

In Du Sable's home, the first marriage in Chicago was performed, the first election was held, and the first court handed down justice. The religion of the first Chicagoan was Catholic and every contemporary report about Du Sable describes him as a man of substance who started the story of Chicago, as well as the story of the African American in Chicago. Now the community leaders and history enthusiasts want Du Sable formally honored every March 4 as Chicago's founder's day when the city celebrates its birthday.

Du Sable has history on his side but until recent years at least, apparently lacked the support to leave his name as widely on Chicago's street map.

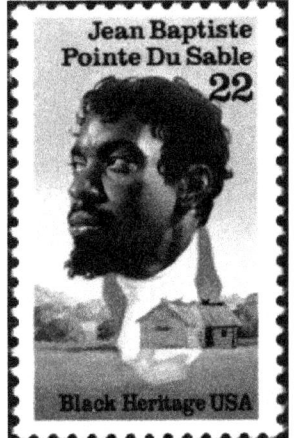

Just two tiny streets were named for du Sable--Jean Avenue, a two block long street on the West Side, and the oddly named De Saible Street, a private, block-long South Side street. Du Sable, though, did get a high school named in his honor, as well as the DuSable Museum, the nation's first African-American history museum, and Du Sable Harbor.

A new park at the mouth of the Chicago River also bears his name, but the site is tainted with toxic waste that needs to be cleaned up before it can be used for recreation. A statue also is being planned in his honor.

Du Sable was said to have been born a free Black in St. Marc, Saint Dominique (Haiti). He was the son of a French mariner and an African-born slave mother. His father took him to France to be educated. In about 1773 he made his way up the Mississippi to the Chicago area. He established a trading post on the North Bank of the Chicago River mouth, at what would later become Peoria. His business prospered and became the center of a permanent Chicago settlement. His trading post was the main supply station for White trappers, traders, les coureurs des bois and the natives. Du Sable made many trips to Canada to bring back furs and it was reported that he was very closely associated with the French in New France.

His loyalty to the French and the Americans led to his arrest in 1779 by the British, who took him to Fort Mackinac. From 1780 to 1783 or 1784 he managed for his captors a trading post called the Pinery on the St. Clair River in present-day Michigan, after which he returned to the site of Chicago. By 1790 Du Sable's establishment there had become an important link in the region's fur and grain trade.

In 1800 he sold out and moved to Missouri, where he continued as a farmer and trader until his death. His 20-year residence on the shores of Lake Michigan had established his title as Father of Chicago. But his admirers say du Sable remains underappreciated.

"He is the founder and the reason we exist," said Antoinette Wright, president of the DuSable Museum of African American History. "He really put an imprint on it, but he wasn't recognized for it."

For years, du Sable was overshadowed in the history books and in local honors--including streets and statues named and created in his honor- by late-arriving, white settlers whose names are still familiar in the city: Hubbard, Kinzie, and Wentworth. "It was the climate of the day," Wright said.

It was only in 1999 that city officials formally recognized du Sable as Chicago's founder--almost 225 years after he and his family arrived at the unsettled, fertile land that would later become the city.

Du Sable, who was married to a Potawatomi Indian woman by the name of Kittihawa (Catherine), presided over a frontier settlement that in some ways mirrored the diversity found in the sprawling city that exists today. His settlement welcomed American Indians, as well as Canadians, British, French and Americans.

"There was an incredible fusion of cultures and languages," said Russell Lewis, director of collections at the Chicago Historical Society.

Despite the existence of slavery in the United States, du Sable was the acknowledged leader of the settlement. "He came here, and he was a leader while others were enslaved," said Haroon Rashid, founder of Friends of du Sable, a community group.

Still, much remains a mystery about du Sable, including when he arrived in the Chicago area, as well as his reasons for selling his property around 1800 and moving away from the region. Even his birthday is unknown, although he is believed to have been born about 1745.

"He's an enigma. There's a lot we don't know about him," Lewis said. "But that lack of knowledge, in some ways, adds to his appeal."

Historians and history buffs are still trying to fill in the gaps about du Sable, which keeps alive interest in the city's founder.

"I meet two or three people a year who have new theories about who he was," Lewis said, calling him "a very powerful symbol for who we are today."

Community leaders, though, say there needs to be more official recognition of the role du Sable played.

DuSable Museum founder Margaret Burroughs is calling for a 20-story arch to be built in his honor along the Chicago River, or even straddling the river near where du Sable once lived.

Lewis thinks, at the very least, Pioneer Court along Michigan Avenue at the north bank of the Chicago River should be renamed in du Sable's honor, particularly because that spot is thought to be near where du Sable settled.

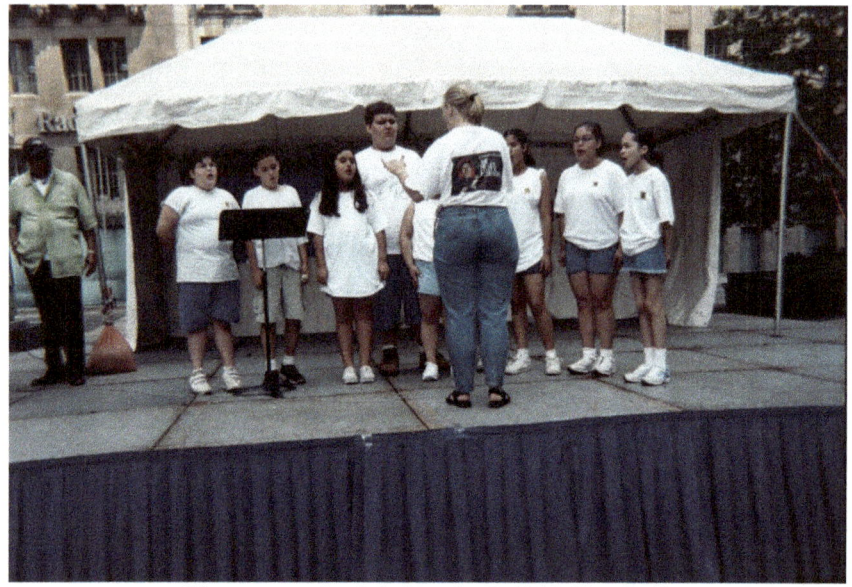

Elementary school choir at the DuSable Now Rally

The event was purposely designed to show a broad multicultural inclusion, from the speakers to the entertainment as a way to convey the reality that the city of Chicago roots was centered in diversity from its Founding Father Jean Baptiste Pointe DuSable. Prior to the Friends of DuSable advocacy, that factor was the one thing that Chicago was not recognizing in its social and cultural history. The schools and, most importantly, the city of Chicago Commission of Human Relations: Advisory Council on African Affairs who I had just become a member of, whom we had a partnership with Friends of DuSable in the event because they wanted to be a part of the leadership in the discussion of Equal Human Rights, as the narrative for The Spirit of DuSable. That was the thinking in recruiting the elementary school that was of Native American and Catholic inclusion.

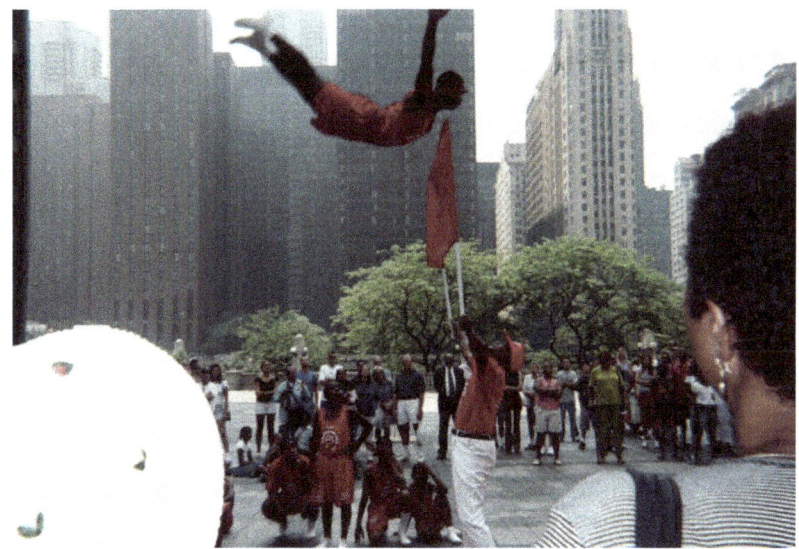

The Secretary of State Jessie White tumblers at the Du Sable Now Rally

The Secretary of State Jesse White was a politician from the State of Illinois; he has served as the 37th Secretary of State of Illinois since 1999. History will record him as the longest-serving and the first African American to hold that position. Prior to his position as the Secretary of State, he served as the Cook County Recorder of Deeds for six years and he also served in the Illinois House of Representatives for thirteen years earlier than that position. It is recoded that in 1959, He founded the Jesse White Tumbling Team to serve as a positive alternative for children residing in the Chicago area. Well over 10,700 young men and women have performed with the team. When we contacted him about our efforts to commemorate DuSable and to get the awareness of DuSable's legacy to the powers to be, Secretary White not only agreed to be a speaker but that he would bring his young Jessie White Tumblers to be a part of the entertainment. We conveyed to him that our goals were to put some visible presence of DuSable in the area of Chicago that DuSable resided in when he was alive: Pioneer Court near the Chicago Tribune building. In the picture of the Tumblers that is the Sectary Jessie White holding the banner those young Tumblers were diving over.

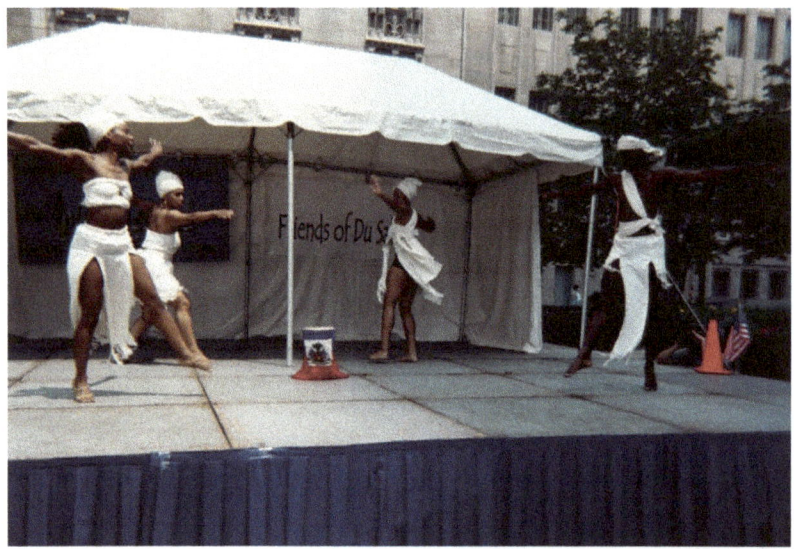

Tambula Haitian Dance team at the DuSable Now Rally

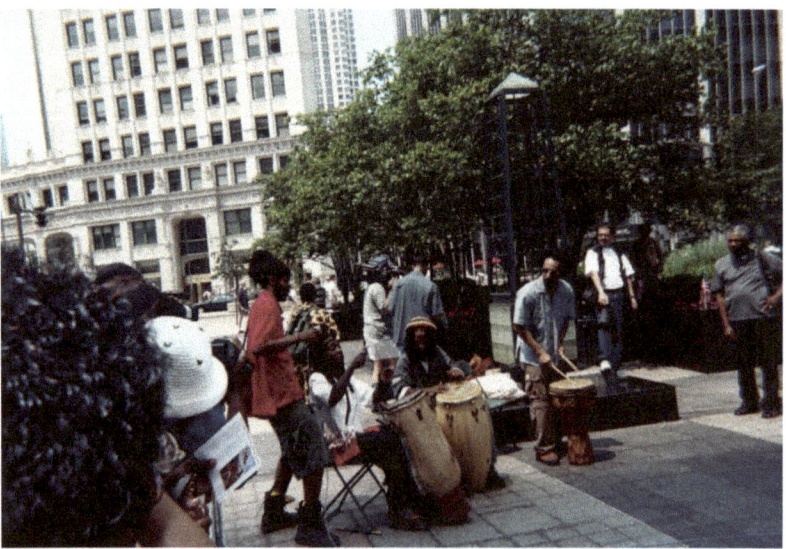

Haitian drum choir at the DuSable Now Rally

The Haitian community had a personal interest in our events in that because says that the founder of Chicago was a Haitian; his legacy represents their heritage and they wanted to proudly represent him in any way they could. One obvious way was to do that was through cultural edutainment in music and dance. The Tamboula Haitian music and dance group became Friends of DuSable's official events entertainment in Chicago.

There gifts of langrage in diversity French, English and Creole, which would help make their performance of entertainment unique to the average American citizens. There was a sense of Afro-Caribbean spiritual spirit in the nature of their presentations.

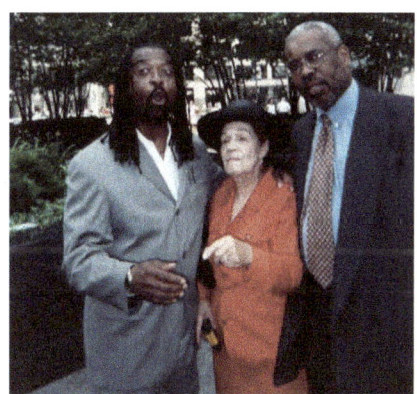 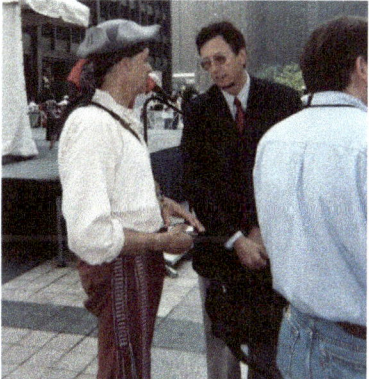

Haroon Rashid, Virginia Julian, Arnold Romeo, Native American Lawyer John Low at the DuSable Now Rally

In the picture with Haroon is DuSable historian Ms. Virginia Julian, city of Chicago Commission of Human Relations Advisory Affairs Director, Mr. Arnold Romeo and in the center picture on the right is Native American Legal Consoler John Low. They both were board members of Friends of DuSable at that time, John being of the Pottawatomi tribe American Indians and Arnold being a Trinidadian from Trinidad. They represented what Friends of DuSable was from the beginning, a multicultural and diverse governing body of social leaders. These are a few of the proposals and suggestions that the Friends of DuSable advocated and partnered with in order to achieve the measure of success that we did.

In 2003 Friends of DuSable made a proposal to the city of Chicago in regards to ways to commemorate DuSable that read like this.

PROPOSAL

In acknowledging and recognizing the rich history of Chicago and the great accomplishments of Chicago's first citizen and founder, we are proposing that the City of Chicago introduce an ordinance that names March 4th as a day of celebration for Jean Baptiste Pointe DuSable Day.

During the week of March 4th, a series of events will be hosted throughout the City of Chicago to honor DuSable and celebrate its beginning. The celebration series will be sponsored by Harold Washington College, the Chicago Historical Society, Chicago Public Schools, and various corporations.

The implementation of a Jean Baptiste Pointe DuSable Day will not only serve as a day to honor and recognize DuSable for his accomplishments, it will serve as a catalyst to bring the people and communities of Chicago together for a day of unified commemoration

DuSable's House: Wood cabin 22 feet by 40 feet, 2 Barns, Horse Mill, 1 Bake House, 1 Poultry House, 1 Workshop, 1 Dairy, 1 Smokehouse, 2 Mules, 30 Cattle, 2 Calves, 28 Hogs, 44 Hens and Equipment: 8 sickles, 7 scythes, carts, saws, copper kettles, axes and other house tools.

Our proposal was ambitious yet comprehensive, which is why we called on all public and private agencies in Chicago to play a role. The DuSable Day project was an on-going collaborative effort with a 5-year projection plan in place to complete its goals which lead to state and national recognition.

Getting to Know DuSable Symposium

The following year, we planned and presented our next major event with one of our board members Miss Elsa Tullos who was also an administrator for Chicago City Colleges. Through her guidance we were able to make plans to work with one of the City Colleges in the downtown districts of Chicago the Harold Washington College to create a symposium centered on the legacy of DuSable. Irony of that was we were well aware that during the life of the former Mayor Harold Washington, who was the person that the new City College was dedicated to and named after, was that he had made attempts during his lifespan in city hall to bring national attention to the legacy of DuSable and it was because of my affiliation with members in his inner circle that I first became aware of DuSable history. It seemed fitting that I should be advocating building a bridge of relationship with the college in his namesake for that purpose.

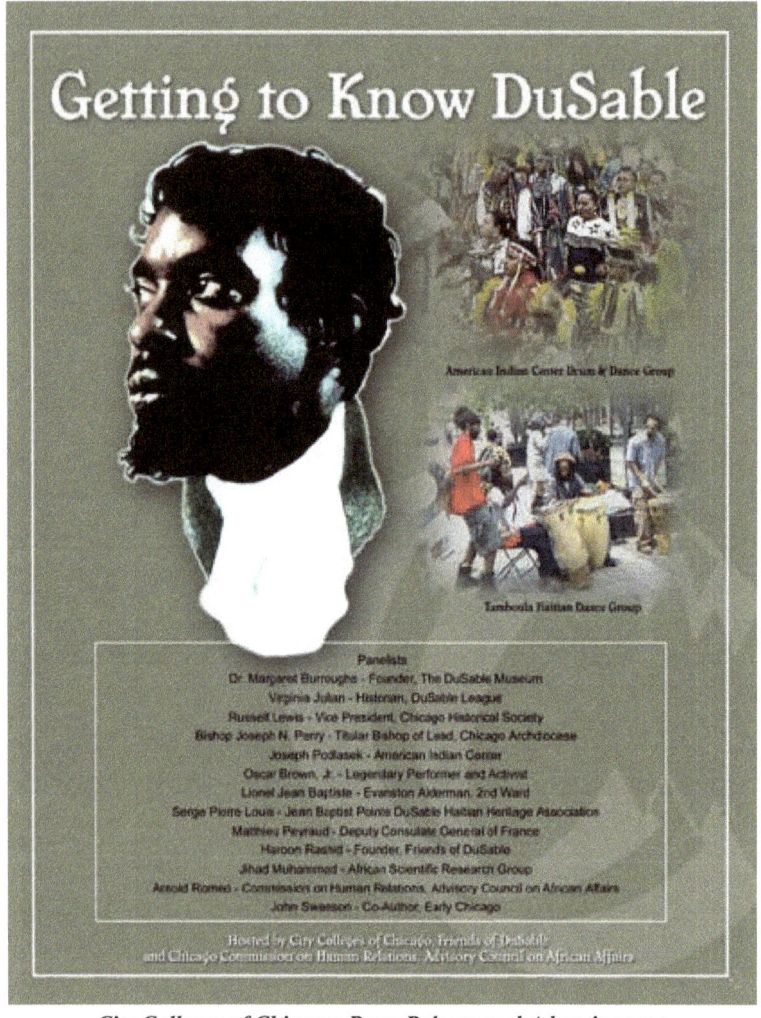

City Colleges of Chicago: Press Release and Advertisement

Harold Washington College Hosts Special Event Honoring Jean Baptiste Pointe Dusable

Chicago, IL (February 25, 2003) - On Tuesday March 4, 2003 from at 11 a.m. until 2 p.m., Harold Washington College (HWC) will be partnering with Friends of DuSable and the City of Chicago

Commission on Human Relations, Advisory Council on African Affairs to host a commemoration on the life and achievements of Jean Baptiste Pointe DuSable. The commemoration is being presented as a symposium entitled "Getting to Know DuSable."

HWC is located just blocks away from Pioneer Court, 401 N. Michigan, where DuSable founded the city. Also DuSable Park is just east of HWC, where the Chicago River meets the Lake.

"This partnership provides a good opportunity for the HWC students and the community to understand that the important aspects of DuSable's legacy are right at their door step and this is just the beginning of the exploration" said Jada Goodlett, Director of Marketing for Friends of DuSable.

Highlights of the event include music and dance presentations by the American Indian Center Drum and Dance Group and Tamboula Haitian Drum & Dance Groups. Special guest panelists will also engage in historical discussions with the attendees. HWC will serve as one of several sites celebrating the life of DuSable, an astute multicultural businessman who was instrumental in the development of Chicago.

Chicago Public Library, the DuSable History Lecture Series

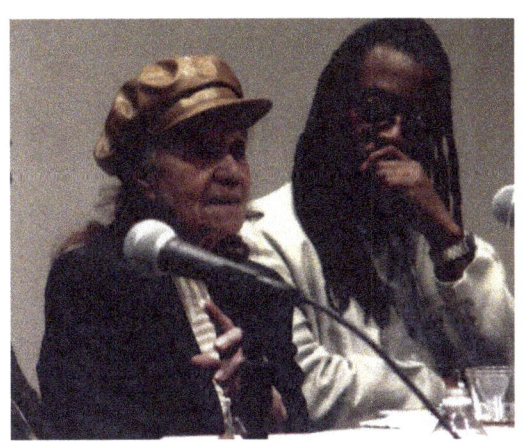

DuSable historian, Dr. Virginia Julian

In 2003, in partnership with the Chicago Public Library, the DuSable History Lecture Series featured notable DuSable historian, Dr. Virginia Julian

During March 2003, the Chicago Public Library celebrated the life of Jean Baptiste Pointe DuSable. Throughout the month, the library featured a variety of programs that highlighted the heritage and contributions of the founder of Chicago. Highlighted Events:

2003 The DuSable Park Coalition

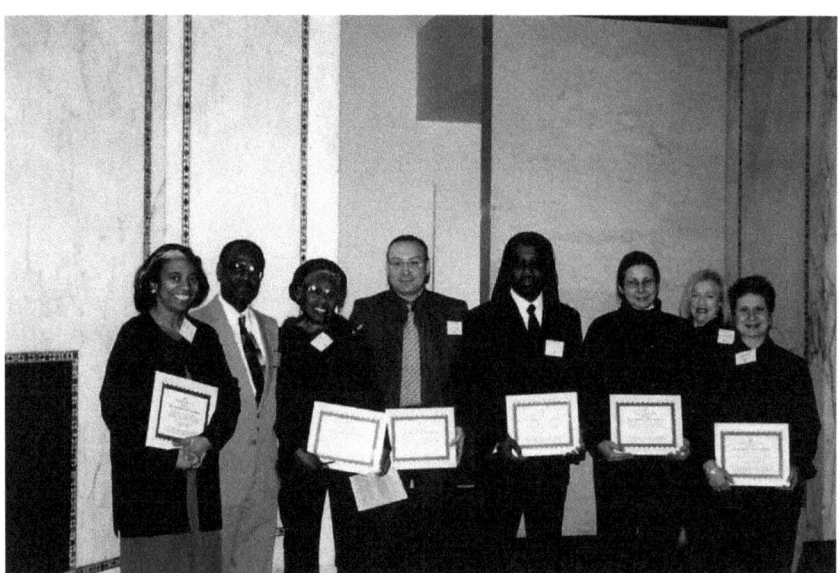

The DuSable Park Coalition Friends of the Parks 2003 Advocacy Award February 6, Left to right: Patricia Holloway, Bronzeville Children's Museum Dr. Serge Pierre-Louis, Association of Haitian Physicians Abroad Bessie Neal, Chicago DuSable League Bob O'Neill, Grant Park Advisory Council Haroon Rashid, Friends of DuSable Susan Urbas, Chicago River Rowing & Paddling Center Eleanor Roemer, Friends of the Parks (presenter) Rosalle Harris, Streeterville Organization for Active Residents.

HISTORY OF DUSABLE PARK

1987 - Dedicated as DuSable Park by Mayor Harold Washington

1998 – Amended Planned Development, including DuSable Park

21st Century:

2000 – Formation of DuSable Park Coalition

2001 – Coalition presents DuSable Park Exhibit and Symposium at the Chicago

Architectural Foundation

2002 - Park remains undeveloped, hidden in plain view

2002 – Coalition meets with public officials and Chicago Park District

2002 - Kerr-McGee commences thorium clean-up, under U.S. EPA U.S. EPA continues to monitor environmental clean-up during park planning process

2002 – Meetings with Artist, Martin Puryear, DuSable Museum, and Chicago

Historical Society

March 19, 2003 – Chicago Park District sponsors Community meeting to begin public process to design and develop DuSable Park

2003 - FOD was approached by other groups to help with their efforts to remember DuSable. One group was working to establish a public park that was designated to be called DuSable Park. This was done under the leadership of former Mayor Harold Washington. Friends of DuSable join in the efforts to complete the erection of the park.

2004 - I was asked to speak at a Chicago Public high school Dunbar High to motivate students; this is the nature of the speech.

DUNBAR HIGH SCHOOL LECTURE:

In The Spirit OF DuSable
Featuring
Haroon Rashid
President/Founder/Friends of DuSable

What is the Millennium Factor?

Reference
    Millennium Factor: American Council for the United Nations University Japan www.acunu.org / futurefoundation.org
    Millennium Project: Logistics Quarterly Magazine volume 5 Dec. 1999 of the Logistic Institute

What are the Definitions for Globalization & Diversity?

Globalization involving the entire earth: worldwide.

Diversity - the fact or quality of being diverse: difference:
    Variety or multiform

I have been studying the effects of society for some time and in one of my searches on the Internet I discovered more information about global changes as it relates to the millennium. How the computer industry in 1999 gave free support to people who had personnel computers to protect them from crashing the first day of 2000. This service was call by Microsoft and others the millennium factor. Also the USA federal government hosted a national and global security watch, based on the so-called millennium factors. Scientists around the world converged at the American council for the United Nations University in Japan and sponsored seminars by global companies and universities like Motorola, Harvard University on the millennium factors. So I feel it is important to tell you in a language that I believe you are intelligent enough to understand. You do not have to agree, just think about it as a possibility. How many of you know what a millennium is and how it is developed?

The year two thousand marked the beginning of what is called the millennium. It is a way of measuring time in civilization. Nineteen ninety-nine ended the way the world would forever be governed, looked at, or judged. Some scientist believes that the old world of so called civilized man agreed, recorded its birth date around the time of Christ, two thousand years ago. It is further believed that mankind, not knowing the rules of governing self with others as he explored the world, created a world of divide. In his quest for power or might among others he developed a fence in, or territorial way of living. That way of life was accepted by global leaders from century after century to systematically program man against man, tribes against tribes, towns against towns, Cities against Cities, States against States, Countries against Countries and Nations against Nations. It became necessary to develop a United Nations as a way to find a civilized solution for Nations to get along.

Math is the only true science. In the language of math there are ten individual numbers -one through ten fractions. When you get to the number ten, it starts all over with a one; of course two ones equal eleven, this is known as the tens. If you continue this method of adding, the fractions become hundreds, or a century in time. Ten one hundreds equal one thousand or a millennium. This cycle is also the method of the measurement of Euro-centric time for the life of mankind, as we know it until now. In nineteen ninety-nine when the number one changed to a two with three zeros behind it; this is what is known as the millennium factor; a century equals one hundred years, so there are ten new centuries to create a new world.

You and I are living in the first decade in the twenty first century. You might ask what does that mean. It means that nothing really matters that happen before two thousand it is a fresh start for every person living to make a difference in the new world. Yes, everything you do today matters, and for the record, you and I are likely to be remembered for at least one hundred years. The first ten to twenty years, these are your youthful years also the critical window of opportunity years for you. Any creditable thing your mind can conceive; you can achieve in this time period.

Computer specialists one hundred years from now will look back to see what you did that was creditable that might seem increditable in that time. That is, of course, if you are able to find what you were born to do, that will complete your ancestors' birthrights of greatness. Otherwise you will likely be forgotten, or erased from history. We believe that every one of you has the potential to succeed and Friends of DuSable, as well as the staff and teachers of Dunbar High, are here to help you fulfill your dreams for success.

So I say to you, if Life is a game, play to win.

My goal is to make my historical mark in the twenty- first century, knowing that whatever I am able to do that is remotely creditable at the beginning of the twenty-first century; I know that it will seem incredible at the end of the first fifty years in the twenty-first century. I believe I must do it for my ancestors and my descendants so that my record is honorable at the beginning of the twenty second century.

So I do all that I do, knowing that I have the spirit of time on my side as we live in the beginning of the second millennium. I believe we are all special people that were born to witness and work in this time, a time of absolute divine change and revelation.

I encourage you and all who live in this special time to step out on faith and do your part in remaking this world community, as a willing instrument of the divine will of the Creator.

2004: The DuSable Founders Way Honorarium

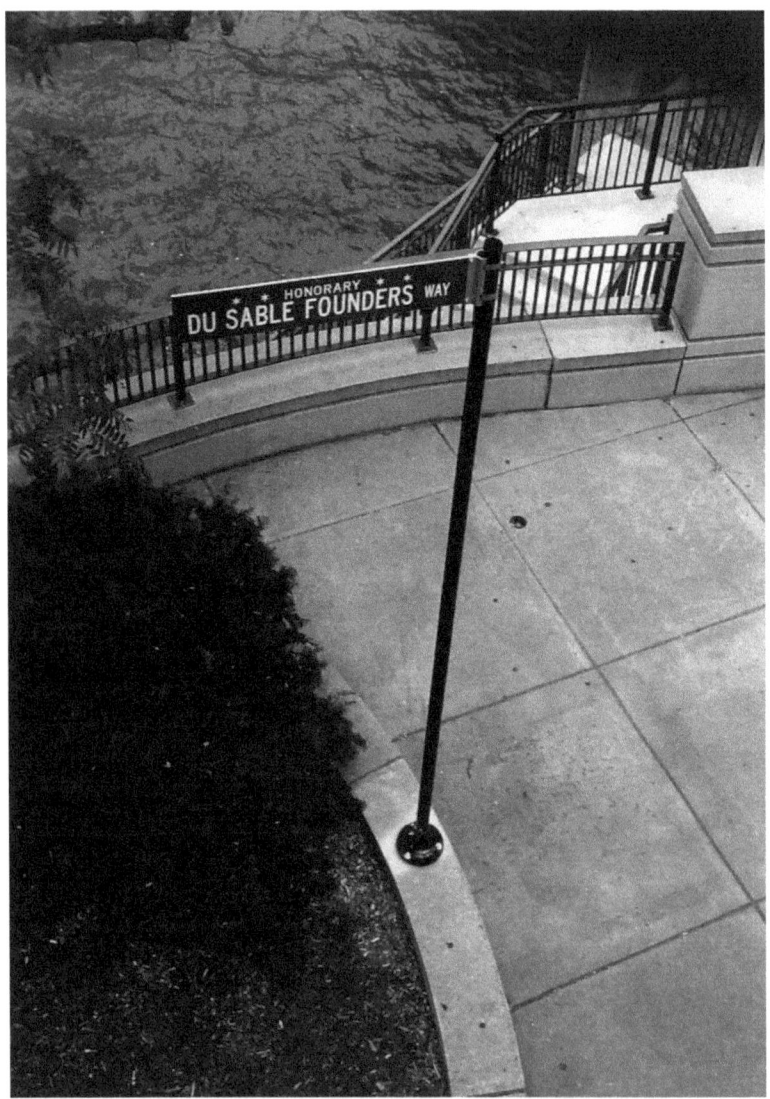

2004 Friends of DuSable along with the DuSable Park coalition and Friends of the Park work with Alderman Burton Natarus of the 42 wards to establish the naming of DuSable Founders Way. It is a strip of the Chicago River walk from the Michigan Avenue DuSable bridge tower to the Lake on the east side of the river.

Friends of DuSable was very fortunate to have established good friends and supporters who believed in what we were doing and that it would make a difference to many in time to come. Lonnie Bunch president of The Chicago Historical Society was one of those friends that guided and advised us in our efforts. He made the usage of the historical Society as a place Friends of DuSable could plan and utilize the facility for our annual celebration of DuSable.

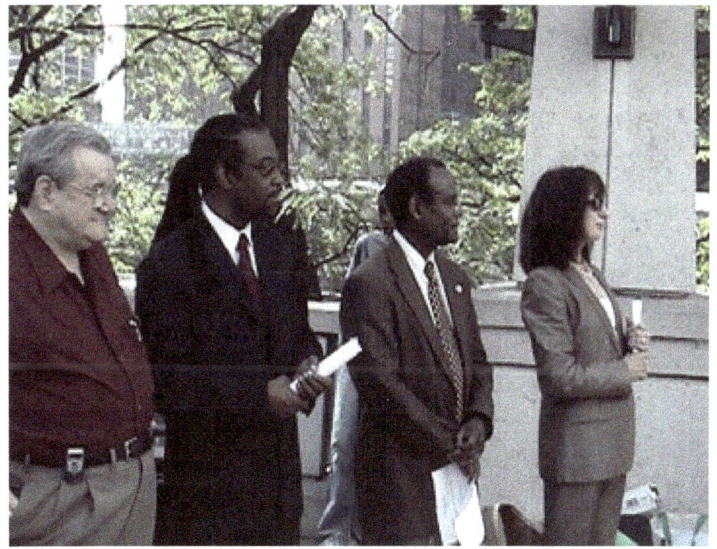

Alderman Burton Natarus, Haroon Rashid, Dr. Serge Pierre-Louis, Erma Tranter

42 Ward Alderman Burton Natarus and the DuSable Park Coalition: introduced and passed an ordinance designating the river esplanade between Pioneer Court and Michigan Ave. on the west end, to the proposed DuSable Park location on the east, as DuSable Founders Way.

The DuSable Park Coalition was represented by Haroon Rashid, President / Founder of Friends of DuSable, Dr. Serge Pierre-Louis President of the DuSable Heritage Association and Erma Tranter President of the Friends of the Park. It was done in conjunction with the Mayor's Office of Special Events, as the City of Chicago celebrates its annual birthday March 4th each year.

In time FOD established a Who's who list of supporters of which without their support none of the accomplishments would have been possible; Dr. Margaret Burroughs, Founder of the DuSable Museum, the City of Chicago Commission on Human Relations

City of Chicago Mayor's Office of Special Events, the City of Chicago Park District Commissioner Timothy Mitchell, the Chicago Historical Society, the United Way Metro Chicago, South African Consulate Chicago, Consulate General of Haiti, Consulate General of France, McCormick Tribune Foundation, Chicago Public Radio, Former Alderman Leonard DeVille, Alderman Burton Natarus, DuSable League,

DuSable Museum, Friends of the Park, City Colleges of Chicago, Chicago Public Schools, Chicago Catholic Schools, Catholic Archdiocese of Chicago, Imam W. D. Mohammed W.D. Mohammed Ministry, Chicago Public Library, Pokagon Band of Potowatomi Indians, Bronzeville Children's Museum, Chicago Tribune Newspaper, Chicago Defender Newspaper, American Indian Center, McGrath Lexus, Chicago Sheraton Hotel, Jessie L. Jackson Jr. U.S. Congress (dist. 2), State Senator Kwame Raoul 13 (dist.), Jessie White Secretary of State , Northwestern University Kellogg Law, Chicago Cultural Affairs Department, American Health & Beauty Aids Institute, Chicago From The Lake, Ltd., Sam's Wine & Liquor Chicago, Architectural and Historical Cruise, The University of Chicago Hospitals , Melanie Span Cooper President WVON radio, Linda Rice Johnson CEO Johnson Publishing Company, the Greater North Michigan Avenue Association, The Chicago Loop Alliances.

2004 Annual DuSable Chicago Founders Day Commemoration

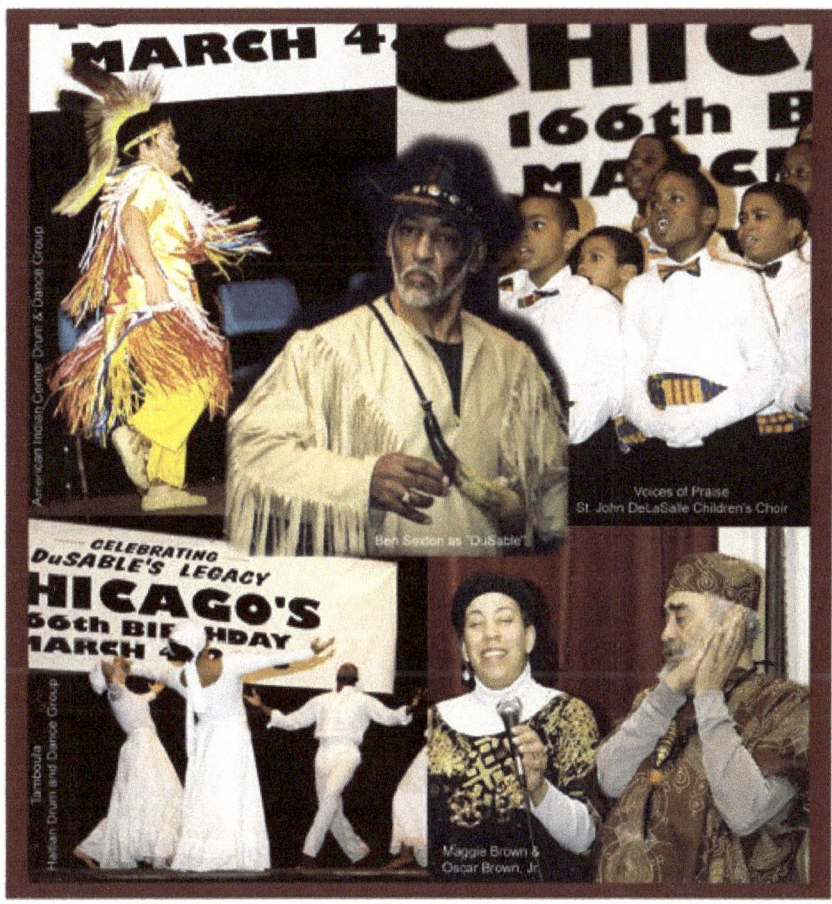

Live Performances by:- Oscar Brown Jr., legendary musician and lyricist, performing a dramatic interpretation of William Goodlett's screenplay highlighting DuSable's life- Maggie Brown, renowned vocalist and Ben Sexton as "DuSable" performing excerpts from Oscar Brown Jr.'s musical "Great Nitty Gritty"- American Indian Center Drum and Dance Group - Tamboula Haitian Drum and Dance Group. - Voices of Praise, St. John De LaSalle Academy of Fine Arts Children's Choir.

Program Supported by: City Colleges of Chicago and the United States Postal Service

The Friends of DuSable is a nonprofit organization, incorporated for the purpose of researching and disseminating the incredible history of Jean Baptiste Pointe DuSable, founder of modern Chicago. In acknowledging the rich and diverse history of the City of Chicago, as well as the great accomplishments of its founder, we have established this citywide commemoration in honor of DuSable. The implementation of the DuSable Commemoration not only serves as a day to honor DuSable, it is a vehicle to bring together communities for a day of unity, in celebration of the origins of the great city we all share.

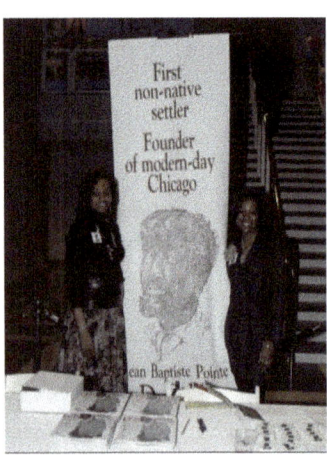

On the right; Erika Summers, Assistant to City of Chicago Mayor Richard M. Daley

Hosted by John Davis, Anchor CBS 2 TV News

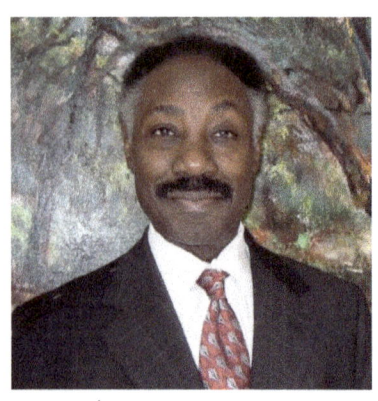

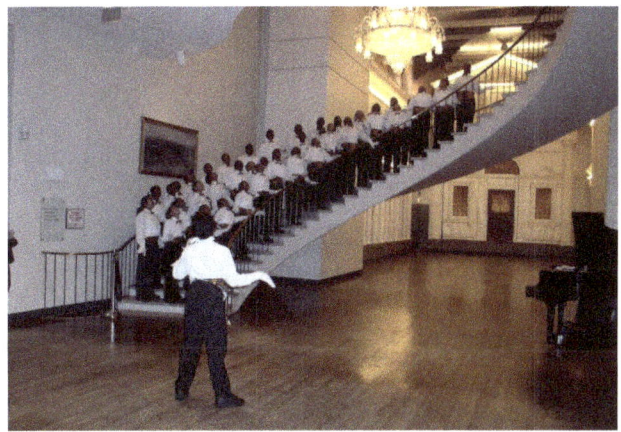

Musical Presentations: Voices of Praise, St. John De LaSalle Children's Choir

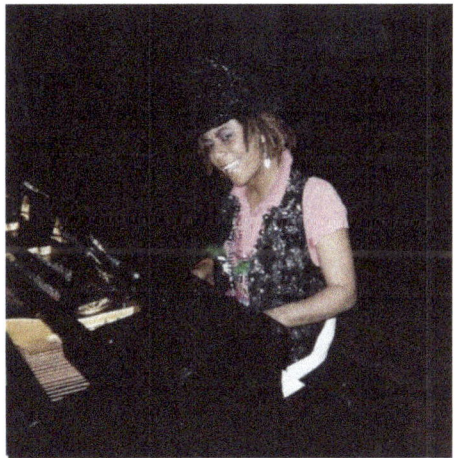

Musical Presentations: Aki Antonia, Jazz Pianist

The Friends of DuSable Second Annual Commemoration Celebration for Jean Baptiste Pointe DuSable: the DuSable Initiative and ensure that the legacy of Jean Baptiste Pointe DuSable is not forgotten.

We were working with the Mayor's Office of Special Events and a collaboration of organizations of like vision organizations to continue an annual Jean Baptiste Pointe DuSable commemoration. This year was the first time the Mayor's Office of Special Events and Friends of DuSable partnered to sponsor the City of Chicago's birthday celebration and our event, Looking Back, March Fourth; The City of Chicago recognized this day as a way to honor Jean Baptiste Pointe DuSable for his accomplishments. This celebration was an overwhelming success.

The Friends of DuSable continued to be a catalyst to bring people and communities together for a day of celebration in the spirit of diversity. With the commitment of supporters, we all agreed to advance toward our dream of making this event a major tourist attraction for the city of Chicago

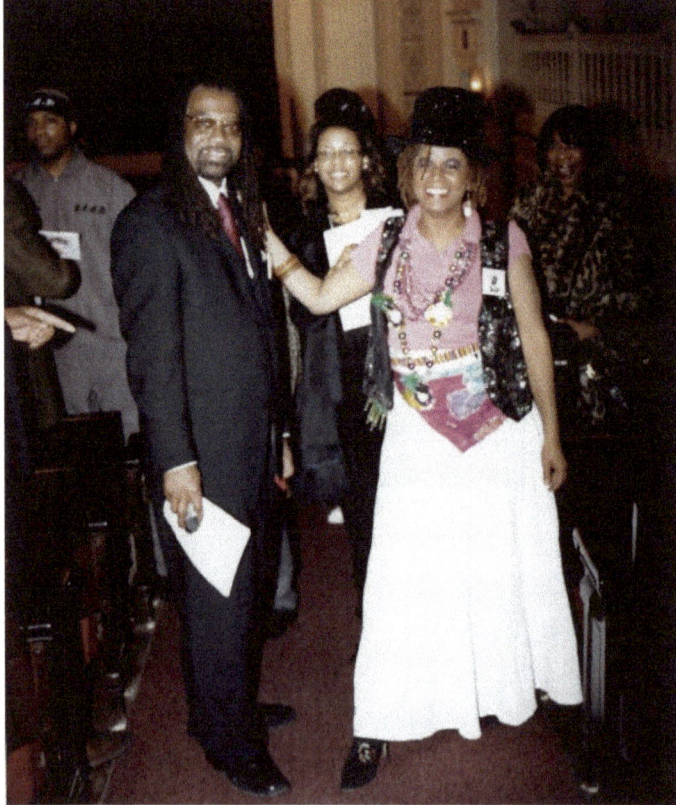

Friends of DuSable board members Haroon Rashid, Jada Goodlet Russell and Aki Antonnia

At this event we had a few of the winning essays read, entitled "How to Celebrate DuSable" in a book, written by Chicago Public and Catholic school students. This contest was implemented by Commission on Human Relations African Advisory Council and Friends of DuSable; the book was published by the Mayor's Office of Special Events.

Also enclosed were program books and the Friends of DuSable t-shirts.

DuSable Founders Day Commemoration & Award Ceremony

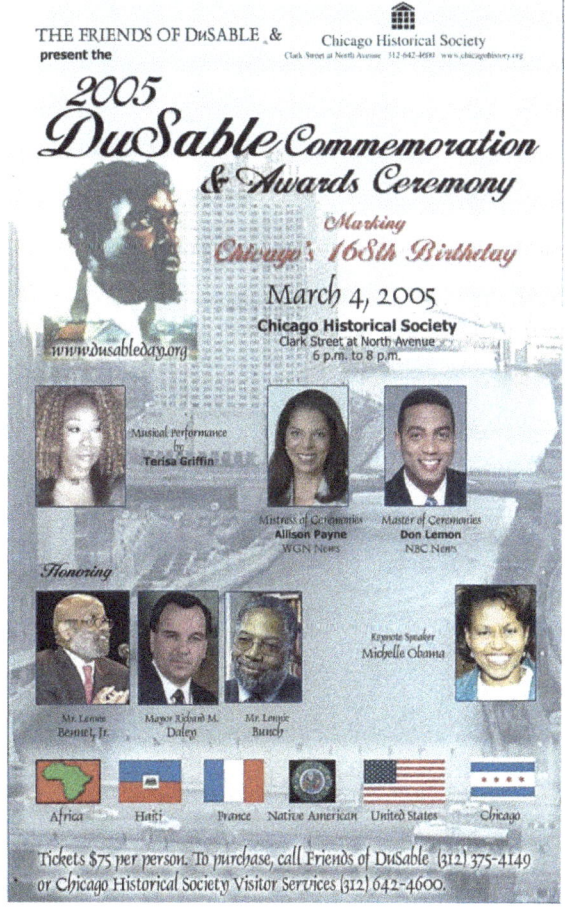

MY CULTURAL BIRTH RIGHTS

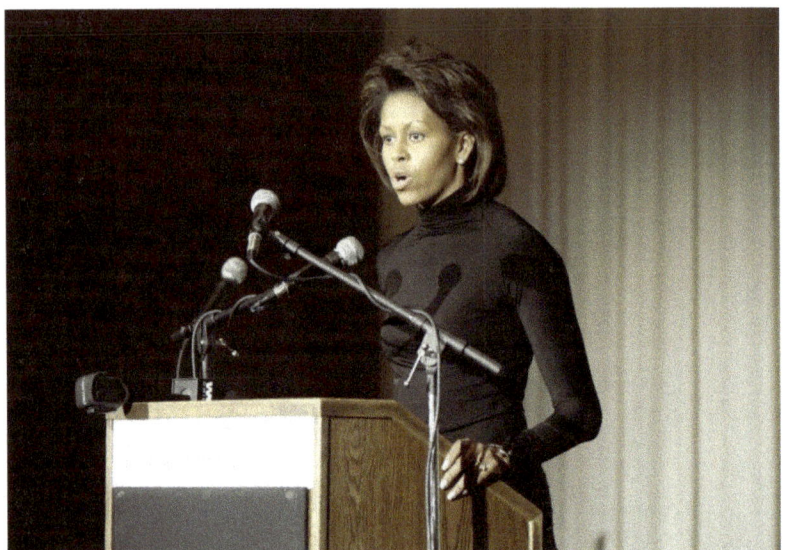

Michelle Obama keynote speaker For the Annual DuSable Commemoration and awards ceremony

On March 3rd 2005 Mrs. Michelle Obama, wife of newly elected Senator Barrack Obama. Mistress and Master of ceremonies were Ms. Allison Payne (WGN TV News) and Mr. Don Lemon (NBC TV News). There were artistic interpretations from all aspects of DuSable's background; including Haitian, French, Catholic, and Native American, and more.

In addition to the event series at the Chicago Cultural Society, the March 3rd 2005 citywide event series expanded from the core programs established in the first year. The City of Chicago shared our vision of a month long effort to celebrate diversity throughout the city of Chicago. Moving forward our programs targeted to bridge the many ethnic and cultural communities and institutions, not only throughout the week, but also for the entire month.

The Mayor's Office of Special events joined with the Friends of DuSable, the Chicago Historical Society, Chicago Department of Cultural Affairs and all of the other 2005 co-sponsors to present a full week of activities throughout Chicago. This partnership was a promise to enhance the citywide recognition of DuSable and would help to forge new relationships throughout the city.

The week began with a variety of activities throughout the city, including the Chicago Historical Society, Bronzeville Children's Museum, DuSable Museum and the American Indian Center, such as: Arts & Crafts Workshops, Lectures, and Films. Winners from the DuSable Essay Competition for grade school students from the Chicago Public Schools and Chicago's Catholic Schools 3rd 4th and 5th grade, which was co-sponsored by the Friends of DuSable and the Commission on Human Relation African Advisory Council, some of the winners read their winning essays as well as ***Cutting the Celebratory Cake*** with Mayor Richard M. Daley.

The week closed at the Chicago Historical Society with a special reception and performance entitled "Celebrating DuSable's Legacy" presented by the Friends of DuSable, also the second "Spirit of DuSable" awards ceremony, featuring keynote speaker:

Friends of DuSable: March 4, 2005 DuSable Founders Day Commemoration & Award Ceremony and the City of Chicago's 168th. Birthday celebration at the Chicago History Museum keynote speaker, **First Lady Michelle Obama** then President of Community Relations at The University of Chicago.

Award recipient of the ***DuSable Leadership award*** was Chicago **Mayor Richard M. Daley.**

MY CULTURAL BIRTH RIGHTS

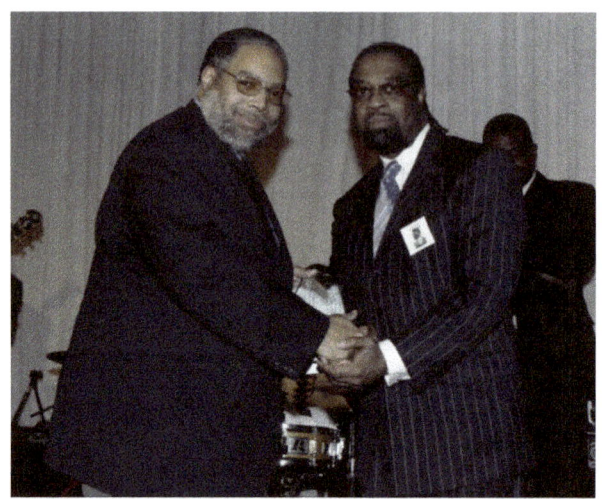

This was Dr. Lonnie Bunch the first and only African American to serve as the President of the Chicago Historical Society before he went on to becoming the first President of the Smithsonian African American History Museum in Washington D.C. receiving the Friends of DuSable, Spirit of DuSable award.

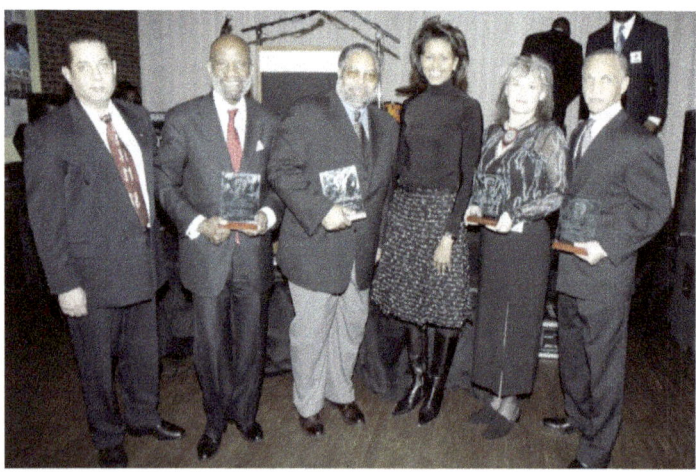

Lesley Conde' Consulate General of Haiti, with "The Spirit of DuSable" award recipients Award "The Power of the Written Word" Lerone Bennett Jr. Journalist Writer, Award "Historical Integrity" Dr. Lonnie Bunch President of the Chicago Historical Society, First Lady Michelle Obama then the President of University of Chicago Hospital Community Relations, Inaugural Award for "Accomplishment In Business" Barbra Jersey President of Native American Financial Consultant Firm and the Inaugural Award "Outstanding Leadership in Government" Mayor Richard M. Daley received by Wayne Watson Chancellor Chicago City Colleges; on behalf of the Mayor.

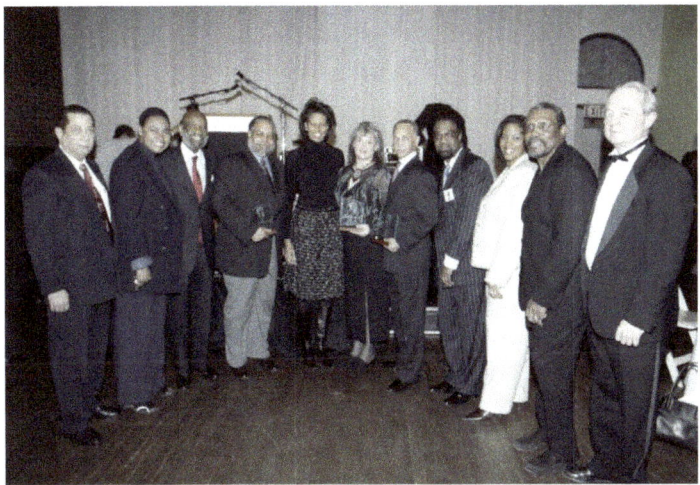

Lesley Conde' Consulate General of Haiti, Elsa Tullos FOD board member, Lerone Bennett Jr. Journalist Writer, Dr. Lonnie Bunch President of the Chicago Historical Society, First Lady Michelle Obama Keynote speaker was then President of The University of Chicago Hospital Community Relations. Barbra Jersey President of Native American Financial Consultant Firm Dr. Wayne Watson Chancellor Chicago City Colleges Haroon Rashid President FOD Andrea Knowles FOD board member Pat Patterson FOD board member Bill Walley FOD board member.

The Jean Baptist Pointe DuSable Founder of The City of Chicago Ordinance

On March 2, 2006 I along with others again testified before Chicago City Council to encourage them to pass a city ordinance that declared all citizens to Commemorate Jean Baptiste Pointe DuSable on and during the city's official Birthday celebration March 4th. This time it was passed unanimously.

Even though we had an ordinance, it was passed without a city mandate. So a year later FOD with the help of the Human Relations Committee for City Council, chaired by Alderman Billy Occasio to organize a public hearing, in the DuSable African American History Museum. The purpose was to have opened public dialog with leaders and citizens to give testimony before the city council that encouraged a DuSable resolution that gave mandate to the DuSable ordinance. One month later the resolution that was drafted by Chicago Commission on Human Relations African Advisory Council, in which I was a proud member, was voted on and approved by a unanimous decision.

That enactment will always be one of the premier actions in Chicago History, wherein it carries along with it a resolution that gives a mandate that all citizens, schools, colleges and universities, businesses, organizations, associations and religious institutions should find ways to commemorate the founder of Chicago Jean Baptiste Pointe DuSable on the city of Chicago's birthday, March 4th each year. After that the ordinance was permanently united into the annual city of Chicago Birthday celebrations.

HAROON RASHID

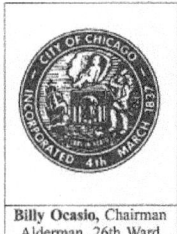

Billy Ocasio, Chairman
Alderman, 26th Ward

—— City of Chicago ——
Committee on Human Relations
121 North LaSalle Street
3rd Floor, City Hall, Room 300
Chicago, Illinois 60602
(312) 744-6853
Fax (312) 744-2766
Email: bocasio@cityofchicago.org

April 17th, 2006

Haroon Rashid
Friends of DuSable
200 N. Dearborn
Suite 1802
Chicago, IL 60601

Dear Mr. Rashid:

It's with great honor that I enclose two certified copies of the ordinance recognizing Jean Baptiste Pointe DuSable as the City Founder of the City of Chicago.

The ordinance, sponsored by nine (9) Aldermen including myself, passed unanimously by the City Council on March 1st, 2006. It represents an official acknowledgement of DuSable's ethnic, economic and cultural contributions through his unparallel leadership and admirable determination.

On behalf of the Human Relations Committee, we congratulate civic leaders like yourself, elected officials, the general public and the organizations involved in making this ordinance a reality.

Should you have any questions or need any assistance, please contact our office at 312-744-6853.

Sincerely,

Billy Ocasio
Chairman
Human Relations Committee

"Henceforth, the ethical motto shall be *live and help to live* rather than *live and let live*."
Alderman Billy Ocasio, 26th Ward

A Cruise for DuSable

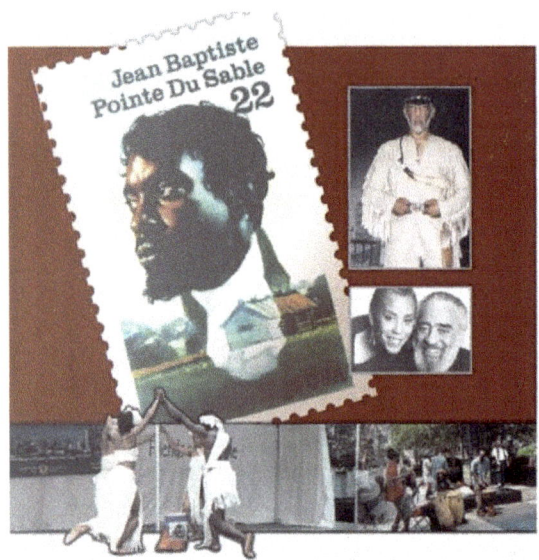

Second Annual Unity Cruise & Fundraiser   "A Success"!!!

Friends Of DuSable NFP: is very pleased by the warm reception it received at the DuSable Unity Cruise and Fundraiser on October 11, 2007. FOD received such welcomed support in favor of the DuSable Welcome Center from all of the prestigious individuals who attended. Such support at the event compelled FOD President, Haroon Rashid to say:

"That the time for honoring Chicago's Founder in this way, has finally come." *He goes on to say that, honoring DuSable in such a way gives recognition to all those who came before and after the Founder of this great city.*

FOD would like to thank all of the individuals who attended

the cruise and ask for your continued support. FOD is aware that a project of this size will require the assistance of many, which essentially requires the need for funding. Our organization relies solely on your contributions. For information on how to make a contribution please call our office at: (312) 375-4149 or email us at: dusable2001@yahoo.com.

Friends of DuSable NFP (FOD) **Second Unity Month Dinner Discussions Will Be An Evening Boat Cruise, Departing from the Chicago River on the Original Settlement Sight Of Chicago's Founder, Jean Baptiste Pointe DuSable .** This year's networking will consists of a pre-event VIP Reception at a River Chicago Restaurant before departure, followed by a Gala Banquet Dinner on the Historical Wendella Boat Cruise line; as well as a tour guide of Chicago waterways and culminating with an after-Party at a popular Chicago Jazz Night Club. The theme of discussions is about Chicago's past and present as a City developed in diversity by immigrants and business pioneers like Chicago's Founder Jean Baptist Pointe DuSable. The DuSable Unity Day Cruise will be focusing on the Continuance of that unique Spirit in today's Chicago growing global community. The program includes elements supplied by FOD that recognize the role DuSable played in welcoming a very diverse group of settlers and traders to Chicago in the 1780's and 1790's.

The event will be taped and broadcast, on a tape delay basis, by Columbia College School of Media and Visual Arts and will be viewed on Chicago Public Television Cable Network channels in over 1.5 million homes. Chicago's most noted celebrities, as well as political, business, cultural and community leaders will be in attendance.

Sponsors and supporters will be recognized at all of the above events through program listings, announcements and appropriate signage. Event publicity, including press releases will also include recognition of major sponsors.

There is a sponsorship and supporters package under cover of this letter that details the levels of sponsorship available with corresponding benefits. I thank you in advance for your time and consideration.

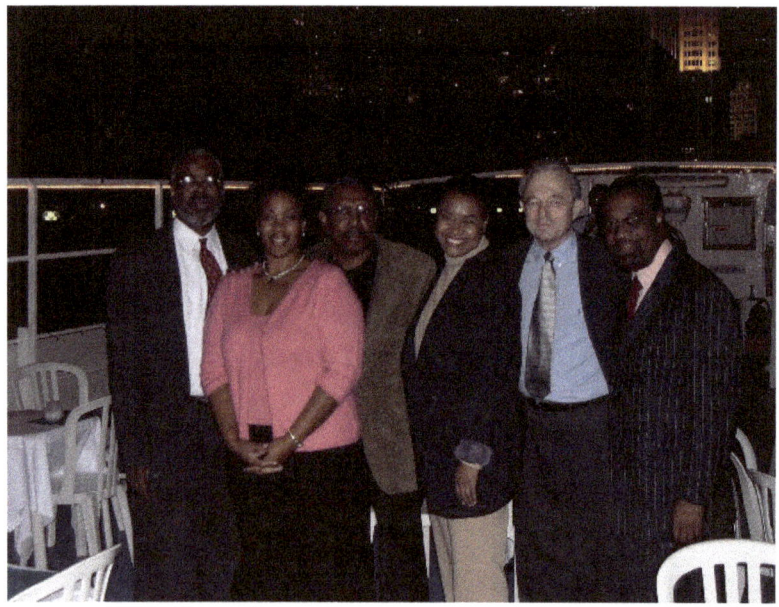

"All Aboard"! Friends of DuSable Executive Board members Arnold Romeo, Andréa Knowles, Pat Patterson, Elsa Tullos, William Walley and Haroon Rashid

The brand new *Wendella MV* for the Second Annual Unity Cruise and Fundraiser, hosted by Friends of DuSable (FOD). This year's cruise featured the unveiling of a proposed new Welcome Center commemorating Chicago's Founder, Jean Baptiste Pointe DuSable. The cruise departed at around 6, but prior to departure Aldermen Brendan Reilly (42nd) and Walter Burnett (27th) spoke great volumes in support of the proposed Welcome Center. The Aldermen both exited for other scheduled events and the cruise was blessed with prayer by Reverend Green of Pleasant

Ridge M.B.C. Bill Walley/Treasurer & Haroon Rashid/President both of FOD spoke and introduced some of the distinguished guests that were on board. The first to speak on behalf of the DWC was Chicago History Museum President, Gary Johnson. Following Mr. Johnson was Phil Levin, Planning Director/Greater North Michigan Avenue Association. He welcomed FOD and the DWC to the neighborhood and is looking forward to assisting in any way possible. Antoinette Wright of The DuSable Museum was in favor of the Welcome Center, as well. Bob O'Neill President of the Grant Park Conservancy was also in attendance and seemed to be the most inquisitive of the guests that evening. Ty Tabing, Executive Director/Chicago Loop Alliance said that the DWC is going to be a place that will be supported from his organization. After the guests gave their say, Jack Kelley and Greg Battoglio of McBride Kelley Baurer Architects, presented the drawings and conducted the presentation. As they spoke of the DWC the cruise headed eastward towards DuSable Park. The park is instrumental in the development of the DWC, as it will be the eastern most point of the river walk. Bill Walley discussed the significance of the park and how key the developmental process is. As the cruise toured downriver, there was a question and answer session that took place. Everyone had great questions pertaining to the development of the DWC.

Overall the cruise was a great success and everyone onboard showed an unbelievable amount of support. Everyone who attended seemed to have an appreciation for the Welcome Center and want to aide in any way possible.

Others in attendance were: Arnold Romeo, Advisory Council of African Affairs, Commission on Human Relations; Rob Rejman, Chicago Park District/Director Lakefront Construction; The Haitian Consul; and Sarah Fleming/Planning Manager, Greater North Michigan Avenue Association.

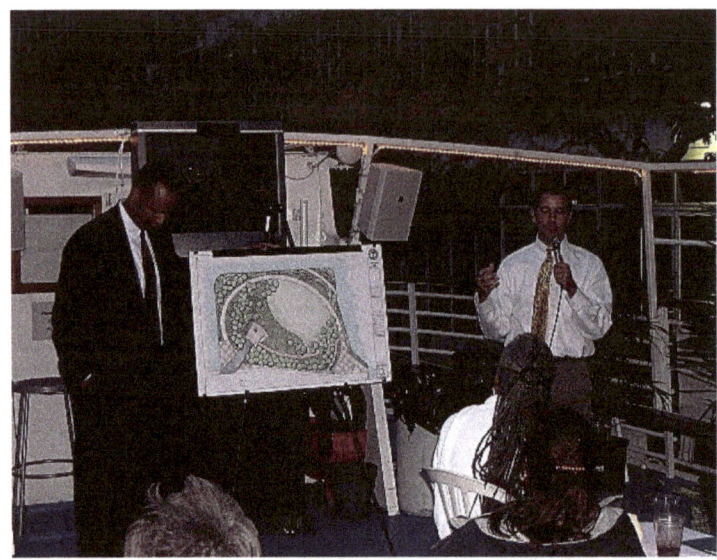

Presentation from the city of Chicago Park Districts and the Chicago Department of Transportation: on a schematic plan to build the DuSable Park and the DuSable Heritage Corridor.

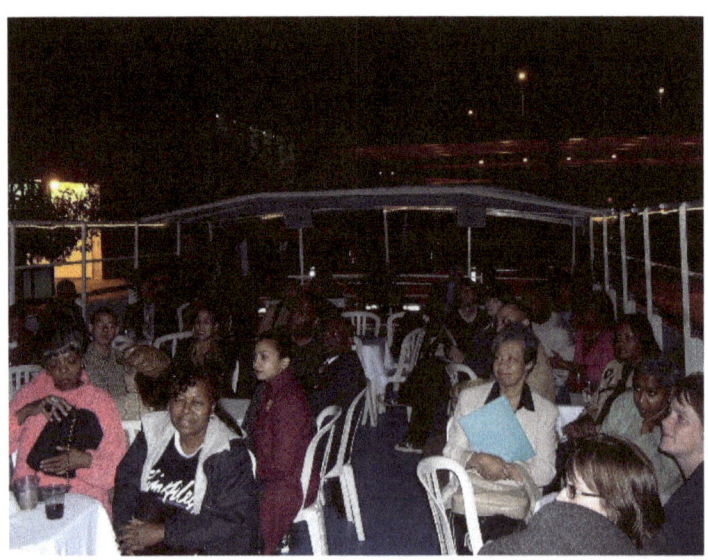

Second Annual Unity Cruise & Fundraiser "Was A Success"!!!

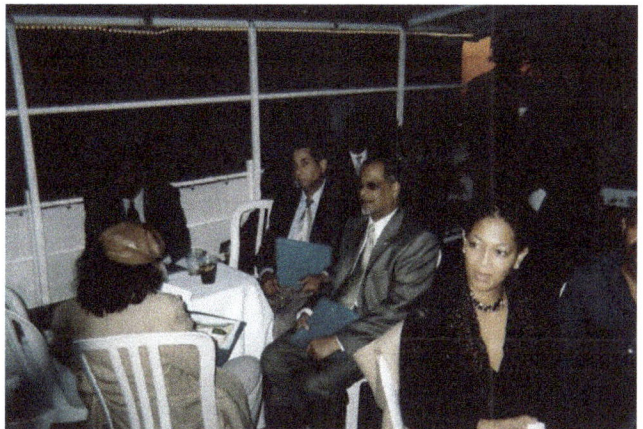

FOD international partners table on the left in the center was Chicago Haitian Consulate General Lesley Conde and Haitian delegates, on the right table from South African representative was Ms. Mbali Mncwabe.

Friends of DuSable NFP: was very pleased by the warm reception it received at the DuSable Unity Cruise and Fundraiser on October 11, 2007. FOD received such a welcomed support in favor the DuSable Welcome Center from all of the prestigious individuals who attended. Such support at the event compelled FOD President, Haroon Rashid to say:

FOD would like to thank all of the individuals who attended the cruise and offered their continued support. FOD was aware that a project of this size that we were committed to do would require the assistance of many, which essentially required the advocating for our DuSable legacy mission. That type of progressive outreaching was instrumental in eventually the lobby successes of the newly elected Alderman of the 42 Ward Brendan Reilly to continue the support of FOD missions.

2008 DuSable Harbor Boathouse Ribbon Cutting

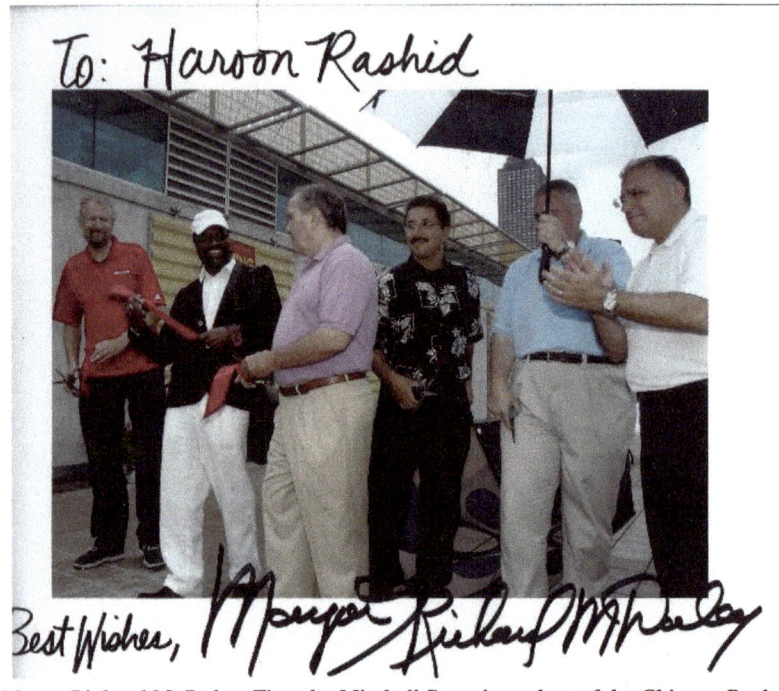

Mayor Richard M. Daley, Timothy Mitchell Superintendent of the Chicago Park District and Haroon Rashid, Friends of DuSable cut the ribbon to officially open the DuSable Harbor Dock and Rest House.

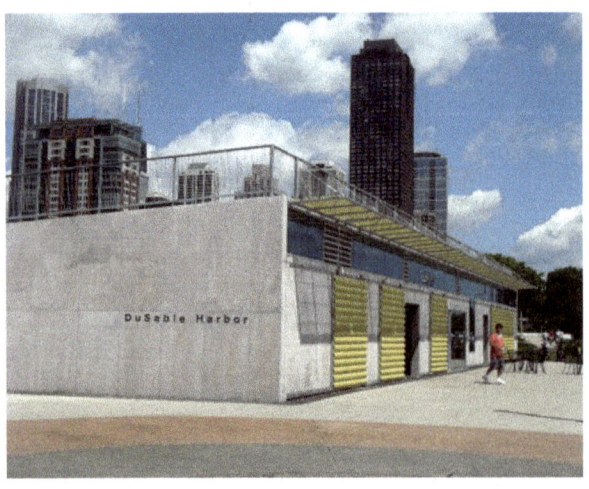

The DuSable Harbor Boat House on the Lake Michigan walkway at DuSable Harbor

In 2008 I was asked by the Mayor's Office of Special Events to participate in the official Ribbon Cutting ceremony to represent the DuSable Park Coalition, the group of private public principles that was responsible for the enactment that lobbied for the continuum of the proposed DuSable Heritage Corridor development plan.

The structural and demographical components of the targeted area included The DuSable Founders Way, the Chicago River Walk on the northeast side of the river from the Michigan Avenue DuSable Bridge to the designated DuSable Park area located just before Lake Michigan. Then on the south side of the Chicago River from the DuSable Bridge to the DuSable Harbor on the far southeast end of the Chicago River and Lakeshore Drive. This area was considered by members of the DuSable Park Coalition as a historical heritage landmark that should be honored as such.

DuSable Bronze Bust Erection Ceremony

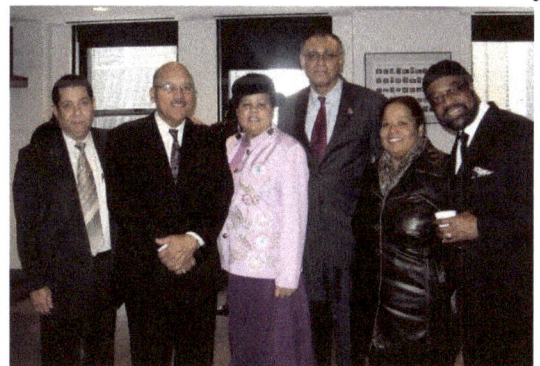

Participants in the honorary DuSable Bust ceremony: Lesley Conde' Consulate General of Haiti, Mr. Lesley Benodin, Ms. Aliette Marcelin, Mr. Harry Fouche, Haitian supporter and Haroon Rashid.

What a great day for the Magnificent Mile! A bust of Jean Baptiste Pointe DuSable, the founder and first businessman of the city of Chicago, was donated by Mr. Lesly Benodin, a Haitian-American businessman who has lived in Chicago for the past forty years. The monument also recognizes the vibrant presence of the Haitian American community in the city today.

The bronze sculpture was received by the Department of Cultural Affairs on behalf of the city, and on Friday, October 16th, city officials, dignitaries, activists, and Chicagoans at large rejoiced in celebration of the historical dedication. The day was of special significance to Mrs. Bessie Neal, the 89-year-old former president of the DuSable League, whose group has been advocating a life-like statue of DuSable since 1928.

Haroon Rashid, founder and president of the Friends of DuSable (NFP) and a member of the Greater North Michigan Avenue Association, said that he was pleased that the language on the monument reflects the city's official acknowledgment of Pointe DuSable as the founder of Chicago. The Friends of DuSable partnered with the Chicago Commission on Human Relations African Advisory Council to co-author the city's DuSable Commemoration Ordinance. Mr. Rashid further expressed gratitude for Alderman Brendan Reilly's (42nd Ward) support and demonstration of civic leadership in his bid to pass through City Council a resolution renaming the Michigan Avenue Bridge the "Jean Baptiste Pointe DuSable Bridge." Special gratitude is also extended to Mr. Harry Fouche of Chicago and Ms. Aliette Marcelin of Evanston, who provided much-needed logistical assistance with the monument.

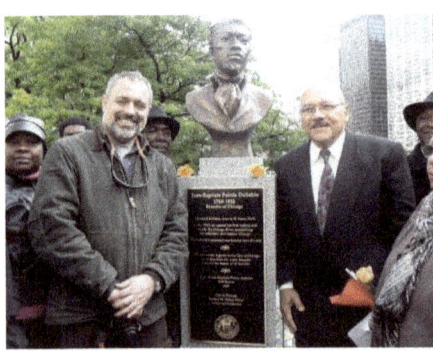

Mr. Erik Blome, and Mr. Lesley Benodin

The Jean Baptiste Pointe DuSable Bronze Sculpture was designed and installed by artist Mr. Erik Blome, in the location of Pioneer Court next to the DuSable Bridge.

The monument was given to the City of Chicago by Haitian-born, Mr. Lesley Benodin, to honor the legacy of its founder.

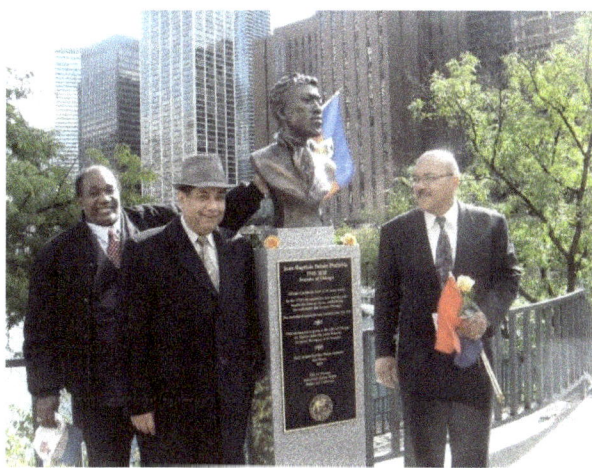

Lesley Conde'
Consulate General of
Haiti, Mr. Lesley
Benodin

DuSable Bridge Naming Ceremony

The Michigan
Avenue DuSable
Bridge

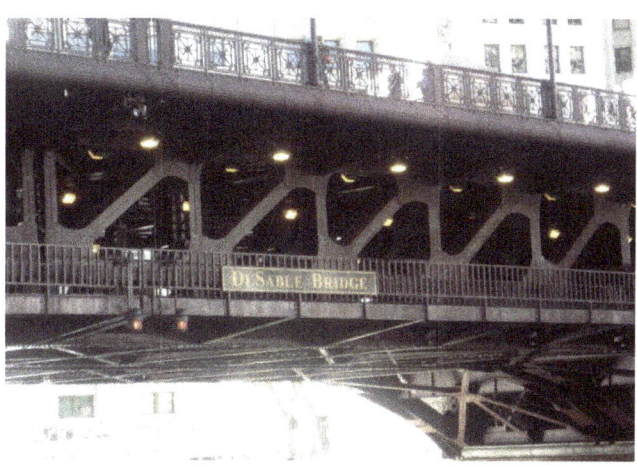

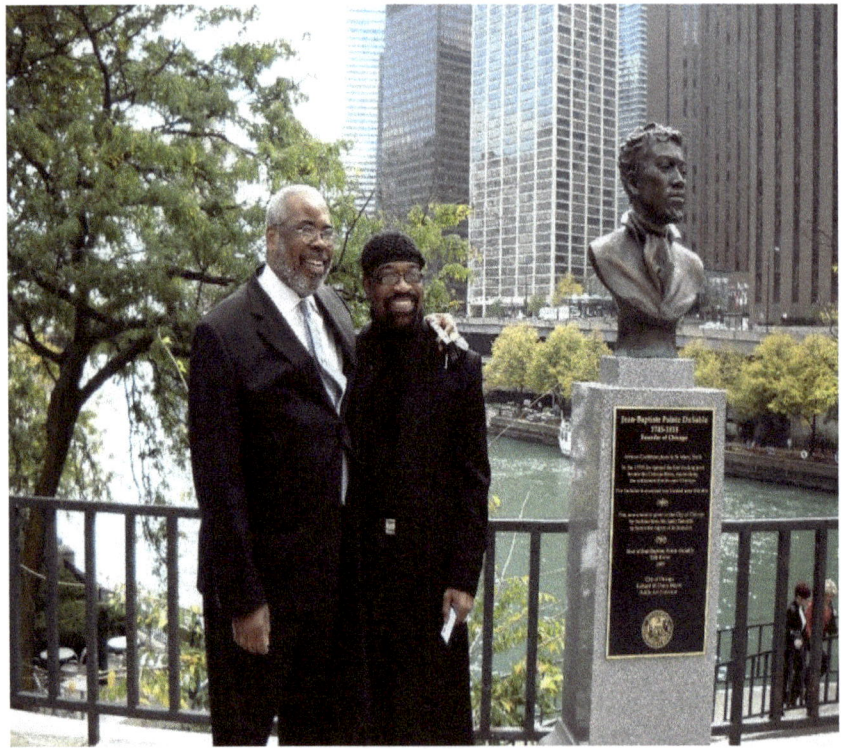

Arnold Romeo: Director of Commission on Human Relations Advisory council of African Affairs and Haroon Rashid.

October 15, 2010 Friends of DuSable encouraged the city of Chicago Department of Transportation to post signs on the Michigan Avenue Bridge and street to rename it The DuSable Bridge in honor of Chicago's first permanent resident, Jean Baptiste Pointe DuSable. An ordinance was introduced by 42 Ward Alderman Brendan Reilly and passed by the Chicago City Council in 2009 for the DuSable Bridge dedication. The ordinance was the result of years of advocacy by the Friends of DuSable Coalition and the greater Chicago Haitian American leadership. This is a copy of that enactment that went into law through the lobbying of the Chicago City Council that was introduced by BRENDAN REILLY, Alderman - 42nd Ward in the form of a City Ordinance.

Authority Granted To Rename Michigan Avenue Bridge: To "Jean Baptiste Pointe Du Sable Bridge".

WHEREAS, The City of Chicago is justifiably proud of its rich cultural and ethnic heritage; its rapid ascent from frontier trading post to major commercial, cultural and education center; and its place among the world's great cities; and

WHEREAS, Du Sable became the first permanent, non-native settler of Chicago when he built a cabin on the north bank of the Chicago River, at the current site of the Tribune Tower; and

WHEREAS, Du Sable became Chicago's first real estate developer and builder in about 1773, when he established a settlement for himself, his wife and about one hundred other Potawatomi; built a trading post; established a dairy farm; and planted fruit orchards and fields of corn, hay and alfalfa; and

WHEREAS, shortly after establishing the settlement, Du Sable established Chicago's character as a haven to immigrants, when one hundred French Canadians arrived seeking refuge from the British and Spanish armies; and

WHEREAS, The Chicago settlement founded by Jean Baptiste Pointe Du Sable was characterized by racial, ethnic and cultural harmony and mutual respect among its diverse inhabitants; and

WHEREAS, in 1833, the Du Sable settlement, with three hundred fifty residents, was incorporated as the Town of Chicago; and

WHEREAS, On March 4, 1837, Du Sable's settlement had grown to four thousand one hundred seventy inhabitants and was reincorporated as the City of Chicago; and

WHEREAS, DuSable is such an important part of Chicago History that DuSable High School was dedicated in 1934 and the Du Sable Museum of African American History and DuSable Harbor are named in his honor; and

WHEREAS, the State of Illinois and City of Chicago declared DuSable the Founder of Chicago on October 26, 1968; and

WHEREAS, It is appropriate that the City of Chicago, in so many ways influenced by the activities, efforts and accomplishments of its first non-native settler, recognize and celebrate Jean Baptiste Pointe Du Sable as its founder; now, therefore,

Be *It **Resolved**,* That we, the Mayor and the members of the City Council of the City of Chicago, do hereby state that the name of the Michigan Avenue Bridge be changed to Jean Baptiste Pointe du Sable Bridge as a memento of the high esteem in which he is held.

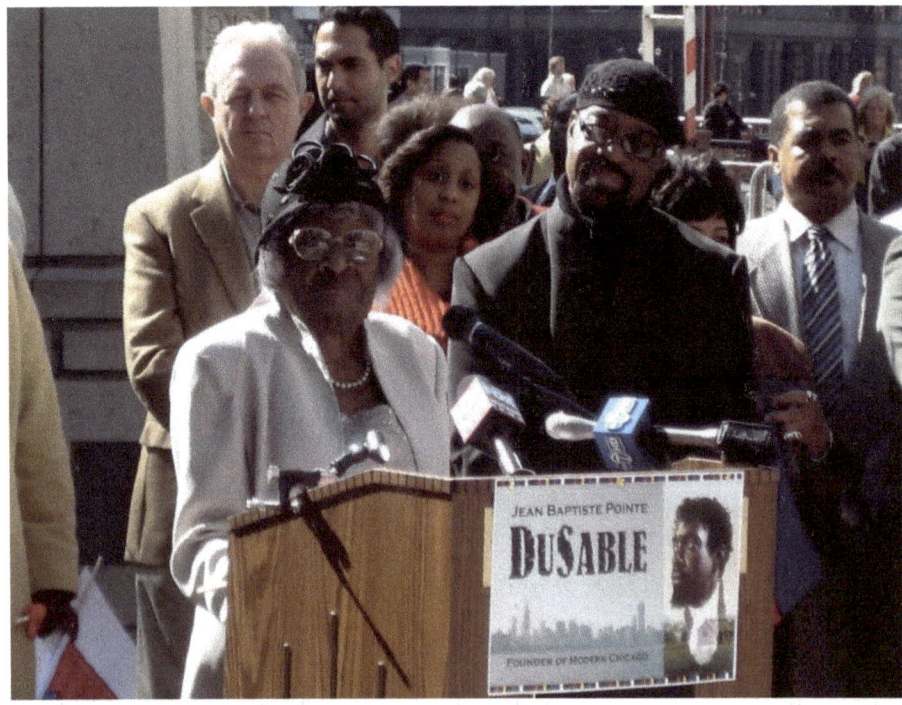

Keynote Speaker Mrs. Bessie L. Neal President of the DuSable League

October 15, 2010
By Alejandra Cancino, Tribune reporter

Alice J. Neal devoted her life to having a street in downtown Chicago named after Jean Baptiste Pointe DuSable, a black man known as the city's first non-native settler. But she died before DuSable had a citywide recognition.

On Friday, her daughter-in-law, Bessie Neal stood before politicians and leaders of various organizations at the ceremony to officially rename the Michigan Avenue Bridge as the DuSable Bridge. It isn't a street, but it is a Chicago landmark.

"Anything that is no trouble to you is no good to you," said Neal, who celebrated her 90th birthday in February. "You are going to have to have some ups and downs; I don't care what it is. And I believe that we had some ups and downs before we got this, but we are proud that we got it."

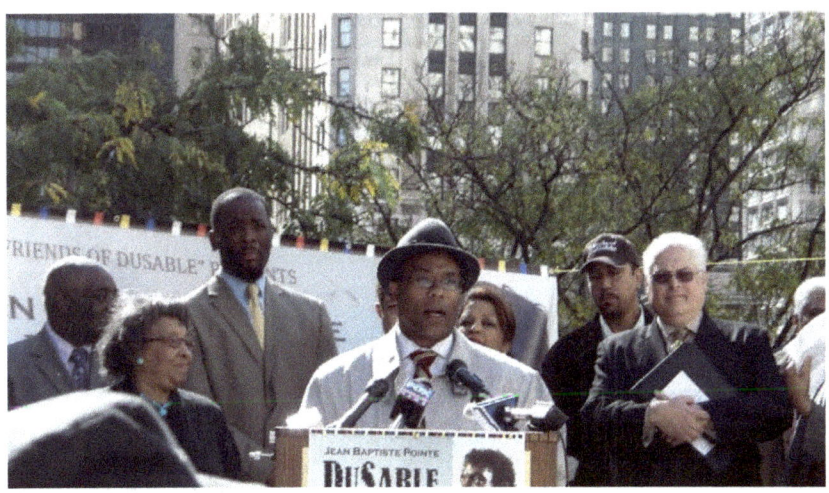

Alderman 24 Ward Walter Burnett & Chairman of the Aldermanic Black Caucus

Alderman Burnett giving a heartfelt speech, talking about the long awaited ambitions of the Black Caucus to do something like the DuSable Bridge enactment that would be a permanent monumental visible sign of the pride of Chicagoans' city Founder Jean Baptiste Pointe DuSable, glorious roots and legacy.

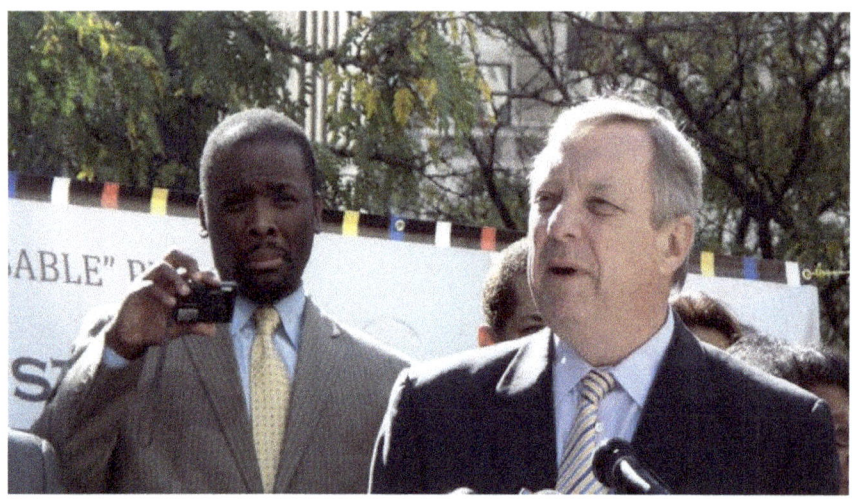

Mr. Patrick Brutus videotaping Illinois: United State Senator Richard Durban speech

The DuSable bridge ceremony drew out the leadership of Chicago and the State of Illinois to partake in the historical enactment. State Senator Richard Durban was in attendance as an honorary speaker to give his support and acknowledgment for the historical renaming of the Michigan Avenue Bridge to the DuSable Bridge located in the heart of Chicago. In the background of the picture is Mr. Patrick Brutus who was then President of the Chicago Haitian American Association.

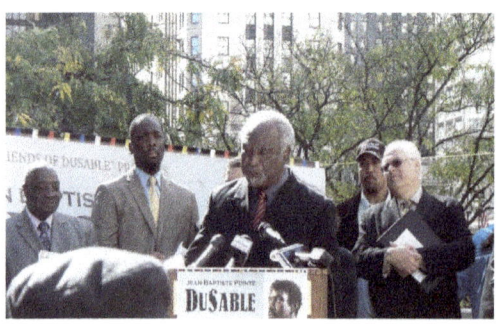

Douglas Pendarvis Vice President of Friends of DuSable, Patrick Brutus Kyle Obllski Public relation Friends of DuSable and John Chicow Ex-Officio President/CE: the Magnificent Mile Association

Long time supporter of Friends of DuSable efforts to preserve the legacy of DuSable United States Illinois Congressman Danny Davis was a key speaker on the efforts to commemorate DuSable in the State of Illinois.

US Postal Envelope

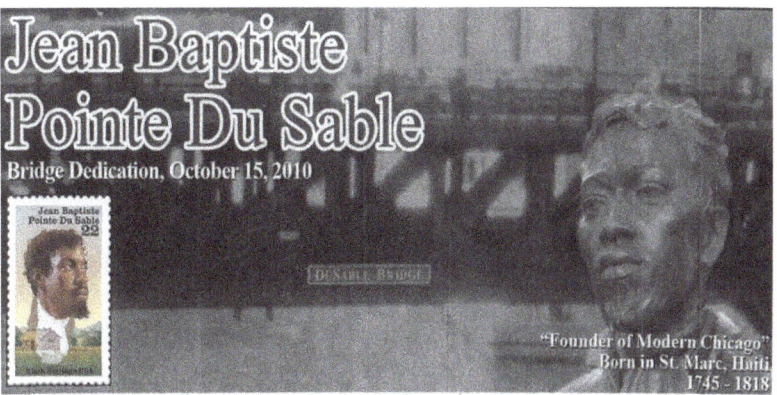

Friends of DuSable: the DuSable Coalition and the United States Postal Services collaborated and partnered in the creation of an honorary DuSable Bridge envelope as a way of instituting a Federal level of importance to the DuSable Bridge dedication October 15, 2010:

I most certainly have lived a Blessed life!

Love is the proper name and character of The Most High, The All & All, and Master of The Universe, and there is only one race, the Human Race existing together as Human Beings. Anything that will attempt to replace that reality is a distraction or an illusion.

Haroon Abdullah Rashid

Part Three

**African American Hair & Beauty Industry:
The Other Black Gold**

Chapter Twenty
Knowledge Is Power

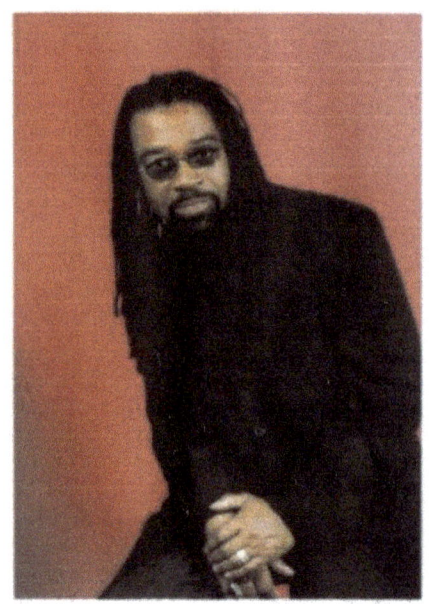

HAROON RASHID SOCIAL ACTIVIST, MASTER HAIR STYLIST AND EDUCATOR

As we all know or should know the African American Hair and Beauty industry has been one of the most lucrative legal economical markets and revenue streams in the African American communities. It has been estimated that the potential buying power in the African American community is somewhere between 300 to 400 billion dollars per year. With that amount of money, it is a common question often asked in the African American community, *where do all the moneys go?* Or simply, where is the money? It is believed by many that we wear it, eat it, drive it or live in it. There has always been economical waste of money in the African American community, partly because of an instinctive desire to be perceived of as ***making it*** or ***moving on up!*** Like the television sitcom version of the Jefferson's theme song says, (**we're moving on up to the top on a deluxe apartment in the Bronx**). This is a direct link to the unhealed psychological fallout of being deprived during slavery conditions of the basic natural human developments of success that a free sovereign citizen simply expects this human to be right because of their sovereignty in America. The reason that African

Americans have been the major target group for marketing of material valuables by the media industry examples; sports, fashion, music, theater, movie or television, basically the field of entertainment, and synthetic products of sensations and pleasure i.e. alcohol, drugs, etc. Unfortunately, this is where too much of our money and potential wealth is spent. The great African American Historian Dr. Carter Woodson in his book **Mis-Education of the Negro;** Dr. Woodson was the first African American to Graduate from Harvard University with a Doctorial degree. In his book he said that when he compared the education of the Negro for higher education to whites he could see it taking on two different meanings and purposes. He said that in his days at Harvard when a white person seeks education most of them were there to gain knowledge to further a project or purpose in their family business or to improve their community. They were connected to their education for a greater cause than a diploma, degree or a job, unlike the Negro. Whites most likely had ambitions to use their education to build or better their own business. On the other hand, most African Americans going to the same school were content to get a diploma with a high degree status that gave them a Sir-title to shop for a so-called good job. He used the example of the Doctors Degree in education; there was no such thing until the USA government agreed to allow African Americans to become presidents or to run one of the select number of Negro Colleges provided by the government. Atlanta University, Morehouse College, Spellman College, Howard University, Fisk University, Tuskegee University, etc.

Not surprisingly, before there became a law that all Negroes seeking the job of a President for a higher institution, they must go back to school and receive a new Doctorial Degree in Education. There was never such a requirement for this type of degree for the white Presidents of Negro colleges, not even for the White colleges that until then and after they presided in those capacities. This new challenge was placed on the Negro after they lobbied the government to allow them as African American educated leaders with Masters Degrees in education to govern these institutions. The President of USA and the government instituted a doctorial degree requirement in Education that only the Negro had to have in order to get the same job that many whites did not need to run the same Schools, not even after the law for the Negro was instituted.

When you think about it, all of this mental excitement that this caused among African Americans' brightest minds in those days just to get a job or training when education is supposed to prepare you to help yourself and others, training prepares you to do a job. Too often the so-called Negro forgets why they were brought to America, it was to work and do a job willingly or unwillingly that was all we as a people were brought here to do. Not govern ourselves and or to be equal with white Americans, which was never in the plans of the original planners or framers in America. Like General Electric, Ford Motors, Sears and Roebuck, the so-called Negro was a product made in America to make others comfortable or rich from our good work. As Dr. Carter Woodson said the Doctorial Degree in education was an attempt to misseducate us from doing for ourselves and staying under the watchful eyes of the so-called Masters training. The irony of that is the so-called Negro leaders did well in the presiding over those schools, in spite of the cynical attempt of the powers at that time to manipulate the race of misguided people by being taught by their former slave masters. Because of the attempt to MissEducate the Negro into psychological dependence, a new criteria or bench mark for higher Education - Doctors Degree - for all has now been accepted as today's standard; we turned water into wine. God makes a plan then the Devil makes a plan, but God is the best of planners.

"The American Hair Beauty & Wellness Credit Union"

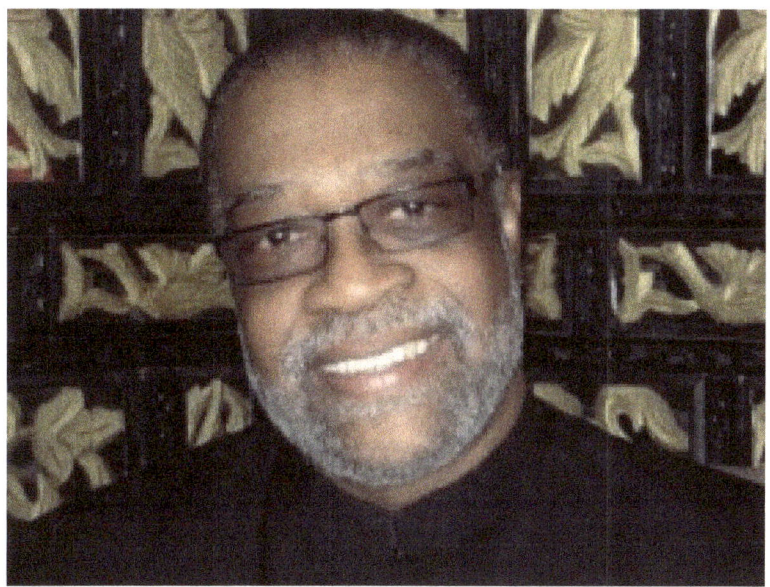

HAROON RASHID - SOCIAL & CULTURAL ACTIVIST

This plan to help address the hair and beauty industries number one histaminic problem

I was a member of the City of Chicago's Commission on Human Relations Advisory Council on African Affairs for twelve years. I am also the Founder and former President of Friends of DuSable, a not for profit organization dedicated to educating the public on the history of the founder of modern day Chicago, Jean Baptiste Pointe DuSable.

In acknowledging the rich and diverse history of the City of Chicago, as well as the great accomplishments of its founder, (FOD & CCHRACAA) have established a citywide commemoration in Honor of Jean Baptiste Pointe DuSable.

The now implementations of the DuSable Commemoration not only serves as a day to honor DuSable, it is a vehicle to bring communities together for a day of unity in celebration of the origin of the great city of Chicago they all share.

I am a devout advocate for human rights that dedicates my free time to political and social causes.

I was introduced to the hair and beauty industry at the age of 15, working as a salon assistant in my uncle's barbershop in Boston, MA. It was there, at Sportsman Barbershop, that I began my interaction with hair care professionals and clients. At the age of 18, I enlisted in the United States Marine Corp. During the last year of my four-year stint, I became the base barber at McAlister Naval Ammunition Depot in McAlister, Oklahoma, as an off duty assignment. That experience exposed me to the multi-cultural and diverse aspect of hair care service. By the age of 22, I had completed Wilfred Beauty College and Vaughn Barber School, in Boston, MA. As you can see, major emphasis was placed on the hair business, well before any formal education began.

Over the years, I built an outstanding reputation as a Hair Beauty & Wellness Specialist. I have traveled and worked in three continents: North America, Africa, Europe, as well as the Caribbean an educator for leading hair care companies. I have been commissioned to do consultant work for top companies such as Revlon, Roux Lab, Clairol, L'Oreal, Johnson's Products, Carson's Products, Deena Corp, Elentee Vitale, and Mc Bride Lab.. In South Africa, I served as an Advanced Educator for M&M Products. In London, England I was contracted as an Advanced Educator at Alpha Beauty Academy. My commercial credits include ad campaigns for Fashion Fair, Isoplus, Duke Men's Products, Shades of you Hosiery, and Ebone Cosmetics. I have received magazine editorial coverage from Working Mother, Rapp

Pages, Essence, Ebony, Bride's Today, Shop Talk, Upscale, EM, Jet, and Black Elegance.

I have owned several hair care businesses nationwide, have trained and employed hundreds of professionals, and know the industry from the top to the bottom. I have said throughout my long tenure, that my biggest disappointment in the Industry is the lack of organization and protection for life service in retirement, insurance benefits & financial security for career professional practitioners.

That being a no secret factual problem in the Hair, Beauty & Wellness industry, it has become a driven ambition for me to find ways to Analyze, Organize, Deputize & Supervise an action plan for individual professional practitioner's sovereignty & security in the Hair, Beauty & Wellness industry. There is a model that is known to be a benefit by other professional industries through the protections of organized unions. The idea is not new and it has roots that go back to Europe, where credit unions gave it birth and have unsuccessfully attempted to implement it in past years, in the American Hair & Beauty industry; unfortunately leaving hundreds of thousands professionals to good fortune or bad luck; but for certain with no organized security or real planned benefits. A couple of similar models of what we know work and that have benefited others like the National Association of Nurses Union, National Teachers Union, and The Professional Screen Actors Guild Union, etc.

That being said, I, Haroon Rashid am launching an exploratory plan to create a national organization of Hair, Beauty & Wellness professionals that will advocate for their own necessary benefits for survival in the twenty first century in the establishment of "**The American Hair, Beauty & Wellness Credit Union**".

To do this, we will first need to establish a non- profit corporation bylaws and a (AHBWCU) board of Directors with a

State by State membership drive plan to organize nationwide via the existing hair beauty & wellness organizations. The (AHBWCU) will be a membership driven organization, for professional practitioners, teachers and students for the purpose of credit union services example; Banking Services-savings-loans-checking & credit development, Insurance- health-property, 401k retirement, Continuing Education funds & network available for regulated licensed professional throughout North America.

There will be a standard monthly dues fee, with sliding options for individual desired coverage, a portion will automatically go into the personal member credit savings, insurance, continued education & administration cost.

Other options: retirement benefits vary on personal choice of value in your desired plan. All fees and regulations will be determined by democratic elected Board and approved vote by majority members.

Members will be of a non-discriminated multicultural bilingual nationwide professional membership.

The American Hair Beauty & Wellness Credit Union Schematic Plans.

A credit union is a non-profit, cooperative financial institution owned and operated by its members. Organized to serve and democratically controlled, credit unions provide their members with a safe place to save and borrow at reasonable rates. Credit unions differ from banks and other for-profit financial institutions in those members of a credit union are also owners. The board of directors is elected in a democratic one person-one vote system regardless of the amount of money invested in the credit union. Not for profit, not for charity, but for service is a credit union motto. Since profit is not a motivation, interest rates have been historically favorable for consumers at credit unions, compared to banks.

Credit Union Membership: To join a credit union, you must be eligible for membership. Each institution decides who it will serve. Most credit unions are organized to serve people in a particular community, group or groups of employees, or members of an organization or association. If you are a relative of a credit union member, you are also eligible to join.

Low-income designated credit unions are a unique form of credit union. They serve primarily low-income members in distressed and financially underserved areas. In the past few years, NCUA has emphasized the benefits these institutions provide to the many people who are often un-served by traditional banking institutions. NCUA also manages a Revolving Loan Fund and provides technical assistance grants to low-income designated credit unions.

American Hair Beauty & Wellness; Health / Savings (AHBWHS)

- Overview
- Details
- Fees

Ensure a Healthy Future with a Health Savings Account (AHBWHS)

With the American Hair Beauty & Wellness Savings Account, you can deposit funds to pay for current or future medical expenses. Funds used for qualified medical expenses, including dividends, are tax-free. Unused funds remain in the AHBWHS year after year, earning tax-deferred dividends.

- High dividend rate of 2.00% APY with an average daily balance of $100 or more

- Easy access to funds via a free VISA® AHBWHS Debit Card or AHBWHS checks

- Free AHBWHS checks

- No fees for account opening, maintenance or transactions

- No initial deposit or minimum balance requirement

Free 24/7 account access:

- Personal customer service

- American Hair Beauty & Wellness Savings <u>online banking</u>

- Self Service Telephone (SST)

Investment Program*

- Available through American Hair Beauty & Wellness Savings Retirement and Investments Services:

SOCIOECONOMIC POLITICS

Let's talk about socioeconomic politics. I believe that by using the glorious heroes and heroines of our past and present, we can build a secure and prosperous future in the new age era of the Millennial. I believe we can and must revive the entrepreneur spirit and forces in the African American, Diaspora communities. I believe we can and must call on, or simply ask our ancestors to bless our efforts to use their great examples for today's success. For me, far too much time has been wasted talking about the past, as it relates to anger over slavery, the slave masters and their children. I believe that we continue to empower those evil acts and people as a legacy, in our lives by the constant acknowledgement of them. However, there are many of our ancestors' histories that must be used again. We will talk about just a few of them later.

We know that if there was an economical support funds system that was available to every African American's community, for example: reparation trust or self-help trust, maybe a joint partnership trust fund. Conditions for success among many in those communities would improve. Many of us are aware of pension funds that are as large as 80 billion dollars, the teacher's union in California, for example.

It has been estimated by some that more than 2/3 of African American elders will retire without funds for retirement. More than 60% of African American youth will not have the opportunity for technical training or advance education for jobs in the year 2000. It is further believed that over 65% of business and personal property in the African American community will be owned by people that do not have compassion, or interest in those communities.

Those statistics set the environment for criminally infested communities that are soundly rooted in apathy and despair, a result of gangster style entrepreneurs and profiting, i.e. drugs, prostitution, racketeering, etc. This has been a major cause and source of job opportunity among the African American youth, far too long, which obviously, culturally robs youth of legitimate leadership opportunities.

I, with others, believe that in just a few short years the tolerance level for the present style of living will be at a ZERO percent level. More African American youth will be jailed or simply murdered, until America has the kind of African Americans that it will tolerate for its future plans. I might be wrong in my vision of America, but just in case I am not, I choose to make plans with those of you that will listen, to prepare for the future.

One other thought is about how many of us felt about the coming of the Millennial, many thought that there would be something horrible to happen on the day of 2000. The predictions for at least one hundred years were that those who lived to see the year 2000 come in, would be devastated by the things that they would witness. However, at the least, if you were of the so-called chosen people, which were just a small number, you were led to believe that you would be spared. We were pleasantly and nervously shocked New Years Eve 1999, but then came the 2000 American elections for the United States of American Presidents. That was the first sign of the ***New World Order*** and the first sign of things to come that was bold and different. A battle of wrong against right; good versus evil, as though the Angels of heaven and hell were released to pave the way for a great spiritual war.

September 11, 2001 brought the greatest sign that all we had been warned about was true, but not as we expected. Two commercial airplanes were driven into the World Trade Center in New York City, another crashed into the pentagon in Washington D.C.

Brave passengers in a remote area of Pennsylvania forced one of the planes down. It is believed, that plane was scheduled to hit the White House. All this was done as a part of a scheme to put fear and to change the comfort of security in America. That tragic incident under the leadership of President George Walker Bush: brought about a fear and anger in America that resulted into a war that was purposely misguided against the wrong nation and their leadership that resulted into hundreds of thousands of Human deaths. Private American companies like Halliburton, who's CEO was the Vice President of the United States were benefiting in that horror by the billions of dollars. Then eight years later the world was ready for the "Agent of Change" under the new world order with the first African American President of the United States of America, President Barack Husain Obama.

This has made the question of economical, political and social values more important than ever in the focus in Americans families and communities.

WHERE IS THE MONEY?

We started this lecture with a statement "where is the money?" Of course money alone cannot change our conditions, but history shows that in the African Americans' past and present, when there was money available to do for selves, and the knowledge to manage it, they did very well. For example, in the days of Madam C. J. Walker, while America was in a financial depression, African Americans within her circle prospered and grew by manufacturing hair and beauty products.

In the city of Tulsa, Oklahoma, again in times when America was struggling, African Americans prospered and grew with the enterprising of oil; until white citizens of Tulsa got jealous of the success of their African American neighbors, they created a riot and encouraged the United States government to perform one of the worst acts of terrorism in the post slavery American History by dropping bombs on its own citizens destroying entire townships within a city in the United States of America. This was done with the purpose of stopping African Americans and destroying their progressive will at that time.

A similar example was Rosewood, Florida whereby hundreds of African Americans were killed; their homes and business were burned down. They own most of the businesses in the city, and were doing very well until white Americans again got jealous, and destroyed them.

In Tuskegee Alabama African American men were given syphilis injections so that U.S. government could test risky treatments as an experiment. Many African American men died from this deplorable act of terrorism.

This pattern of racism, envy and home grown terrorism can be seen from the beginning of American history, throughout, up until today. There are stories of European settlers bringing diseased blankets to kill the Native Americans for the land. Because of greed and insecurity, genocide was acceptable for far too many, and marks America with a shameful and disgraceful history to its victims.

In Washington D. C. where the black population is over 70 %, minorities are dependent on the government and/or white non-residential businesses for jobs that too often have failed their progress.

Gary, Indiana and Newark, New Jersey are other examples when minorities take control of local government, national, federal government and the corporate businesses move out or lose interest for supporting the local administration and the communities.

Mr. Joe Dudley, said in his book entitled "The Fact Book," in the African American community the main source of income is the hair and beauty industry. I personally would like to see some percentage of that money come back to the African American communities to help rebuild them with pension funds, housing and community business investments. It is said that among the Korean community that when one of them comes to America they are helped by their government, as well as their new American community to invest, or work in the beauty supply and nail service business. It is also said that they put their money back into their own communities, and country; we should learn from them and follow their example.

If we look at the hair industry there is an incredible story that I want to share with you. In the early American civilization among the upper class especially in the north, fashion, style, and image was important so that the new settlers could establish a so-called aristocratic society. Therefore, hair was an important way of classifying one's status, and having a hairdresser with artistic skills to help enhance the beauty of a person was considered a high standard.

Chapter Twenty-One

The History Behind The Hair Industry

From A Hairstylist, To A Saint

History has shown that there have always been African Americans who were great hair stylists that were even well respected by European Americans that were wealthy, and contributed great value in their time. As written in the book "Slave from Haiti: A Saint for New York". The book is about the life of Pierre Toussaint, written by M. L. Couve de Murville, Archbishop of Birmingham, England. (Quote) In New York there was a black man named Pierre Toussaint that moved from Haiti August 21, 1797 as a slave, for a well-off French businessman named Monsieur Jean Jacques Berard. Mr. Berard arranged for young Pierre to learn a trade when he arrived in New York, that of hairdressing. It is important to note that the French people in 1789 fought and won a revolution and the declaration of the Rights of Man was proclaimed, but the plantation owners of Haiti had no intention of the slaves benefitting from those rights. So in 1791 there was a slave revolt, and the blacks took up arms against the whites and the great African Hero Toussaint L'Overture became the first leader of African descent to liberate his people and country, the Island of Haiti in 1797. It is my belief that Mr. Berard felt that it was to his best interest to leave Haiti that year for him and his family's safety. So Mr. Berard came to America with their slaves, that experience of the war in Haiti scared the thinking of both the so-called master and slave. The so-called masters had a deep respect, or hate for the Haitian people, because to be defeated by their former slaves had to be a humbling experience.

On the other hand, it must have been a great sense of pride for the slave to know that your people fought and won independence from their former owners. This pride gave Pierre a sense of dignity that later shaped his career with great inter-personal skills. As one of his clients used to say; "Some of the most pleasant hours I pass are in conversing with Toussaint while he is dressing my hair. I anticipate it as a daily recreation." Many of his clients were French ladies in exile, but an increasing number belonged to what was called rudely WASP Society (WASP standing for white Anglo-Saxton Protestant).

Another quality was bilingualism; this understanding of the importance in education and especially of bilingualism is something that marks Pierre out from many other white or minority immigrants in his time. Most of those that came to the United States wanted their children to learn English only, so as to get along in their new country.

In Pierre's will, in 1842, he mentioned explicitly his belief in 'the best advantages of education, and instruction, far exceeding in importance the accumulation of property.'

Pierre not only made sure that his niece had lessons in French and in English; he also set her a practical exercise every week by making her write two short letters, one in French and one English.

More than any other quality among African American immigrants, and African American slaves that made a difference in their lives was the right to be educated, to maintain their language and culture. Of course that kind of liberty was only tolerated for the few that were able to acquire wealth.

Pierre Toussaint was so good in his trade that, when Monsieur Jean-Jacques Berard died, hard times fell on the Berard family. Pierre became the breadwinner in the estate and he took over the responsibilities, and continued to care for his former owner's wife as a token of gratitude for the trade opportunity that was given to him. Marie Elizabeth Berard was a kind woman. Knowing she could not afford to care for Pierre, she had her friends pay Pierre to fix their hair, to which many of them treated Pierre as a confidant and consultant. Elizabeth became ill and as a show of appreciation she freed Pierre; shortly after that she died. Pierre had most of the upper class white women request his service and his council; he became wealthy, and used his wealth to build a Catholic parish and a charm school for African American girls.

Pierre's social contributions were well-respected in his time, in 1787 a group called the New York Manumission Society was founded and it achieved success when its first president, John Jay, became Governor of the State of New York. In 1799 he signed the abolition bill, which provides the progressive abolition of slavery in the State by 1827. The colored people of New York organized a celebration in 1800 to mark the passage of the abolition Bill the previous year and Pierre Toussaint was invited to take a prominent part of the procession.

The catholic Archdiocese has considered him as a candidate for a Saint. So in my opinion the Hair and beauty business has always been a good alternative for independent entrepreneur and social leadership because it serves a need that can transcend race, and if you are really good it does not matter.

However, when the first group of women that decided they wanted to organize themselves to uplift their race as it was said at that time, suddenly race did matter and the need to establish regulations and laws came to America for the beauty industry. The African American hair and beauty companies and organizations have always been different from the white or European hair companies and organizations because, African Americans' goals and objectives were designed to empower professionals and themselves racially.

As the story, and life of Madam C. J. Walker clearly shows, this spirit of empowerment lasted for a while, among the African American beauty professionals and then the curse of greed and lack of entitlement took over. I believe because of this we now witness, at the beginning of the millennium, a full bloom takeover of the major African American Beauty Companies. There presently is a decline in the economical growth of the African American hair industry, organizations, and ultimately the community. I personally do not think that it is too late to bring some of the glory, and good times back again into this industry.

WHAT HAPPENED TO THE AFRICAN AMERICAN HAIR INDUSTRY?

I am going to tell you my version of what I think happened, and how it came about.

In the early eighties I was a local television producer in Atlanta, Georgia. I aired a show called Professional Hair Care and the Fashions. This show came on twice a week on Cable Atlanta television. It was at one of those shows that I hosted a series of interviews, with celebrity hair stylists at the annual Bronner Brothers Hair and Beauty show in Atlanta, Georgia. At this show I also created a forum debate between the presidents of the two largest professional organizations that represented the white, and the black professionals, National Hairdressers and Cosmetology Association President, Alexander Neweea and the National Beauty Culturalist League President, Dr. Katie Whickham. At that forum several things happened, but right away you could see that the professional beauty business, at that time, was and is segregated; and based on race, these are some of things that I observed needed attention:

1. A need for discussions on leadership for the young African American professionals in the industry in regards to trend setting. Since the European professional organization was organized and well-respected as the trend setter for everybody, and to be frank a lot of the styles were not designed with the African American in mind.

2. The discovery that the (African American) National Beauty Culturalist League had in their bylaws, that only women could lead their organization, which I believed prevented many brilliant potential leaders; for example, Nathaniel H. Bronner whom at that time was a member from helping the organization to grow. It also maintained a sense of gender dualism that need not have been, which put the organization to a disadvantage to other organizations that did not have those rules in their bylaws or problems to their organization's potential leadership.

3. The need for mentor, and motivation, by Master Stylist to junior stylist. With the elimination of an apprenticeship program among stylists, the hair industry had become a highly competitive one, whereby junior stylists took the attitude that they were just as good as senior stylists. So the respect among most junior stylists for experienced senior stylists to this day does not exist. Because of this, clients and the African American community are short-serviced to the culture of the hair and beauty industry.

4. The discovery that the African American Hair and Beauty professional organization was started before the European American professionals in America through the majority influence of the Madam C. J. Walker Beauty Culturist

Union. This opens the question of race in the beauty industry on the basis of controlling the money in the two different communities from Madam C. J. Walker's day until now.

5. It also shows how the white hair and beauty professionals were inspired by the success of the black professional hair and beauty unions.

6. How, at the beginning, America was the only country that had a need for the government to regulate hairdressers and to make mandatory schools and testing before receiving a Hair or beauty license. Which brings up the question of whether regulating had a hidden agenda to monitor the cash flow in the industry, and piggyback off the success of the organized African American unions.

7. There was a lot of talk about the control of the black dollar and ethnic product loyalty by the black manufacturers. To make African American hair stylists and consumers feel obligated to buy from the black companies, attend their shows, and support their growth, so that the dollars generated from sales and services would stay in the African American community.

8. Need for community responsibility, and accountability on the part of African American hair stylists. To take leadership in regards to the culture among our clients, and social trend settings.

It is important to know; at that time, I was a member of both organizations. This was strenuous at times, because too often I was the only man in the room. First of all, at that time there were not that many male Stylists who had a national status that were not gay. I can recall many times that I felt that because I was not gay, many of the opportunities that could have enhanced my carrier were kept from me because of the exclusive network among the gay community. Also as a member of the National Hairdressers and Cosmetologist Association in Boston, where I joined, I stood out being an African American straight male hairstylist; I was technically a double minority. I was asked after the interview by Dr. Whickham to be the official representative, or spokesperson for her and the National Beauty Culturalist League, in regards to the African American Company's support to sponsor my idea of an African American trend release. It was a known fact, at that time; young African American hair stylists were attending the white shows and joining the white organizations over the blacks. We felt strongly that in order to attract the young stylists to the black organization they had to compete with the white organization Fashion forward approach in trends.

During that time, there was a lot of talk about African American companies organizing, with the intent of controlling the so-called black dollars to stay in the African American communities. The American Health and Beauty Aids Institute was formed under the leadership of Mr. Lafayette Jones. He founded AHBAI in 1980 and served as its President until 1986 when he then joined Johnson Publishing as the Vice President & General Manager of Johnson Supreme Beauty Products.

Lafayette was a brilliant young man whom I knew as a friend and colleague, and with whom I had many discussions with at that time. This organization had most of the then known African American owned manufacturers in their membership, with a collected value of 200 million dollars or more.

My friend, mentor and industry leader, Mr. Nathaniel Bronner was a past important Chairman, but not the first. A short list of AHBAI Chairmen and the order of their Chairmen is as follows, each serving two-year terms: George Johnson, Johnson Products (1980-82), Cornell McBride Sr., M&M products, McBride Research Laboratories (1982-84), Comer Cottrell, Pro-line Corp (1984-86), Edward Gardner / Gary Gardner (1986-88).

AFRICAN AMERICAN BEAUTY TREND RELEASE

Dr. Whickham brought me to Washington DC at the corporate headquarters of the National Beauty Culturist League as the official spokesperson in an effort to help generate much needed income for the organization and create a program to increase memberships. The goal for the meeting was also to prepare me to speak with Mr. Lafayette Jones of AHBAI on behalf of his organization and so we then drafted a letter and sent it to this prestigious group of men.

I convinced Dr. Whickham that we could create our own trend release, so the letter was asking them for their support towards our efforts in creating a first-time African American trend release. In the hair industry there was a time when hairstyles and fashion where coordinated by the Caucasian hair and fashion organizations two times a year in the Fall / Winter & Spring / Summer for annual fashion forward trend releases events. These events were very popular for fashion forward progressive stylists.

In the meantime, I was calling and collecting support from the top African American hair celebrities to put together a trend release committee that would select a team and create the looks. The matter of developing and executing a "Trend Release" was one of many potential execution tactics in AHBAI's vast marketing tool kit that could be a priority of a host of other proven tactics in their list of "to do's". We all learned that a trend release was important among some professional industry members and sophisticated stylists who might want it to be; it was not as much needed to the then priorities of the National Beauty Cultural league and the American Health and Beauty Aids Institute administration at that time.

Even though we were not able to achieve our initial interest in the African American Trend release during that time, I learned that Lafayette on behalf of the AHBAI administration, met with Dr. Katie B. Witcom many times at NBCL Washington D.C. headquarters. They showed high regards and respect for Cosmetologists and the NBCL. Under the leadership of Mr. Lafayette Jones' administration, AHBAI made many financial contributions to NBCL to keep them solvent and not go bankrupt. They sent plane tickets for their leadership to attend important industry meeting. Unfortunately, near the end, Dr. Witcom was aging rapidly, losing her eyesight, mental agility and decision-making authority. The NBCL was subsequently undergoing significant leadership changes and its membership began to decline rapidly.

Mr. Bronner, and I were both members of NBCL and had love and loyalty for their efforts to progress and stay afloat. He told me in one of our many talks that he would have gladly taken over the reins when I asked him to consider it, if not for the known fact among fellow members about the bylaw that states that only a female could become the leader or president of the NBCL organization.

The one thing I can say, for sure, that Mr. Bronner showed extreme genuine interest in his relationship with the AHBAI efforts during that time and in the campaigns that AHBAI launched called

"Black on Black Love". He felt that was a needed and worthwhile cause to promote African

Americans loving one another, rather than hurting each other, and he encouraged it.

Let me talk about The Revlon boycott spearheaded by AHBAI and the African American leadership in the eighties, which had to do with trying to get African American consumers to buy Black-owned products. It was also about delivering a message to Mr. Irving Bottner, President of Revlon Realistic division hair products. At that time, Mr. Bottner made some very unfortunate and disrespectful remarks about black-owned beauty companies.

One of those comments was publicly quoted in a national news magazine called Newsweek. AHBAI was appalled and took its rebuttal to the streets in the top 40 US cities. Prior to that, the Federal Trade Commission (FTC) declared that Johnson's Ultra Sheen relaxer must carry a warning label that coincidentally had the exact same ingredients as Revlon Relaxer. Although it had the same chemical ingredients, Revlon was not required to carry the same labels on their products. This was unfair tactic and really a restraint of trade or an antitrust matter.

Then Revlon's President Irving Bottner exploited the situation, using unfair marketing techniques by telling African American stylists that Ultra Sheen was declared inferior by the US government by referring to the warning that was just on the African American owned Ultra Sheen relaxers. Many African American stylists went for the okey-dokey and believed Revlon was a superior product to purchase. As a result of that enactment, Johnson Products lost millions of dollars and in the interim lost its premier relaxer category market share leadership.

Mr. Lafayette Jones was brought on the scene in a leadership position, first as Vice President of Marketing and Sales for Johnson Products, then President of AHBAI (American Health and

Beauty Aids Institute) He was responsible for its activities. struck back with a massive national campaign at Revlon in 40 US markets, placed their product in coffins, and publicly buried them.

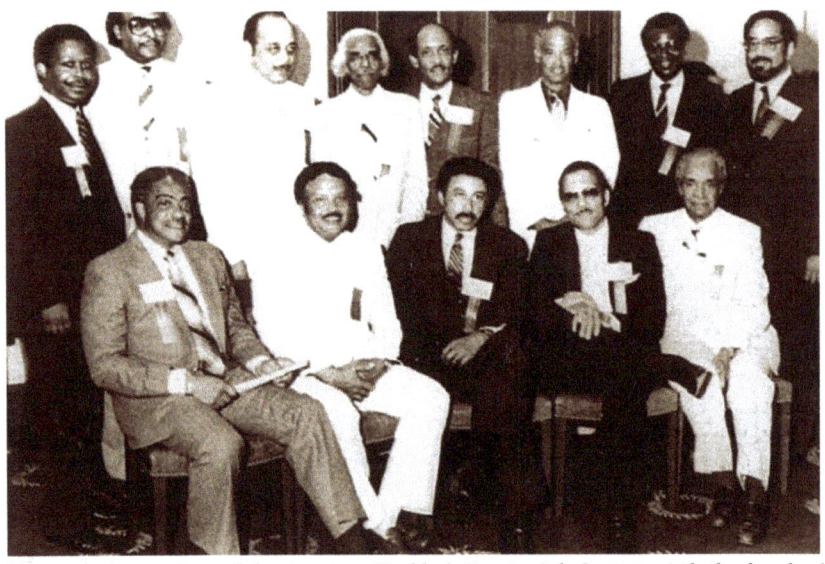

These are the members of the American Health & Beauty Aids Institute, with the founder Mr. Lafayette Jones on the upper far left side.

AHBAI asked for a community boycott, which was led by Reverend Jesse Jackson. AHBAI supplied the marketing template and supplies to the leaders in the 40 markets. Later Revlon's board of Directors asked for a peace treaty and agreed to clarify Mr. Bottner's statement, and the rest is history.

After that no one, no other industry, Beauty company, or competitor ever denigrated AHBAI in any way because they spoke serious truth to power; and they put some people on the street and in the media to tell their story. AHBAI taught their business competitors to respect African American Beauty Business owners. It also held them to a higher standard of providing new opportunities for Black people employed in their companies.

Bottner's comment was prophetic, only in that M&M products, Soft Sheen Industries, and Pro-Line International were acquired by major beauty domestic and international companies.

Later Mr. Irving Bottner apologized and Revlon appointed its first Vice President, Essie Barnett.

THE BEGINNING OF VIOLATION

I believe today that the beginning of violations is best described in this previous information of how the Caucasian competitors systematically use unfair tactics to discredit the great accomplishments of organized African American entrepreneurs.

This type of injustice is not new as we can easily relate to the American history destruction of Black Wall Street in Tulsa Oklahoma, which was done by evil jealousy of Caucasians because of the insecurities and rise of African American businessmen.

I named this chapter of the book the Other Black Gold in tribute to the phenomenon. It was because the wealth from the oil industry owned by African Americans was called Black Gold, which infuriated some so-called humans.

Also something closer to home is the African American hair and Beauty industry again systematically destroyed as was the wealth and great progressive enterprising in the hair industry that was unmatchable during the days of the great late Madame C. J. Walker in her heydays with the rise of African American wealth in the Hair and Beauty industry the new Black Gold.

It is telling, that some of the very same evil techniques that were used in the past was again used to hinder or stop the rise of the Black Gold.in America.

But Yet We Still Rise from the people that built the WHITE HOUSE for others, to an African American family in the 21st century that now has the occupancy of that historical monument.

EMPOWERMENT-ENTITLEMENT

1. This brings up the subject of Empowerment, Entitlement, and the business of Reparations.

2. Empowerment is a very broad statement, so I want to personalize it to self-empowerment.

Self-empowerment, to me, means to be in a state of control of your life and style. I've got to tell you, nothing gives you a greater sense of that than having an entrepreneurial spirit; especially if that spirit comes from money markets, stocks, bonds, small business, or personal / commercial real estate. When you make a personal and career decision, based on calculated risk and sacrifices, that is the kind of action that gives you self- empowerment.

Entitlement is a feeling of inclusion, a right to an opinion, a sense of ownership, and leadership. In a democratic society these characters are called human and civil rights. I believe the African American community, Native American and the Latin American -Hispanic more than any other in American lacks the spirit of entitlement. All of us think about this subject have theories and opinions as to how this came about. However most agree that the lack of self entitlement probably does more harm to the development of children than any other human rights issue.

Reparation; much has been said about the debt, which is overdue to the descendants of the African American slaves. To be brief, in my opinion, they were the laborers who were treated like slaves that built America without a paycheck. Too many people have benefited from the so-called slaves' labor and their descendants. The builders, (African Americans) feel left out of that legacy. I, along with others, think the Federal Government should do something similar to what was done for the Asian community,

Native American community, Jewish community in Europe and others for so-called wrongdoing. Too many African American's share stories of descendants whose ideas and accomplishments were stolen, or conveniently hidden. Reparation is a way of healing some of that pain.

I want to thank Mr. Lafayette Jones for some of his clarity of the times, detailed in this section.

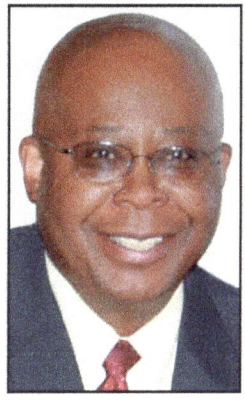

Marketing chief executive and publisher Lafayette Glenn Jones was born on February 17, 1944. He credits his parents, who managed a small landscaping business, with his own entrepreneurial drive. Jones received his B.A. degree from Fisk University in 1965, and went on to attend executive management programs at Dartmouth College's Amos Tuck School of Business and Stanford University's School of Business.

Jones first worked for the Job Corps and the YMCA as a program director in the mid-1960s. He then directed client promotions at the Washington, D.C. radio station WOL from 1967 to 1969. From 1969 to 1974, he worked as a sales and marketing executive for Lever Brothers, Pillsbury Company and General Foods. From 1974 to 1979, Jones served as a marketing manager for Hunt-Wesson, where he created the Orville Redenbacher Gourmet Popping Corn and Hunt's Manwich strategies. In 1979, he was appointed as vice president of marketing and sales at Johnson Products Company in Chicago, Illinois. In 1981, Jones founded and served as executive director of the American Health and Beauty Aids Institute (AHBAI), the trade association of black hair care companies. He also founded Smith-Jones & Associates, an association management firm.

In 1988, Jones was named vice president and general manager of Supreme Beauty Products Company, the hair care subsidiary of Johnson Publishing Company. He then joined Sandra Miller Jones' Segmented Marketing Services, Inc. (SMSi) in the early 1990s, where he went on to serve as president and chief executive officer of SMSi-Urban Call Marketing, Inc. and publisher of the company's *Urban Call* magazine. Jones also became publisher of SMSi's *Shades of Beauty* magazine in 1998.

Jones has authored articles for numerous publications including *OTC Beauty Magazine* and the *Beauty Industry Report*. He authored a column in *Sophisticate's Black Hair Styles and Care Guide* and the 1999 Green Book's special section on ethnic hair care. Jones also wrote a column for *ShopTalk* magazine for fifteen years. He is a frequent speaker at conferences and has guest lectured at Harvard University, Dartmouth College, Duke University, Wake Forest University, and Howard University. Jones has also served on the boards of several organizations including Urban Getaways, the Mardan Institute and the Promotion Marketing Association.

Chapter Twenty-Two

Ancestors That I Admire

There are many that I could mention, past and present, but this is just a few that I have chosen that I look at their life story for guidance. I have the belief that there is nothing that I can do to change my past, there is no promise for me that I can experience a future, and there are no guarantees. Therefore, I can only live my life as it unfolds and use what I have gained in life's lessons from the past and present of myself and others, and prepare for what ambitions I have for tomorrow. I am in full awareness, knowing the only thing that I have been given is the life and love from the Most High that He gives to me day by day.

That being said it is incumbent upon me to treasure my life, respect my past and be grateful for the opportunity to see and live tomorrow if it pleases God. As I was taught, live every day as though you are going to live forever, and by the same breath, as though you might die at any moment.

These are two of the many heroes and mentors that I admire and have chosen to highlight first, as you will see others in a chapter to follow. It is because I spent the majority of my career in the same field of operation as the great **Madam C.J. Walker** the Beauty Culture business and I grew up in the same city – Boston, Massachusetts - that another unsung hero of African American descent, **Mr. Crispus Attucks,** who is rarely mentioned or researched, I felt it appropriate to highlight some measure of their great history in respect to my African American research. I have chosen parts of their life missions as a hypothetical narrative for a formula for success in the following chapter.

MADAME C. J. WALKER

Madame C. J. Walker is an African American Hero. She, along with Pierre Toussaint, Crispus Attucks and Jean Baptiste Pointe Du Sable, to me, has done more to legitimize the African American patronage, and entrepreneurial spirit, in my opinion more than many of the African American Heroes in their perspectives that I am. Which makes you wonder what if the African Americans were not constantly manipulated or intimidated and off message from then until now, where could we be in America today?

The great Madame C. J. Walker changed the image of a housekeeper, wash women, nanny, mistress, and people with no culture, class, etc., into a financially secure, independent entrepreneurial group of women, she made the so-called Negro women and girls look beautiful in her life time. With the money she and her well-trained women earned, enabled them to help their mates with their plans and goals to be uplifted in American society from overt slavery, suffering and death. Because of their economical success they were able to gain the respect of white men and the envy of the white women of culture in their times.

The African American women that were beautified by Madame C. J. Walker, in her day, had a mystique, as did the women in the days of the African Moors. That class of people whom dazzled and fascinated all of Europe and Asia in its day. Josephine Baker dazzled them also when she went to Europe from America as a product of Madame C. J. Walker's time.

Mrs. Walker took her ideas, products and skills on the road with her and trained women from coast to coast. She preached in churches and lodges all across America and internationally. She convinced African American preachers that by helping the African American women and girls to become more cultural and beautiful the whole race would be better off for it.

It is said, because an "African American woman" named Madame C. J. Walker did those things, she is dated as one of the first people in modern history that is credited for a crusade to beautify an entire race of people. For her efforts, she became recognized as the first woman in America to earn a million dollars or more. With her money she helped finance African American colleges such as Bethune Cookman College in Florida. She also helped fund the NAACP, YMCA, and YWCA She further helped fund the Honorable Marcus Garvey back to Africa movement and "Black Star line" ships.

The Harlem Renaissance and colored social society sprung its roots from Madam Walker in her Mansion in upstate New York, with renown figures as neighbors, such as the Rothschild's, the DuPont's and the Getty. She entertained the sophisticated people of color and was a pioneer introducing to America legendary entertainers like Langston Hughes and leaders like Fredrick Douglas that she financed with her money. Mrs. Walker built one of the first independent movie houses in America where African American film writers and producers could showcase their talents in a respectful manner. She sponsored fashion shows to teach the African American women how to dress like the rest of so-called cultured American women. She also helped change forever the image of African American women that Hollywood was presenting to the world in her day as Aunt Jemima and referring as Nappy head coons or Pickaninnies.

Madame Walker said that she noticed when white women put attention to their hair; they were looked at in a higher light in the eyes of society. White women were using curling irons and permanent curling machines to change their hair texture to curly, the opposite of its natural texture. With her hair oils and hot comb, she gave the African American women the same options as those of the whites expanding their options for change. Simply using the law of attraction in hair artistry, the opposite attracts and like repels.

She lifted the consciousness and self-esteem of African American women to a level that they would be willing to openly compete for America's attention as serious business leaders and as a new beauty contender for the world community. Because of those things she stands out as a twentieth century leader, and mentor.

Little is said about Madame Walker's patriotism, but it is written that she was the guest of the President of the United States on many occasions and she was asked by the Negro leadership to lobby for African American men to fight in World War two, so that white America would give respect to the so-called Negro efforts to sacrifice for America. Even though history shows us that white America was not ready to respect African Americans in her day, as they should have. She would visit African American troops at their training camps to encourage them that what they were doing was good for future race relations in America.

As Mrs. Golda Meir, Israel's first Prime Minister wanted Israel to work for the Jewish people in her day, so did Madame Walker want America to work for the African American community in her time.

The two sayings she preached that still mean so much today are:

1. I GOT MYSELF A START BY GIVING MYSELF A START.

2. DON'T SIT DOWN AND WAIT, GET UP AND DO SOMETHING FOR YOURSELF.

CRISPUS ATTUCKS

Another leader and African American ancestor that is of great importance was Crispus Attucks. I grew up in Boston and I have always found it of particular interest the legacy of Mr. Attucks as a part of the African and Native American history that is seldom mention by far too few in Boston that are even aware of his increditable legacy and that he was a patriot in early American history. That is why I share some information of him as a way to give some transparency to his untold story. This person was born in Massachusetts. His Mother was a Native American from a tribe called the Natick Indians that later after being converted into Christianity were called the Praying Indians in the New England area. His father was the son of a West African chief, which made him a Prince in his father's native land. In America he was just another slave on a white political leader's Crispus plantation.

When Crispus was a young teenager, after listening to what was known as field slaves. In Crispus' time, a field slave was the most rebellious of the slaves. Even though Crispus Attucks' father was treated well and his master was considered a kind person, the influence of the field slaves made Crispus know he did not and would not be a willing or volunteer slave. As much as he loved his father he vowed he would not be subjugated to following in his father's footsteps as a house slave or servant, so he became a runaway slave.

Soon after running away, he found work as a sea whaler. After learning this craft, he distinguished himself as a master in his craft. He then went on to be considered and to consider himself a free person. Even though on the plantation that his father worked, and he grew up on, he was still considered a runaway slave.

One of the most important factors of Crispus Attucks' life was, one day as Crispus Attucks was visiting Boston from a sea journey he became angry over the way the British police were interacting with a young white man; a scuffle between large gatherings of colonial citizens began. Because of that, he took a position and acted as their leader, to take a stand against the police. Things got out of control and he consequently was shot and killed. That act of courage motivated the citizens to protest the ending of British colonization. The original New England patriots saying, *no taxation without representation*, and the war between British and the America Patriots that led to independence from England and British control. That blind act of courage comes from men or women when they feel they're free to demand their Human Rights, this action impulsively gives them respect from any people.

Throughout history, leaders have cross- racial and social barriers on the strength of courageous leadership when it is needed. In the twenty-first century, former General Colin Powell is an example of the spirit of Crispus Attucks. When he stood, as America's first African American Secretary of Defense, during a time when America was attacked at home, America's response to him was that he was considered as a serious contender for the Presidency of the United States.

I would like to summarize my thoughts with plans for our future. You might have noticed that I had made a suggestion that there was something coming in the year 2000 that some called New World Order, New age, Millennium, etc. It had been predicted by some that in 1999 there were celebrations planned in Egypt that only a select group of leaders were invited to. Most of us had not been invited. It is said there were plans that would change the way America is viewed and the world we live in for 1000 years. If these things might be true, it does not look, as though the African American, community is a part of the good changes. When you look at the cities where the majority of African Americans live, the fact is we see a decline in progressive growth among them.

Chapter Twenty-Three

Formula for Success

I want to take a position that I may not be included in the success of America, but that I have a window of time to call on the spirit of our ancestor the Honorable Madame C. J. Walker. Her motto was **I got my start by giving myself a start.**

We can use some of the formulas that she used in her time to generate economical growth in our community today.

I ask you to join me in the spirit of another of our ancestors, the Honorable Crispus Attucks. His example of blind courage should encourage us to become leaders in our communities; he paid the ultimate price but his name is still remembered. In Boston there is reenactment sponsored by the Bostonian Society every year on May the 5th. Which is the day he was shot that leads to the Boston massacre, it is held in front of the old State building that is still there; all this is done as a reminder of the courage of Crispus Attucks and others. There is also a statue that is in Boston as a further show of gratitude of this great African American Hero.

We must become outraged over where America is leading our community and stand up for our Human and Civil rights to that crime.

Jean Baptiste Pointe DuSable was a Free Black; when others were enslaved he was a businessman, a religious leader, a peacemaker an educator. It has been said he spent all his wealth freeing Africans and African Americans from slavery and as the founder of America's third largest city and the true Black Mecca of America. His example is one that we can emulate and encourage our children the value of speaking multiple languages, as he spoke five and became the ambassador and chief negotiator in the Mid-West region for five nations. What he did we should do and produce world leaders from Chicago and America of African Descent by promoting his noble spirit among us all.

Madame Walker took the Negro women and trained them in the churches and lodges to beautify the black community. She said **don't sit down and wait.** We must do the same thing today!

In Madame Walker's day she helped finance black colleges, created jobs in our neighborhoods, and she helped finance cultural growth in the black communities. If she could do it in her time, I know we can today. I am telling you, if we get the courageous and sacrificial spirit of Crispus Attucks, we can rebuild Gary, Washington DC. Chicago, Detroit and wherever our people need our help. I believe the Beauty Culturist can play a role and can do it again, using our barbershops and Beauty Salons to campaign for this noble cause.

You might ask how? The answer is by using a formula for success that has been used by secret organizations for years. I have been telling people about this formula for years. It is to **Analyze, Organize, Deputize, and Supervise.**

ANALYZE:

- Where is the money in the community, banks, trust, insurance, businesses etc.?

- Where or who are our leaders?

- What is needed for and of the African American community?

- What is needed of the African American spiritual leaders?
- What is needed of the African American business leaders?
- What is needed of the African American politicians?
- What is needed of the African American educators?

ORGANIZE: Campaign to financially secure businesses, private property, and commercial real estate. Develop a $1-$10 a day sacrifice drive. The money will sit in trust for year-to-year investments in our neighborhoods, etc. Fund drives through businesses, politicians, and churches to buy our community without Federal or local government restrictions.

DEPUTIZE: Identify managers in all areas or divisions of our concerns in the communities that we live. Give them guidelines, rules, and regulations and let them use their creative skills to do the job.

SUPERVISE: Develop a board of trust. Take responsibility of every major interest and managers in every aspect; give them our support and resources to be successful, but be responsible for their successes.

Again you might ask the question, why me? I believe that the hair and beauty industry is a spiritual arm and hands in the body called our community.

I believe metaphorically that when our arm and hands are not tied behind the back of our communities, but freely operating, we can build very successfully as was done in Madame Walker's day. I believe that many people in, and out, of our community have benefited by our state of arrest.

I further believe that I am one of many that have been given this mission to liberate us, to unlock the shackles and help lead us to our future. For those of you that might ask *is this a **BLACK THING?*** No, this is a community thing and we just happen to be **black.**

The industry that has made so many people successful, and famous, it is a real shame, that so many African Americans are seeing the profits from their service leave their community into another. It reminds me of the parable in the bible about the people who lost their birthrights to strangers.

HISTORY OF CULTURAL GROOMING

It is easy to see how the business of grooming hair, body, and fashion came from the African people. History shows us that the Egyptian people that were clearly a black African civilization (Nubians) are the mothers and fathers of beautification. The records of their greatness as culturists are still being dug up around the world as hieroglyphic images on vases, pyramids, and statues of early dynasty writings, and visuals.

The hair decorations, faces make over, tattoo or body painting, nails painting, and colorful artistic garments are all some of the world's oldest art works with roots in people of African descent.

The skills and talents that were preserved in many Africans, Asian, and Indian traditions, can be seen throughout civilized history. A birthright passed down through the ages of time is seen in the emergence of the European civilizations. As these European or so- called white race became more exposed to people of African Diaspora. From Asia, the Mongolian Khan dynasty's direct lineage to the African migration in Asia and the interracial mixing that developed: from their travels and conquest of Europe and the richly colorful traditions of India and Hindu culture, etc., and then of course the last people of Diaspora to rule over the Europeans was that of the African Moors. These people influenced most of the known societies and governments of Europe for 1000 years. It is through "that" influence we see great attempts to preserve cultural tradition in secret societies.

In America, there was a colossal attempt to take away all traces of African culture, or birthrights, of the African labors that were brought to America. This stealing of birthrights happened by giving the people of African descent the worst holocaust or slavery known to modern man. Not exclusive of the Native American, East Indians, Asians, Arabic, Jewish, or Irish people. As noted, all peoples at some time have had an experience of the humiliating treatment of slavery. Many believe the worst was done to the so-called Negro, taking away all knowledge of self, history, or culture, from the African looking slaves, everything including his dignity. He was made to feel ashamed of his own biological anatomy, culture, and customs. Then to make things worst was the stealing of their spiritual birthrights, or culture, away from them such as religion, law, family values, social order, and certainly beauty /fashion.

These people secretly admired people of the African Diaspora, so they established private clubs or associations to learn and practice the African Diaspora cultures and traditions in secret. Mason, Eastern Stars, Shriners, Illuminati, etc. claim their Eastern or Egyptian roots in their ceremonies, just as though it is their own.

Tanning of their skin, curling or cutting their hair, painting faces with makeup lipstick, ear and body piercing, hips, lips, buttocks or breast increases, all to look like other than their biological selves. The ancient Egyptian noble men and women of royalty often shaved off all of their body, and head hair to distinguish their selves from the so-called lower class. They would wear headpieces, and wigs in public. These people certainly were African people of color. The Moors rediscovered the art of cutting and shaving head and facial hair. As well as body oils, body scents. Daily baths were exposed to Europeans that came from the ventures of the African Moors. In those days and now: wherein Muslims were required baths five times a day before their daily prayers.

STEALING OF CULTURAL BIRTH RIGHTS

What we are talking about is the stealing of cultural birthrights, and again people of African Diaspora were cheated or robbed in some way, to make the present world leaders of Europe appear to have class, and culture that they might not have had otherwise.

Example the first American European settlers were crude uncultured people. In fact, it is said that most of them came from prisons and were of the lowest classes of citizenry, exiled in primitive nations to be governed in the colonial territories of North America and Australia under the restricted control of their host mother countries and given time of seven years before they would be permitted to go home. To me that explains why most of them were so wicked and evil toward another race; it had become part of their nature while in Europe. There is a saying that *if you put a suit of a man on a monkey, you will not make a man*. What you will make is a monkey in a suit. So the private secret societies that were established in America were to teach them how to be civil, and how to govern themselves, in an expectable way. Many of these secret societies promoted, and supported racism because they were insecure, and jealous of those noble or smart people of color, even though they were using their culture in their rituals.

Even though every human being is connected to the other spiritually, there has never been a time in history that this fact has benefited humanity. Too many people of modern times use their personal nationalism as another means for a cultural divide among each other. The continent from which they arrive becomes a factor in how much or little culture a person has.

Another example, India has rich cultural history; unfortunately, the flaw in that culture is racism, through the Hindu religious caste system. The Hindu Caste system produced the worlds largest and maybe the first cultural racist society. The so-called untouchables are still victims of that class of have, and have not, based on shades of color. It has been told that it was a custom that, if an untouchable walks the streets, he must carry a broom that is attached to him or her from their rear as a way to erase their dark shadow, as they walk among the elite; or be cursed or punished if they do not. It is also said that a Hindu Prince that was so dark he was treated in this low inhumane manner, rebelled and went to Asia and preached against the treatment, and founded a way of life known as Buddhism. So we see Buddha gave a lot to Asian culture based upon his inhumane treatment of racism.

Of course the Europeans in their great hunger for knowledge, and culture learned a lot from Africans, Asians, and the Indians. However, they became closer to white caste Indians, and less toward Asians, or Africans; again color conscious attitude.

The European Spanish people a mixture of White Europeans and Indians/African produced the Hispanic and Latino culture with roots deeply influenced by African and Indian traditions and customs. When you look at the Spanish-speaking people though, you can see the same effects of racism that is among the Indian, Asian, or Caucasian people.

The amazing mating relations are worth looking at, as well, (African- Indian -Latino), and (Caucasian- Hispanic -Asian) these groups seem more naturally attracted to each other in their personal interracial relations. Of course, each group has its own percentage of cross-over relations and racism.

I strongly believe that Indian, Hispanic, Latino, Asian and the Caucasians all have their cultural beginning in Africa, and they all, at some point, have been about the business of concealing that knowledge to their benefits, for as long as they had the power to do so.

Dr. Ivan Van Sertima, a historical scholar and professor at Rutgers University wrote in his book the "Golden Age of the Moors." (The world changed dramatically in 1492, not only because Columbus stumbled in the direction of the Americas, using the magnet of a myth to draw millions behind him, but also because that was the very year the Moors were defeated. It is not an accident that it is Spain and Portugal that spearheaded the movement in this direction. It was on Jan. 2, 1492 that the African leader, Abu Abdi -Llah, otherwise known as Boabdil, surrendered to the Spanish.).

Jan Carew said. 'At a time when the most provinces of Moorish Spain contained libraries running into the thousands of volumes, the cathedrals, monasteries and palaces of Leon, under Christian rule, numbered books only by the dozen.

Van Sertima says again, quote: "The narrowness of vision this produced among leaders of the church and state was to have catastrophic effects. It led to the massive burning of African and Arab books under the order of Cardinal Ximenes de Cisneres. It inspired a similar barn fire of books of Native Americans." Bishop de Landa exhorted his followers in the Yucatan "Burn them all - they are works of the devil." Van Sertima says, "The destruction of the Moorish libraries was particularly vicious because it was not only inspired by religious narrowness and bigotry. Hatred of the dark invaders kindled the barn fires." End of quote!

So it is that historic backdrop that set the stage for the secret societies, and stealing of people's natural birthrights. When you look at the African American, imagine a people that believe that they have nothing to contribute in society but labor. Maybe that is a reason for celebrating in America on Labor Day, with so much enthusiasm by African Americans. Logically it should be considered an insult that most African Americans were brought here by force to labor for white America and treated as slaves. To me the difference of slave or laborer is economics. A slave's work was free, and they could only benefit by the mercy of their master. If his master was primitive and uneducated as most of the European people were in the first place, at that time, the less likely he or she would be considered as a laborer to get paid for their work.

African Americans were not the first people that the Europeans tried to enslave, the Native Americans encountered their evil ways first as the host in America to those new European settlers. History shows that Native Americans resisted and fought many battles, and because the battles were fought in their own lands they won enough, to make the Europeans look elsewhere for their servants or slaves. But the hatred that the European settlers developed for the Native Americans drove them to practice genocide on the Native Americans, and stealing of their land. That is why they turned to China and Ireland for slaves, but nowhere could they get that which would take the cruel evil they were capable of for building the infrastructure of America, but from the African Exiles.

When you look at early American settlers from that prospective, one cannot help but say what a lazy ignorant sneaky society that fathered and mothered this land. We know that this low life mentality took place all over the world, in South America, the Caribbean, Africa, India, and Asia. North America, however, is of special importance to the African American.

In Chicago, at the Museum of Natural History, there was an exhibit called the African Holocaust. It spoke to the effect of white America having two hundred years of uninterrupted free labor, and the jump-start advantages that America had over other so-called civilized nations that had to pay for their labor. Imagine how quickly you could build a company if you did not have to pay for labor.

Secret societies were helped by the Bible that was launched in 1555 to the then new world, by European leadership in particularly King James of England. This revised interpretation under his authority is the backbone for their teaching and stealing of the dark nation's birthright.

Example; there is a myth of Ham laughing at his father Noah, because he, Noah was drunk and naked. The so-called curse of God on Ham that made him and his descendants black, therefore cursed to labor for Shem, his brother and his descendants, the Shemites. It is said Shem covered his father's naked body and drunkenness, and therefore was not cursed, which leaves us to believe he remained opposite of black, which is white. This

Convenient story fit neatly into the scheme of taking whatever blessings the descendants of Ham had.

Also the offspring's of Ham, willingness to be servants and give up all they had from a false spiritual guilt complex. It is easy to see how a people under the influence of another can be made to believe that they had nothing to give but shame, disgrace, and labor. I say that is just what the framers of these secret societies had in mind.

How else could they have persuaded people of color to give up their culture, and take what was given to them so willingly?

Again many have asked the question. What if the African Americans had the same opportunity to develop with their earned income and uninterrupted cultural growth as others did? This might have happened if there was not such an immoral attempt to take away the dignity of the African labor by classifying them all as just slaves.

I believe, like many others, that African Americans and Africa would be much further ahead in the world community if this had not happened.

I believe African Americans were spiritually blessed by the wise ancient elders of Africa, who saw the evil plan of the European mind, and hid a lot of African culture in ceremonies, traditions language and music.

This is why, regardless of how enslaved they were, there always has been someone that has had enough of the puzzle, to figure their way out of blind leadership by their oppressors. Let's reflect on some of these great African American heroes and their successful contributions; we shall see a formula, and a common similarity among them all.

Chapter Twenty-Four

African American Mentor Biographies

It has been said that African Americans, at one time in history, were so hungry for knowledge, particularly about their own great leaders and accomplishments, that they would risk dying in order to read and do research because it was prohibited by their former slave masters for fear that the negro would develop some measure of intellectual equality with them.

It is now a common joke among many African Americans with a sad measure of reality to it that African Americans in these days would rather die than to read or do any research about themselves for their much needed knowledge of self and heritage.

With that in mind I have developed in this book a limited collection of micro bios for your further research and your future reference regarding the characters that are mentioned in this book.

However, by no means, are these all the people from the past and present that we should do research and encourage the young generation to discipline themselves to read and write about and comprehend the progressive leaders and mentors who among the African Diaspora.

For me, there is nothing more insane than people that will give a blistering argument about a subject, based on hear-say, without even doing any research. That kind of ignorance most certainly was not what our ancestors fought for and died for; but to be educated and knowledgeable was and is the aim.

I am content that just as we will read a Webster dictionary, Google, or Wikipedia search on the Internet for information that might be available for your use when it is needed, I give to you this limited list with some information for your record when needed.

I might add a strong recommendation that you read or familiarize yourself with every one of these brilliant people.

To name a few past and present examples:

St. Augustine of Hippo (354-430) the man, which the first city in America was named after by Don Pedro Menendez de Aviles a Spanish explorer, who had royal permission under King Philip II. While celebrating Feast day on a ship August 28, 1565, which was St. Augustine's death in the year 430, the coastline of Florida appeared. A few days later, Don Pedro Menendez de Aviles and a fleet chaplain had outdoor mass on the shore land of Florida that marked the beginning of continuous Christian presence in the new land he found and named St. Augustine. This famous man St. Augustine was born in Africa; his mother St. Monica was a devoted Christian. His father's was name Patricius, (who died about 371). St Augustine; is considered by the Catholic Archdiocese as one of the most intelligent men who ever lived.

Isabella (Sojourner) Truth (1777-1883) very little is known of her early life. It is said she had five masters up until the time of her emancipation. Before her liberation` in 1817 she had been married and her five children had been sold into slavery. It is said that Isabella prayed for a name that had spiritual meaning because she had a wandering spirit she was given "Sojourner" and "Truth". Because she felt herself called to preach the truth about slavery and because she felt, "God is my Master and his name is Truth, then Truth shall be my abiding name until I die."

She was a very soulful, eloquent gospel teacher in her day, the kind that moved people naturally in a way that was untouched by the eloquence of what they learned. Even though she could not read or write, among her most important personal possessions was a small autograph book, with names of distinguished persons and testimonials, such as: For Aunty Sojourner Truth, Abraham Lincoln, and October 9, 1864. Sojourner Truth was talked of very highly by General U.S. Grant, March 31, 1870.

She lived to be over 90 years old. Her life ended November 26, 1883 in Battle Creek, Michigan where she lived and labored for more than twenty-five years.

Reggie Lewis, (Wall street investment tycoon, owner McCall patterns, Beatrice Foods the only African American who has an international law department building built in his name at the prestigious Harvard University). A man that as a boy was poor and came from a single family home in Baltimore, Maryland; later he was considered one of the wealthiest black men in America before his early death.

Jessie Owens (Olympic gold medal winner an American Hero. A native of Chicago Illinois and in his time he was considered the proud product of the Chicago Public Schools. He went on to Ohio State University; and as a student at Ohio State University, Owens had broken five world records competing in the big ten championships in Ann Arbor, Michigan, in 1935. Combining great skills as a sprinter, low hurdler, and broad jumper, Owens won Olympic gold medals in four events at the 1936 games: 100 meter, 200 meter, long jump, and relay. Hitler refused to present Owens with his four medals. Jessie Owens proved that Hitler's theories of Aryan superiority were false, and the African Diaspora is equal to, if not better than so called pure white people.

Mary McLeod Bethune, (1875-1955), the daughter of former slaves, originally planned to be a missionary to Africa but she was rejected because of her race. So instead she became an educator, teaching in mission schools in Georgia and Florida and founding the Daytona Educational and Industrial Institute for Girls in 1904. The school merged with Cookman Institute in 1923 to become the Bethune-Cookman College, where she served as president of the National Council of Negro Women, she led battles for federal anti-lynching legislation, job training for rural women, and the admission of black women into the military service. Bethune won the Springarn Medal in 1935 and was appointed the director of the Division of Negro Affairs of the National Youth Administration under President Roosevelt. The statue of Bethune, erected in 1974 in a public park near the Capital building, was the first statue in Washington DC to honor either a women or an African an American.

Marcus Garvey, (1887-1940) "Back-to-Africa" leader, was the most widely known of all the agitators for the rights of the Negro and one of the most phenomenal. He was born in Jamaica, West Indies, of very humble parents. Leaving school at sixteen, he went to work as an apprentice in the printing plant of P. Austin Benjamin in Kingston. Six years later, he was a foreman. In the meantime, he had been organizing the printers of the city and soon afterward led them in a successful strike for better pay. In 1911 he went to England, where he attended London University. In 1917 he came to America. His addresses on the race problem aroused the so-called Negro until by many he came to be regarded as another Moses. In March 1917, he organized a movement, calling it the Universal Negro Improvement Association. He bought a fleet of ships, and he founded the Black Star Line. He established factories in the United States; the raw material of Africa and the West Indies was to be brought to America, manufactured there, and shipped back to those lands. These ships were also to be used to transport migrant Negro settlers, to the so-called new world in

Africa. His contributions were so impacting that it is said, the Black Star Flag' as the symbol for the new independent Country of Ghana in West Africa, was given by the Country's first President Dr. Kwame Nkrumah, because of Garvey's influence of his life.

Frederick Douglass, (1817-1895) An ex-slave, who rose to be a mighty champion of freedom. Born in one of the darkest periods of slavery on an estate owned by Colonel Lloyd in Talbot County, Maryland, his life was one of worst kind toward a slave; his life was one of extreme hardship from the beginning. It was forbidding for him or any slave to read when he was a boy. After watching his slave master scold his wife and forbid her to teach him to read, it made him realize as nothing else could have the value of education. So he became a self-taught man. Although President Lincoln and Mr. Douglass both had similar educational learning experiences, they differed that Douglass was forbidden, as a slave to read, and Lincoln was not as a free man. Maybe this is why Lincoln had such great respect for Mr. Douglass' great intelligence. It was known that they both had different views and opinions of the future of the so-called Negro in their days. Example; in the publication that was owned by Mr. Douglass, called The North Star, later Frederick Douglass' Paper, Douglass reported the speech made by Lincoln at Charleston, Illinois, September 18, 1858. "I am not, nor have I ever been, in favor of making voters or jurors neither of Negroes, nor of qualifying them to hold office. Mr. Douglass was given the position of the U.S. Ambassador to Haiti, and he spent the remaining years of his life fighting for the Human Rights amendment of the Negro.

George Washington Carver, (1860-1943) agriculture Wizard of Tuskegee. The son of slave parents, he knew neither his father, nor his mother. All three had been captured by nightriders and taken from Diamond Grove, Missouri, to Arkansas. He later wandered on to Minneapolis, Kansas; he entered high school, and graduated. Later he entered and graduated from Iowa State College, where he received his M. S. degree in agriculture. In 1896 he joined the faculty of Tuskegee Institute, where he taught and directed agricultural research. He was a pioneer in promoting crop rotation as a means of soil conservation. He is perhaps best known for developing innovative uses of the peanut, sweet potato, and soybean. Carver donated his life savings in 1938 to form the George Washington Carver Foundation. Carver National Monument near his birthplace in Missouri was the first national monument to honor an African American. He was a modest man.

Dr. Ivan Gladstone Van Sertima (26 January 1935 – 25 May 2009) was a Guyanese-born associate professor of Africana Studies at Rutgers University in the United States.[1]

He was best known for his oleic alternative origin speculations a brand of pre-Columbian contact theory, which he proposed in his book *They Came Before Columbus* (1976). While his oleic theory has "spread widely in African American community, both lay and scholarly", it was mostly ignored in Mesoamericans scholarship, or else dismissed as Afro centric pseudo history to the effect of "robbing native American cultures".

Lerone Bennett, Jr. (born October 17, 1928) is an African-American scholar, author and social historian, known for his analysis of race relations in the United States. His best-known works include *Before the Mayflower* (1962) and *Forced into Glory* (2000), about President Abraham Lincoln.

Bennett was born in Clarksdale, Mississippi on October 17, 1928, the son of Lerone Bennett, MR. and Alma Reed. When he was young, his family moved to Jackson, Mississippi, the capital. He attended segregated schools as a child under the state system.

Bennett graduated from Morehouse College in Atlanta, Georgia. He has noted this time was integral to his intellectual development. He also joined the Kappa Alpha Psi fraternity.

After graduate studies, Bennett became a journalist for the *Atlanta Daily World* in 1949, continuing until 1953. He also served as city editor for *JET* magazine from 1952-53.[1] It had been founded in 1945 by John H. Johnson, who first founded its parent magazine, *Ebony,* that year.

In 1953, Bennett became associate editor for *Ebony Magazine*, serving as executive editor beginning in 1958. He served for decades as editors of this prominent magazine. It has served as his base for the publication of a steady stream of articles on African-American history, with some collected and published as books.

He was noted in 1954 for his article, "Thomas Jefferson's Negro Grandchildren,"[2] about the 20th-century lives of individuals claiming descent from Jefferson and his slave Sally Hemings. It brought black oral history into the public world of journalism and published histories. This relationship was long denied by Jefferson's daughter and two of her children, and main line historians relied on their account. But new works published in the 1970s and 1990s challenged that position. Since a 1998 DNA study demonstrated a match between an Eston Hemings descendant and the Jefferson male line, the historic consensus has shifted (including the position of the Thomas Jefferson Foundation at Monticello) to acknowledging that Jefferson likely had a 38-year relationship with Hemings and was the father of all her six children of record, four of whom survived to adulthood.

Cheikh Anta Diop (29 December 1923 – 7 February 1986) was a Senegalese and French Afrocentric historian, anthropologist, physicist, and politician who studied the human race's origins and pre-colonial African_culture. Cheikh_Anta_Diop_University, in Dakar, Senegal, is named after him.

Born in Thieytou, Diourbel_Region, French_Senegal, Diop was born to an aristocratic Muslim Wolof family in Senegal, where he was educated in a traditional Islamic school. Diop's family was part of the Mouride brotherhood, the only independent Muslim fraternity in Africa according to Diop. He obtained a bachelor's degree in Senegal before moving to Paris for graduate studies, where he ended his scholastic education. His great book The Origin of African Civilizations and video lector on "The African Origins of Humanity-The Historical and Scientific Evidence!

J. B. Fuller, one of the greatest salesmen of modern time, the father of door to door sales his products were the Fuller brush and household products out of Chicago IL. His product was so popular that many Hollywood productions and shows were named after his company. The early 50s Lucille Ball, who played the Fuller brush girl on a TV show, Sid Caesar also played a role as a Fuller brush boy. This shows the great popularity of Mr. Fuller and his Brush Company. Mr. Fuller was a man that most of the African American old money millionaires in Chicago say they were either directly or indirectly influenced by.

Benjamin Banneker (1731-1806) was the first black man to issue an almanac. His series continued until 1797. Mr. Banneker was born in Maryland, where he became a tobacco farmer. He was a brilliant mathematician, and mechanic that led to his invention of the wood or striking clock in about 1752. Under the commission of President Thomas Jefferson, he surveyed, and helped architecturally design the nation's capitol Washington DC. Because he was too sick to do his work in the field, he consulted as an assistant to George Ellicot, in the survey of the ten-mile square of the District of Columbia.

It is said that his brilliance was so respected in London England that the powers to be at that time so name the towering clock in Westminster Abbey Big Ben, as a tribute to him.

Josephine Baker, (1906-1975), Entertainer, Humanitarian, born Freda Josephine McDonald in St. Louis Missouri. In the Broadway musicals "Shuffle Along" (1923) and "Chocolate Dandies" (1924) she gained prominence in New York, but her career became legendary after she moved to Paris in (1925). It was there in La Revue Ne'gre and at theatre des Champs-Elysees she won acclaim for her dramatic jazz singing and dancing and her exotic costumes. Baker became a naturalized French citizen in 1937 and spied for the French Resistance during World War II. In the 1950s she and husband Jo Buillon, an orchestra leader, adopted twelve orphan children of different races and nationalities; Baker called them the "Rainbow Family".

Honorable Elijah Muhammad, Black Nationalist/Spiritual Leader Born 1897 in Sandersville, Georgia as Elijah Poole, his father was a Baptist preacher. It was from that youthful exposure that the Honorable Elijah Muhammad began to shape his mission. While living in Detroit, he met a man that became his mentor and guide. This man was referred to by Honorable Elijah Muhammad and many others, then and now, as Master Fard Muhammad. Master Muhammad taught Honorable Elijah Muhammad the mysteries, and secrets of Islam. He was the leader that did the most to make African Americans feel proud of being called Black people as opposed to being called colored, Negroes, or Niggers. He and his organization built self-help programs for African Americans. Through those teaching the Nation of Islam was born.

The Honorable Elijah Muhammad raised hundreds of thousands of followers and millions of listeners all over the world. His teachings effected many people from Malcolm X, Muhammad Ali, Wallace Muhammad, or Louis Farrakhan. All of these men had something in common; they were all his leading representatives. And men like Jessie Jackson, Martin Luther king, King Nassir of Egypt and many more important men and women council with this great man about the African American communities and the world. His basic teaching was that the African American is a descendant of the original man.

Wallace Muhammad, A spiritual leader. Wallace is the next to the youngest son of the Honorable Elijah Muhammad with his wife Clair Muhammad. Wallace grew up watching his father as a very busy and important man. There were many times he was not with his father because of the restraints of his father's leadership. But because he was given the best teaching available at that time, he grew up very smart and very fast. He spoke Arabic fluently, and by the time he was 25 he was the minister for the Muhammad Mosque in Philadelphia PA. He was the one man that Malcolm X. and Minister Farrakhan would seek advice and counsel from other than the Honorable Elijah Muhammad. He was the first leader in the Nation of Islam to openly teach and practice Orthodox Islam. He called it world Community of Islam.

Al Hajj Malik Shabazz a nationalist, revolutionist and spiritual leader. He was born in Omaha, Nebraska; his father was a follower of Marcus Garvey; his father was murdered by a white mob of racists. As a child he was discouraged by his teacher from trying to get a higher education and was told he would have a better chance at getting a vocational skill because he would do better working with his hands. Little did he know that might have been enough to motivate him to work with his intelligence and become a leader? After joining the Nation of Islam he was made the spokesperson for the Honorable Elijah Muhammad, he then called Malcolm X. It was Malcolm that started the first newspaper to the Nation of Islam. But he left the NOI over disagreement with policy within the NOI. He started his own movement and organization; it was called the Organization of African American Unity. The motto was "by any means necessary, the ballot or the bullet." The influence of men that he met in the Holy City of Mecca, Wallace Muhammad, inspired him spiritually to become a committed orthodox student and teacher.

President Dr. Kwame Nkrumah: President, of the first independent democratic government in the Republic of Ghana Africa. President Kwame Nkrumah was also the founder and CEO of the Organization of African Unity. The (OAU) under the instructions of President Nkrumah commissioned one of my mentors, Malcolm (X.) Shabazz created a chapter of (OAU) in America, it was called the Organization of African American Unity (OAAU) his mandate and instructions was to go before the United Nations and speak on the issue of Human Rights on behalf of all people of African descent. Dr. Kwame Nkrumah was a student of the New York University (NYU), he received his PHD in Law while attending.

Katherine Dunham. (1910-1963) Was the first black choreographer to work at the Metropolitan Opera House; A dancer, choreographer, school founder, and anthropologist, she was born in Gyln, Ellyn Illinois, and graduate from the University of Chicago and Northwestern University. Dr. Dunham incorporated her training in anthropology and her study of African and West Indian dances into her own techniques and dance instruction. She and her work had been seen in many Hollywood musical films as a dancer and a choreographer.

Dr. Martin Luther King (1929-1968) Dr. Martin Luther King was the oldest son of Alberta King, a school teacher, and a Baptist minister Martin Luther King who he was named after. His youth was in the sweet Auburn district of Atlanta. At 15 years old he entered and in 1948 graduated from Morehouse College in Atlanta, Ga. with a BA. In 1951 he graduated with a BD from Chester, PA.

1953 Dr. King married Coretta Scott they had four children together. In 1957 Dr. King became the leader of a group of black ministers known as the Southern Christian Leadership Conference. King was to be named the president later. 1959 Dr. King went to India, there is little doubt the admiration that Dr. King had for Mohandas K. Gandhi's spirit of passive resistance helped to shape the techniques for his civil rights movement, and it's successes.

1955 Dr. King received his Doctoral PH.D. Degree on June 5th from Boston University.

1962 King met with President John F. Kennedy to urge support for civil rights; less than a year later he was arrested in Birmingham after demonstrating in defiance to a court order. It is believed that the letter he wrote from jail was widely circulated and became a classic of the Civil Rights Movement. In August of that same year 250,000 civil rights supporter's march on Washington and Dr. King delivered his famous "I have a dream" speech.

1968 April 4th Dr. King was assassinated in Memphis Tenn.

Booker T. Washington, 1856-1915, Born in Virginia as a slave, he became an educator and first black American depicted on a US postage stamp. Booker Taliaferro Washington was the foremost black educator of the 19th and early 20th Centuries. He also had a major influence on southern and race relations and was a dominant figure in black public affairs from 1895 until his death in 1915. After a secondary education at Hampton Institute, he taught school and studied briefly, law and ministry. In 1881 he founded Tuskegee Normal and Industrial Institute on the same model of the college that he went to, Hampton Institute in the black belt of Alabama.

Washington was an educator; at the time he was teaching; there were different schools of thought for African Americans in the North led by a group called the Talented Ten. Their attempt was to bring the so-called Negroes into mainstream politics and white-collar education. The other group was the self-help agriculturist and technical labor tradesmen that Booker T. Washington would teach at Tuskegee. Mr. Washington's approach to educate the so-called Negro for vocational trade education inspired many to work with his school. The United States Government partnered many times with Tuskegee from agricultural techniques to training airplane pilots, to fights in America's war as the Tuskegee Airmen.

Carter Woodson, Historian, (1875-1950) Organized the first learned social society devoted to the professional study of African American history, in Chicago Ill. September 9, 1915 at the YMCA, on Wabash Avenue. Mr. Woodson was born in New Canton, Virginia. He was educated at Berea College (Kentucky) (lit.), the University of Chicago (B. A. -MA) and Harvard (Ph.D.). He is considered the founder and Father of Negro or African American history. The organization he founded sponsored in 1926 Negro History Week. (It is now called Black History Month) one of his many great books that he wrote is "Mis-Education of the Negro".

J. A. Rogers, African American anthropologist and historian. He was a pioneer in black studies and was little appreciated in his lifetime. He did years of extensive research on the influence of African leadership around the world. It is said that his books and writings played a major role on many of the great African studies philosopher's opinions, then and now. His books are "From Superman to Man", "Sex and Race", "World's Greatest Men of Color" one & two, "Five Black Presidents". His books were mostly circulated among the so-called radical blacks in his day, but he was respected by most.

Honorable David N. Dinkins, 106th **Mayor** for the City of New York from 1990 to 1993. He was the first African American Mayor in New York City's history. Dinkins entered office pledging racial healing, and famously referred to New York City's demographic diversity as a "gorgeous mosaic. Under Mayor Dinkins' Safe Streets, Safe Cities program, crime in New York City decreased more dramatically and more rapidly, both in terms of actual numbers and percentages, than at any time in modern New York City history. The rates of most crimes, including all categories of violent crime, made consecutive declines during the 36-months of his service as the Mayor.

Harold Washington, Mayor for the City of Chicago. He was the first African American Mayor in modern Chicago's history. Many believed that he lived in the spirit of his great hero Jean Baptiste Pointe DuSable. Harold Washington attended DuSable High School he was a habitual reader; some say he could finish six books in a weekend. It is believed that is how he learned about the history of the man DuSable and decided he wanted to be like DuSable. Harold, like DuSable, was a highly intelligent statesman, and negotiator, as the State Senator of Illinois, and later Mayor of Chicago. He brought diversity in government and fair play in contracts and business for all people under his leadership

Harold Washington was known all over the world as the great African American leader in Chicago. Under Harold Washington's reign Chicago became the City for people to want to live in. Thanks to Harold Washington, the population of Chicago grew and the reputation of Chicago as being a Diverse fair city has been the popular theme ever since.

Harriet Tubman, (1820- 1913) the first twenty-five years of her life was spent as a slave on a Maryland plantation. She was a revolutionist and leader for the Underground Railroad. She had the courage of a commander, and strategy of a general. She was called Moses because of her success in guiding her people out of the land of Egypt. As a woman General Moses was unusually strong and muscular. After making her own escape she successfully made those trips (thirteen) times back and forth over a network of sympathizers to conduct four hundred slaves to freedom. She did that with a $12, 000

Reward for her capture, she was also called the "black shadow". She was well known in New England and Canada as one of the first African American leaders in the equal rights for women's feminist movement.

Oscar Micheaux, (1884-1951) was born near Metropolis Illinois, the son of a freed slave. He worked in Chicago as a shoeshine-boy. He was a porter on a Pullman railroad car, before moving to South Dakota to become a farmer. It was there he started his true passion for writing, and he wrote several novels. Micheaux formed his own publishing company and sold his books door to door. Micheaux started his own motion picture company, because at that time the white silent film industry did not welcome black film writers. He was the father of the black film industry. When blacks were not considered photographical he pioneered the industry by writing, producing, and directing his own movies.

N. H. Bronner Died in (1993) he was the founder of the largest black hair and beauty show in the world. In 1947 Dr. Nathaniel H. Bronner, Sr. with the help of his sister, Emma Bronner began teaching cosmetology at the Butler YMCA in Atlanta, Georgia. Subsequently the first Bronner Brothers Trade Show was born with 300 people in attendance. The show attracted many well-known speakers Jackie Robertson, Benjamin Mays, Dr. Martin Luther King. Mr. Bronner always incorporated positive motivational speakers to the show. At present Bronner Brothers employs over 300 people, operates two manufacturing facilities, two beauty stores, one hair weaving studios, public relations office, and a corporate headquarters in Marietta, Georgia.

Ronald E. McNair, 1950-1986 Physicist/Astronaut Ron McNair was the first African American Astronaut in Space. He was also one of seven that died when the space shuttle Challenger exposition exploded in Space Jan. 28th. 1986. He was born in Lake City NC, to Carl and Pearl McNair. His mother taught elementary school and his dad was an automobile mechanic. Ron was one of those unique African Americans that excelled, in spite of the obstacles. He was named valedictorian of his high school and went on to attend North Carolina Agriculture and Technical State University. In 1971 he graduated magna cum laude with a B.S. degree in physics. Ron then enrolled in the prestigious Massachusetts Institute of Technology, where he earned a Ph.D. in physics at the young age of 26. He was a Presidential Scholar and a Ford Foundation Fellow. He was named Omega Psi Phi Scholar of the year and Honored as Distinguished National Scientist by the National Society of Black Professional Engineers.

In 1978, NASA selected him for the Astronauts corps. To commemorate his lifetime of accomplishments, the U.S. Department of Education established the Ronald E. McNair Post Baccalaureate Achievement Program, to encourage and prepare low-income, first generation college students for doctoral education.

Arthur Ash, 1943-1993 a political Activist, Champion, the South African awareness of the oppressive style of apartheid to the world, by his call for expulsion from South Africa from the tennis tour and Davis Cup play, and was supported by numerous prominent individuals and organizations. He was the First black man to win at Wimbledon Tennis professional tournament. He was born in Richmond, Virginia.

Charles Drew, 1904- 1950 was born in Washington, D.C.; through experimenting with Blood Plasma he discovered that it (BP) could be used instead of whole blood. It lasted longer and was less likely to become contaminated. He was the farther of the term blood banking. Charles Drew was named director of the Red Cross Blood Bank and assistant director of the National Research Council, in charge of blood collection for the U.S. Army and Navy.

Thurgood Marshal, 1908-1993 Is one of the most well known figures in the history of civil rights in America and the first Black Supreme Court Justice. Was selected by President John F. Kennedy and served on the Court for 24 years until June 28, 1991 when he announced his retirement due to advancing age and deteriorating health. He passed away January 24, 1993.

Scot Joplin, 1867-1917 He was born in Sedalia, Missouri, he grew up in Texarkana, which is city that straddles the border of Texas - Arkansas. It was in St. Louis in 1880 that he became popular for ragtime music. In 1907 Scot went to New York, composed an opera, the score was considered the most American opera ever composed. Many consider him as the greatest ragtime piano player that ever lived and the first black to play on Broadway.

James Weldon Johnson: born June 17th 1871 in Jacksonville, Florida. He was the musical writer, of the national black anthem ("lift every voice and sing"), a school teacher and a principal at a school in Jacksonville, Florida and he was a civil activist. In 1895 he founded a newspaper, the Daily American. He studied law and became the first African American to pass the Bar exam in Florida. In 1906 he secured a position as a Consulate in Puerto Cabello, Venezuela, from there to Corinto, Nicaragua in1909. Before his death, he wrote three anthologies: "The Book of American Negro Poetry" (1922), "The Book of American Negro Spirituals" (1925), and the "Second Book of Negro Spirituals" (1926). During his final years, he wrote a history of Black life in New York that focused on the Harlem Renaissance; it was called Black Manhattan (1930).

Paul Robeson, 1898-1976 was born in Princeton, New Jersey; his father was a clergyman, and his mother was a schoolteacher. He was a graduate of Rutgers University A.B. (1919), Columbia University, LL.B., (1923), Admitted and employed in a law firm; actor appearances include "Simon the Cyrenian", 1921; "All Gods Chillun Got Wings", 1924; "Show Boat", 1928; "Othello", 1930 – 1943: "Toussaint L'Ouverture", 1936.Films include: "Body and Soul", 1924; "The Emperor Jones", 1933: "Sanders of the River", 1935; and "Show Boat", 1936. As an athlete while at Rutgers, he was the first all-American in Football. While going to law school, he played professional football on the weekend to earn a law degree. He was a staunch supporter of the Soviet Union and was censored for his frankness and views.

Adam Clayton Powell Jr., 1908-1972 was born in New Haven, Connecticut, He moved to New York at the age of three. His father was a minister and developed the largest congregation in the United States, at the Abyssinian Baptist Church. He was a graduate with a B.A. from Colgate University in 1930 and M.A. degree from Columbia University in 1931. In 1941 He was elected as an independent to the New York City Council. He married the famous singer Ms. Hazel Scott. He was the Publisher and editor of The People's Voice, which was a weekly newspaper, from 1941-1945. He was elected in 1944 U.S. Congress representing New York District 22. In Washington, Powell challenged the informal regulations forbidding black representatives from using Capital facilities. Powell would take black constituents to dine with him in the whites only House restaurant and ordered his staff to eat there, whether they were hungry or not.

Shirley Chisholm, First African American woman elected to the House of Representatives, was from Brooklyn New York, and was the first woman to seek nomination as the Democrat's presidential candidate. Even though the women's liberation movement did not support her for the President, she was considered one of the greatest and intelligent female political pioneers in modern history. She became famous for the saying (quote) "I was the first female to run for the President of the United States and I just happen to be a Black woman" (unquote).

Muhammad Ali, Olympic gold medalist, US Ambassador, humanitarian. Ali was the first African American boxer to draw a multimillion-dollar gate for his performance. He refused to go to war during the Viet Nam crisis, and went to prison as a conscientious objector. He created the saying in the peace movement "Hell Know I won't go!" He was a hero in the peace movement among young Americans that did not believe in the war. He was stripped of his championship Heavyweight title; after he was exonerated he regained his title and became the ambassador for sports in America. He also was a minister; National spokesperson in the Nation of Islam under Elijah Muhammad.

Oprah Winfrey, first black woman to host a nationally syndicated weekday talk show, The Oprah Winfrey show. She was the first African American woman to earn a value of a billion dollars. She purchased her own television production studio, Harpo Studio. She published a monthly home and fashion magazine called *O magazine*. Oprah has given away much of her wealth to help many people. She started a national book club to create literacy awareness. She is the most popular woman of color in her time; most women of any color want to be like Oprah, a true hero.

John H. Johnson, in 1918 published the *Negro Digest*, the first magazine devoted to summarize the weekly events. That further led to launching of the now famous *Jet* magazine, then later *Ebony* Magazine. He also owned the largest global ethnic makeup line called Fashion Fair, as well as the Fashion Fair fashion show. Johnson expanded his business interests to areas other than his magazines. He became chairperson and chief executive officer of the Supreme Life Insurance Company. He developed a line of cosmetics, purchased three radio stations, started a book publishing company, and a television production company, and served on the board of directors of several major businesses, including the Greyhound Corporation. There has not been a president elect that has not invited Mr. Johnson to the Washington DC inauguration from President Roosevelt to President George Bush, because of his clout in the African American community as one of the "who's who" in America.

George Johnson, the founder of Johnson Products Company. His was the first black firm to be listed on a major stock exchange when it was listed on the American Stock Exchange in 1971. Was one of the largest black companies in America, and the first to have its own research laboratory that studied and produced hair care products for people of color. Johnson Products produced the first no base relaxer system Ultra Sheen. Johnson also pioneer advance educational Hair retreats for professional hair stylist at the famous prestigious Hilton Head Island in South Carolina; it was the first African American company to bring groups of African Americans to Hilton Head Island annually. Johnson Products was always ahead of the curve in the hair industry.

Al Washington, Senior Marketing Executive: at Max Private Label Personal Care Solutions for hair and skin from May 2009 to the present. Former President and Chairman of the Board of Afam Concept Inc. from June 1979 to January 2001 (21 years 8 months). Afam is the maker of Elentee and Vitale hair products; one of the most successful ethnic product lines in the 20th century. The products are available internationally in 50 countries. Mr. Washington managed to stay successful and relevant in the African Diaspora as a progressive African American entrepreneur in the professional hair and beauty industry, when most African American Executives and CEO fell out of the market altogether. In doing so, he remained an example for young entrepreneurs of the ethnic persuasion to persevere and become a leader in the markets of their personal ambitions.

General Colin Powell, 1937 was born in New York City; he is a product of City College of New York (B.S.1958). He attended George Washington University (M.B.A.1971) and the National War College in 1989. He was a four star general, the first African American National Security Advisor; Chairman of the joint Chief of Staff, the mastermind of Desert Storm, and the man the country has said it would like to see as President. 2001 he became the first black to become the Secretary of Defense under President George W. Bush.

Minister Louis Farrakhan, Religious leader; mastermind behind the successful Million-Man March, a great mentor and orator student; and too many believe successor to the Honorable Elijah Muhammad's teachings that the black man is the father of the universe, the maker, owner, and cream of the planet earth. Minister Farrakhan came from and grew up in Boston, went to Winston Salem Teachers College in North Carolina. Met his wife and started a career as a professional calypso singer and violin master to provide for his new family. After meeting Malcolm X. in New York he became a Muslim and dedicated his life to the teachings of Elijah Muhammad. He created and played in a Broadway caliber musical production called, "A White Man's Heaven Is a Blackman's Hell" in such prominent places as the Boston Symphony Hall. After Muhammad Ali went back into boxing to regain his stripped title, Minister Farrakhan became the National Spokesperson for the Nation of Islam, until the death of Elijah Muhammad his lifelong mentor.

Tiger Woods was the youngest man and first African American to win the prestigious master in golf. He created the theory of diversity as a good plus and refused to choose one over the other as to who he was. He called his self a Cabalasion, which represents his roots of Caucasian Black (African American and Asian. Tiger Woods, in his success, carried the reputation of a great athletic role model for young celebrities from any community.

Berry Gordy, The founder of Motown Records one of the largest recording companies for African American music, with more major acts and hits than any other.

Maynard Jackson, The first African American Mayor in the city of Atlanta, who is credited for demanding contracts for people of color in all city projects Like Hartsfield International airport.

George Wilder, The first African American elected Governor for the State of Virginia, and in America.

Spike Lee, Filmmaker, Producer, and Director, "Malcolm X" story, "Do the Right Thing", "School Days", "Jungle Fever", "Bamboozled", and many more. Spike Lee is responsible for the careers of more African American actors than anyone else in filmmaking.

Vanessa Williams, First African American Woman to be elected Miss America; she was stripped of her title, came back to launch a successful singing, acting career.

Winton Marsalis, Trumpeter, Composer, Bandleader, was the first black instrumentalist to simultaneously receive Grammy awards as best classical and jazz soloist.

Michael Jordan, the best basketball player of the nineties, made Nike shoes a popular brand name and one of the wealthiest in the country. He was the most popular athlete in the world with the Chicago Bulls. He also was one of the most successful businessmen in his time.

Magic Ervin Johnson Basketball legend and great entrepreneur helped lead the Los Angeles Lakers to six NBA championships, after retiring became part owner of Lakers. He also owns part of a franchise in Starbucks coffee company, he owns a chain of movie theaters, a chain of restaurants, shopping malls, a Financial investment agency and more.

Johnny Cochrane, the first African American lawyer to win a murder trial case against a white person, an active civil rights lawyer, the famous OJ Simpson case. Johnny Cochrane won more major celebrity cases for people of African descent than any other lawyer.

Reverend Jessie L. Jackson was a part of Dr. Martin Luther King's Civil rights movement. He was the first African American to be a non-symbolic candidate for the presidential nomination. He is the founder of Operation PUSH, a Baptist Minister, political leader in the Democratic Party voter's registration and a syndicated talk show host; he is also known to be the lead person that lobbied for the official name reclassification of the term Negro gender unto the widely accepted new term as African American gender in America.

Olive Lee Benson the First African American to become a member of the prestigious Inter Coiffure hair and beauty organization, the first Since Madame Walker to have an international signature line of products sponsored by L'Oreal of Paris called the Olive Benson Line relaxer system. A creator of her own hair training system and center called the Hair metric system.

Joe Dudley, founder, and owner of Dudley Hair products, and Dudley Beauty School. Has one of the most successful sales force in the hair and beauty business, has the largest national educational beauty school program for men and women of color in the United States. He was also the owner of the famous Fuller Products line

Patrick Kelly, the first African American to been recognized as an international Fashion designer in Paris, was known for his usage's of buttons in his design, And the rag doll.

Willie Smith the First African American to launch a successful men line of close the Willie Wear line of clothes from America that went international.

James Harris Hair stylist James Harris was born on October 20, 1948, in Boston, Massachusetts, to Emma J. Jones-Harris, a supervisor for the Boston City Hospitals, and Grover Harris, owner of a demolition and trucking company. His aunt was a hairdresser and his uncle was a barber. By the time Harris was twelve years old, he knew that he wanted to become a hair stylist. Harris attended the Newman Preparatory School High School for Boys in Boston, Massachusetts. He and a friend purchased wigs wholesale and sold them while in high school, and at the age of eighteen, Harris had his first paying client.

After graduating from high school in 1967, Harris started a career as a hair stylist. He toured the United States with Summit Labs, an African American hair care manufacturing company. In

1972, Harris was a member of the first African American team to win an International Beauty Show. Harris earned a degree from La Newton School of Beauty in Roxbury, Massachusetts, developed products with Revlon and opened his first salon, the Libra Studio, in Mattapan, Massachusetts, all in 1974. In efforts to revolutionize the hair industry, Harris established the Hairmetrics hair care training center with stylist Olive Benson that same year. Hairmetrics was the first advanced hair training center in the world. Shortly after the opening of Hairmetrics, Harris sold his Boston salon and moved to New York in 1977 to become the styles director for Soul Scissors, the country's first chain salon operation. In 1980, Harris helped create Shear Energy, an advanced hair designing system for excessively curly hair. That next year, he started working with Glemby International Beauty Salons as president of the Black Hair Is line. In 1991, Harris became the first African American male member of Intercoiffure, an organization of elite hair stylists and salon owners. He stayed at Glemby International Beauty Salons until 1997, when he opened the Mahogany Door Beauty Center & Spa in Harlem. After three years, he left the salon and started working at L'Oreal in a variety of capacities. He remained with L'Oreal until 2007, when he decided to return to the salon industry and established the James Harris Salon in Boston and New York.

Harris is the founder of the African American stylists' organization, Hair Fashion Group. He participated in fashion shows in South Africa, Cote d'Ivoire, France, Italy, Spain, Brazil and other countries. He has collaborated with celebrities such as Diana Ross, Tyra Banks, Nancy Wilson and Patti LaBelle, as well as designers Patrick Kelly, Betsey Johnson and Gucci.

President Barak Hussein Obama, the first person of African Decent to be the leader of the free world and President of the United States of America. A man of mixed race, half black and white, his father born in Africa of Kenyan descent and his mother in America of Irish descent, he embodies the full reality of multicultural global diversity. In the minds of many his inaugural enactment represented the signal of a New World Order at the beginning of the twenty first century and as a new global Agent of Change.

Michelle LaVaughn Robinson Obama (born January 17, 1964) is an American lawyer and writer. She is the wife of the 44th President of the United States, Barack Obama, she is the first African-American First Lady of the United States. Raised on the South Side of Chicago, she was a graduate from Princeton University in Princeton, New Jersey and the Harvard Law School in Cambridge, Massachusetts. The early part of her legal career was working at a law firm that was called Sidley Austin LPP, which is where she met Barack. Subsequently, she worked as part of the staff of Chicago Mayor Richard M. Daley, and for the University of Chicago Medical Center.

Throughout 2007 and 2008, Obama helped campaign for her husband's presidential bid. She delivered a keynote address at the 2008 Democratic National Convention and spoke at the 2012 Democratic National Convention. She and her husband have two daughters together. As the wife of a senator, and later the first lady, she has become a fashion icon and role model for women, and an advocate for poverty awareness, nutrition, physical activity, healthful eating and equal human rights.

Chapter Twenty-Five

Let's Get Positive!

Of course there are many more heroes that I know, and don't know, that are not listed here. This is not to say that there are not others outside of the African Diaspora whom deserve recognition and respect, as well; but I believe that pride begins with self, first.

With so many individual accomplishments, you must ask yourself, "What prevents the rising of African American conditions?" African Americans can cash in on all of their talents at any time if they had the mind to. Furthermore! Knowing this how can we still accept the second-class treatment regardless to money or power conditions?

We seem to fall into some kind of in, and out sleep, with a feeling that the opposite of what we are is better. Like the Biblical story of the sleeping lion of Judea, this parable is definitely speaking of the African American people. When the lion wakes, it will roar and rule his kingdom and all the other predators will surrender.

SELF HATRED

SELF HATRED example, what is commonly considered a pretty, or beautiful, baby among many in the African American community is generally mixed with White, Asian, or Indian, blood. Light skin, keen features, curly to straight hair. On the other hand, it appears when a dark skin person or baby is compared to a light skin baby, it is common for many African Americans to make comments on how good, or not, the dark skin person's child is, or going to be. Many predict dark skin children to have a bad future, but a good future for light skin children. In certain parts of America, it is frowned on if a dark skin person, will date, or marry a light skin person. In Louisiana, Creole women are so- called set aside, to be kept by a light skin or white man.

In many parts of the mid-west Chicago, Detroit, Cincinnati, Indianapolis, Milwaukee, Minneapolis, light skin people are still considered better looking, regardless of their age, intelligence, or status, unless of course the dark skin person has fame, power or money.

We have seen in the fashion industry over the years that most of the African American models are light skin models. In the nineties, though, we have seen a change where a showing of dark skin models was the trend. Even the African American media agencies, manufacturers, and publishers, in particular Midwestern and western companies when interviewing for a job as an image model, light skin models are generally chosen first.

I believe these are signs of a subliminal control over people of color's conscious, as well as a formula of self-hatred. There is a carefully grafted, then supplanted mental tradition that affects the product of America (Negro) that is deliberately designed by secret societies. These societies' goals were to make people of color not think of their dark skin as beautiful or their culture as good, but in fact see other than self as better. Maybe it's the results of the bible myth of Ham (Hamites-black), Shem (Shemites-white), how else can we explain this unnatural self-hatred, denial of self and inferior complex.

These deeply rooted phobias must be brought forward and systemically eliminated through seminars, consulting, and motivational facts, sharing sessions using African American social workers and psychologists. We must find ways to take back our culture.

Look at the music industry. African American musicians, except for a few, are controlled by other than self, with intent of managing our social activities. Hair, makeup, clothes, through musical lyrics and musical science, our dance, personal character, and perception of self is being fashioned by others.

Rap, Hip Hop the resurgence of musical poetry, brought with it, not only spoken words, but also a factious life style, based on a rough talking, down dress looking, and limited musical talent. I can remember the music and entertainers before rap, when entertainers had to be able to read music, play an instrument, dance well, have a fashion wardrobe, stay out of trouble, and above all, have vocal talent.

FASHION INDUSTRY

Fashion and style of the nineties was a product of systematic marketing, using the science of music, so people's lifestyles definitely are being controlled in this matter.

Taking the matter forward into the millennium fashion industry is tied into this to be blunt, brainwashing people of color. After all there are lots of profits to be made in controlling society, style and taste. I am talking about billions of dollars.

The music can be some time very vulgar, with lyrics that display no intelligence at all. The trend of using former hits, melodies, and sometimes lyrics (sampling) send a clear signal to the fashion industry or any alert industry, that at any given time, this society can be had, because it lacks imagination.

How else can you explain men, not just boys, volunteering to shave their heads like the bible myth of Delilah, telling Sampson (cut your hair and you surely will be strong). Or the opposite of *let it grow* and *let it go* without any limits or concerns of cultural esteem.

Dressing down, as if we did not have over two hundred years of not having, means to dress up to our true potential as people of a Great lost culture, and to know that many of us are descendants of a people that were lost from Royalty and Royal behavior. Once we come to that understanding, we should behave as people of the highest dignity and class; that quality was in our ancestors' history, and is in our genes.

There are very few African American designers that are allowed to get media blessing, somehow in the nineties, most of the designers that conformed to the musical trend designers like Karl Kani, [black] or Tommy Hilfiger [white] who manufactured styles that look like they were meant for babies or young children were very successful. To think a shoe, sneakers that could be purchased for at tops, fifty dollars, are now being sold for two hundred dollars or more, over-sized tee shirts and shorts, worn-looking or torn blue jeans as dress wear, and pants that sag below the waist to allow one's underwear to be seen. What hype! We have been bamboozled, been had, run amuck, as Malcolm X said.

Then there is the media music video that gives a constant fashion show of nude or nearly nude women or girls acting and dancing like sexual strippers and the so-called fashion forecast to what is perceived as the trend. Some call it urban looks, hip, cool, phat, all that, or whatever. All of these are the formulas for controlling the culture of the modern young mind to operate on the lowest level humanly possible.

FINAL COMMENTS ABOUT THE HAIR INDUSTRY

I believe the hair industry is more than a fascinating field. It is also a very important social and political part of a society, nation, and the world community to respect that knowledge and using the skills of the professionals in the business can help develop and maintain a modern progressive cultural society. The industry deals with art, paramedical treatment, fashion, cosmetic beauty, science, and finance. Each of these divisions has its own unlimited margins of growth and career satisfaction.

It has been said by some that there is a subtle bonding effect on people that is caused by touching, particularly touching the head. People have the tendency to talk about their private and innermost thoughts, and so many of the activities that take place in most communities, the professional hair stylists are constantly being informed, with as many views as their skills allow them to service cross- racial and sexual clients. From leaders, to followers, trend setters, to no style at all. People from all walks of life are constantly sharing their thoughts. If they pay attention, a Hair Stylist, Barber, Beautician, Esthetician, Etc., can be a positive culturist to help keep their clients in tune with the times.

Unfortunately, far too many so-called professionals put so much time into gossip, back biting, and jealousy; the majority of information or intelligence is not used for networking, or for uplifting the communities, and in most cases, not even to help them. All the elements are there, and also the freedom to pioneer.

The hair and beauty industry is one of the most unregulated industries in America in particular when compared to the amount of money that is generated and the easy access to independent entrepreneurship. That is why cross-cultural entrepreneurs have done so well, in particular white business people, with black products. From K. K. K. [King Kong Konkoline] hair straightener that was manufactured in the 1950's, until African Pride products made the 1990s. With the acquisition, most of the top hair and beauty companies: Johnson, Carson, Soft Sheen, Dark and Lovely by L'Oreal of France, the beginning of a new era starts as the old end multi-cultural take over.

As a Hair artist, I see the baldheaded hairstyle as a definite sign of character attack on African American diversity in hairstyles. There is a saying that if an individual raindrop falls into a puddle of water or ocean, it immediately loses its identity. To me if you look in a room full of baldheaded persons it is hard to see any individualism in that view. It is as if someone has cloned these people, or brainwashed them into an image and classified it as hip, cool or stylish and many bought into it.

Unless bald is a style that has been chosen, because of conditions i.e. hair loss, scalp disease, or disorder. There is not much imagination or individualism on the part of the person to shave his head. Unless it is a part of a cult, there is the right of passage ceremony among some African boys and girls, in Africa as a sign of preparing for maturity customs. There is also an ancient Egyptian custom of the royal class people's Kings, Queen's, etc., shaving off all hair on their body as a status symbol.

But for me, I still see skinheads as a group of racist angry white men that shaved their heads as a sign of strength or hardness, as one of the first groups to start the baldheaded trend in America. Any way you look at it, you can just about guess what we see through the eyes of a barber, or beauty culturist in one word, boring.

GIVE BACK TO THE COMMUNITY

Personally, I have no problem with the advertising industry taking advantage of a marketing opportunity. However, I must admit that I am disappointed with the lack of professional respect that is practiced or given by most of these marketers and profit seekers toward the educated licensed professionals, and the community they service.

I believe that the hair and beauty industry should make a better effort to give back to the communities that they are profiting from, African American, Latino, Hispanic, Asian, Polish, Italian, French, etc. They can do this by sponsoring cultural activities and programs that highlight Fashion, Arts, Dance, Music, Theater, Literature and Cuisine in the various communities, not just product advertisement.

Organizations must be held accountable to better support community relations in the Multi-Cultural Diaspora, to bridge the divide and better network for Americans.

This can be done in our lifetime by getting involved as individuals in progressive projects in our communities.

There are sororities, fraternities, lodges, public and private social groups that if they were to dedicate, or pledge to change our social status, with their resources instead of maintaining secret pledges to help their elite members or groups, we would all be better off for that in America and abroad.

It is no secret that among the African American athletes and entertainers, and businesses that individually produce over a million dollars a year, there is enough wealth collectively to help us lift African Americans up by their own bootstraps and we should do that. We cannot forget that we are the pioneers for African American recovery so the economical sacrifices that have to be made must come from this pool of wealth. This is the only reason that God gave us these blessings of economical and intellectual success, to uplift our race. We have to think like others do about their race and community that we can do away with despicable conditions of despair and hopelessness. As I stated in the beginning, we were not included in the success of the American dream for the millennium. No one invited us to the party. God has been preparing us for this day, we have what it takes among us to make it for ourselves; it is part of a divine plan. I believe those of us that will not help to make the sacrifices to uplift the race, should beware when the (sleeping lion of Judea does awake) it could be unforgettable and brutal. Now is the time to be heroes and sheroes in America.

WHEN PRESIDENT NELSON MANDELA CAME TO CHICAGO

In the mid eighties I was in South Africa: it was at the time when Mr. Mandela was still in the Robbins Island prison and I, like most activists, had strong unsettling feelings that he might never be released from prison; and there was absolutely no vision or belief that he would one day be released and become the President of the country that had previously incarcerated him. I dreamed of the chance to hear him speak freely without the restrictions that I witnessed on him, when I was in South Africa.

I can remember that I was filled with great joy and excitement when President Nelson Mandela, after being released from prison, came to Chicago. I was there.

He spoke at the Illinois Institute of Technology University campus auditorium. Mr. John Davis, the anchor newsman for NBC Channel 2 was the narrator.

That lecture was part of a tour that Mr. Mandela was on right after he became the President of the South African government. The topic was America has the skills and resources to help South Africa recover and she should do that. He also said that African Americans have the intelligence and resources that if we were willing to bring it to Africa, we alone could save our motherland. He said that we were taken away from Africa, and we have prospered in this land; but the time has come to go home, and help our people as others do in their homeland.

Mr. Mandela pleaded with us to come to Africa, visit and help in the developments that will come out of new leadership. I had many questions for him and he did the best that he could to give me the message for the need of us to return to South Africa and for others to visit, now that apartheid had been lifted. I was so proud and felt special that I had lived to witness in real time on the ground such a miracle and historical world phenomena in my lifetime.

I believe he spoke the truth, but I further believe that before we can be effective in Africa we must first do something effective for ourselves; right here in America. We should put to test how to improve our communities, and people's conditions; so that when we are ready to make an exodus to the motherland, we would have built a much-needed spirit of trust, and respect for ourselves in America. I believe the world is watching, and waiting on us to grow up and truly take that challenge. They know we have what it takes, so they watch and wait for us to wake up and take control so that we might give back to the world our leadership.

WE CAN DO IT AND WE MUST!

I have suggested that African Americans' gift to America and the world is its culture. Art, fashion, beauty, music, dance, poetry, movies, theater, sports, and literature; since we have been in this country under the wicked control of our former slave masters, and their children, we have become a crafty people. When you travel throughout the world, you can see the influence of African American culture, and one instinctively asks the question, *why do we not market our gifts as others do and promote them as our trademark to profit and help ourselves?*

Another thing that really gets under my skin is the attitude of our artists that we must get the approval of white organizations (example Oscar, Emmy, ASCAP, Grammy, etc.) or we do not feel we have made it. Validate your own awards like the Ebony, Essence, NAACP, etc. and be even more proud of those recognitions than the ones from someone other than us might give. Like the old saying goes, *no one will like us, for us, but us.* So we should stop whining and be happy to get the Oscar Micheaux producers and director's award, Paul Robertson theatrical or performance award, Billy Holiday, Scot Joplin, Lena Horne, Louis Armstrong, Sidney Porter, Harry Belafonte and Katherine Dunham Oscar Brown Jr. There are enough Artists from our past that were so great in their day that if we took pride in honoring them today, other communities would envy our awards.

As individuals, we have excelled and others have used our gifts to serve themselves and control the direction of the masses of our people, a modern high tech. master slave relationship. No one is prepared to admit that this situation fits them, but as the old saying goes *if the shoe fits wear it.* We can fix this problem and we must, I challenge you to help rewrite our past from a people that gave it all unto someone else, to a people that pick themselves up and did something for themselves.

In Conclusion

Peace Unto You That Reads This Book.

Haroon Abdullah Rashid

Love is the proper name and character of The Most High, The All & All, and Master of The Universe, knowing that there is only one race, the Human Race, coexisting together as Human Beings. Anything that will attempt to replace that reality is a pure distraction or an illusion!

About The Author

HAROON RASHID
Social Activist, Master Hair Stylist and Educator

In 1999 Haroon Rashid became the Founder and former President of Friends of DuSable, a not for profit organization dedicated to educating the public on the legacy of the founder of modern day Chicago, Jean Baptiste Pointe DuSable.

In 2000 he became a member of the City of Chicago's Commission on Human Relations Advisory Council on African Affairs for 13 years.

In acknowledging the rich and diverse history of the City of Chicago, as well as the great accomplishments of its founder, (Friends of DuSable & Chicago Commission on Human Relation) was responsible for establishing a citywide commemoration in honor of Jean Baptiste Pointe DuSable.

Because of the social activism by Haroon Rashid, the now implementations of the DuSable Commemoration not only serves as a day to honor DuSable, it is a vehicle to bring communities together for a day of unity in celebration on March 4th each year centered on the origin of the great city of Chicago that they all share.

Haroon Rashid was introduced to the hair and beauty industry at the age of 15, working as a salon assistant in his Uncle John S. Jones barbershop in Boston, MA. It was at **Sportsman Barbershop**, that he began his interaction with hair care professionals and clients. At the age of 18 he enlisted in the United States Marine Corp. During the last year of his four-year stint, Haroon became the base barber at McAlister Navel

Ammunition Depot in McAlister Oklahoma as an off duty assignment. That experience exposed him to the multi-cultural and diverse aspect of hair care service. By the age of 22, Haroon had completed Wilfred Beauty College and Vaughn Barber School, in Boston, MA. As you can see, major emphasis was placed on the hair business, well before any formal education began.

He worked as a advance stylist and educator in Boston at the prestigious Olive Benson Beauty salon on Boylston Street before moving to take over the Olive's Beauty Salon in Atlanta Georgia, that he changed to Rashid's Hair care Center. At Olives Beauty Salon he joined the National Hairdressers & Cosmetology Association (NHCA).

Over the years, Mr. Rashid has built an outstanding reputation as a Hair Beauty & Wellness Specialist. He has traveled and worked in three continents as an educator for leading hair care companies.

1. Africa: In South Africa, he served as an *Advanced Educator* in every major city throughout the country.

2. Caribbean: Bermuda, Trinidad, Barbados, Curiosa, Jamaica, St. Lucia Puerto Rico Bahamas

3. Europe: every major city in England & France.

He lived in London England and was contracted as an advanced educator at Alpha Beauty Academy.

Haroon's commercial credits include ad campaigns for:
- Fashion Fair
- Isoplus Products
- Sensitive by Nature

- Duke Men's Products
- Shades of you Hosiery
- Ebone` Cosmetics
- Van Cleef Salon
- Visionary Day Spa
- Gazelle Day Spa.
- Stay Soft Fro
- Elente` Vitale
- Design Essentials

He has received magazine editorial coverage from:
- Working Mother
- Rapp Pages
- Essence
- Ebony
- Bride's Today
- Shop Talk
- Upscale
- EM
- Jet
- Black Elegance
- Honey
- Source
- Beauty Trade
- Shades of You
- Salon Profiles

He has been commission to do consultant work for the following top companies that have contracted his services.
- Revlon
- Roux Lab.

- Clairol
- L'Oreal
- Johnson's Products
- Ebone`
- Duke
- Carson's Products
- Deena Corp
- Afam Products
- Mc Bride Lab
- M &M Products Company

He has owned several hair care business in Boston the Vice President of **Sportsman Pyramid Cosmetics Company/Natural U** hair product and nationwide was the Midwest Distributer for **Carson Products Sensitive by Nature** hair products and **Efalock Professional Tools**. Haroon has trained & employed hundreds of professionals' and know the industry from the top to the bottom. As a former member of the Atlanta chapter of **National Beauty Culturist League**, Haroon served as a personal consultant to former president Dr. Katie Wickham for the proposed NBCL African American Trend Release and he had a seat on the board of the **Chicago Cosmetology Association** - NHCA.

Haroon declares that he is an advocate for human rights and dedicates his free time to political and social causes. His view of the America and the world is one that respects Equal Human Rights as the only expectable narrative and advocacy for the 21st century and beyond and in that spirit he will often quote that;

I Am Haroon A. Rashid!

www.ingramcontent.com/pod-product-compliance
Lightning Source LLC
Chambersburg PA
CBHW062056290426
44110CB00022B/2606